Stress
in Health and Disease

Edited by Bengt B. Arnetz
and Rolf Ekman

Further of Interest

J. Licinio, M.-L. Wong (Eds.)

Biology of Depression
From Novel Insights to Therapeutic Strategies

2 Volumes
2005
ISBN 3-527-30785-0

Stress
in Health and Disease

Edited by Bengt B. Arnetz and Rolf Ekman

WILEY-
VCH

WILEY-VCH Verlag GmbH & Co. KGaA

The Editors

Prof. Dr. Bengt B. Arnetz
Division of Occupational
and Environmental Medicine
Wayne State University
101 E. Alexandrine
Detroit, MI 48201-2011
USA, and
Uppsala Science Park
Social Medicine
75185 Uppsala
Sweden

Prof. Rolf Ekman
Institute of Neuroscience and Physiology
Neurochemical laboratory
Mölndal/SU
43180 Mölndal
Sweden

Back cover
Photo of Bengt B. Arnetz with
courtesy of Robert Stewart
Photography Ltd.

Cover Design
Grafik-Design Schulz, Fußgönheim

■ All books published by Wiley-VCH are carefully
produced. Nevertheless, authors, editors, and
publisher do not warrant the information
contained in these books, including this book,
to be free of errors. Readers are advised to keep
in mind that statements, data, illustrations,
procedural details or other items may
inadvertently be inaccurate.

Library of Congress Card No.: applied for

British Library Cataloguing-in-Publication Data:
A catalogue record for this book is available
from the British Library.

**Bibliographic information published by Die
Deutsche Bibliothek**
Die Deutsche Bibliothek lists this publication in
the Deutsche Nationalbibliografie; detailed
bibliographic data is available in the Internet at
⟨http://dnb.ddb.de⟩.

© 2006 WILEY-VCH Verlag GmbH & Co.
KGaA, Weinheim

Printed in the Federal Republic of Germany.
Printed on acid-free paper.

Typesetting   Asco Typesetters, Hong Kong
Printing   betz-Druck GmbH, Darmstadt
Binding   Litges & Dopf Buchbinderei GmbH,
Heppenheim

ISBN-13 978-3-527-31221-4
ISBN-10 3-527-31221-8

Contents

Stress in Health and Disease. Edited by Bengt B. Arnetz and Rolf Ekman
Copyright © 2006 WILEY-VCH Verlag GmbH & Co. KGaA, Weinheim
ISBN: 3-527-31221-8

Foreword

The discovery of the stress syndrome by Hans Selye 70 years ago has had a great impact on many areas of biomedicine. The present volume presents a multicolored picture of this complex phenomenon in a series of chapters authored by a large number of eminent experts in a variety of stress-related fields. It will no doubt prove useful as a source of information on various aspects of stress and stimulate further research to deepen our knowledge of this field, which is so important for our society.

Living organisms are constructed to increase the chances for survival of the individual and the species. They should thus be able to cope with various unfavorable environmental and internal conditions. If the resulting stress on the system exceeds a certain level, damage will ensue. On the other hand, if the coping machinery is understimulated, damage may likewise ensue. A fundamental problem in stress research is thus trying to define the limit where stress starts to have a negative impact. Unfortunately this is not easy. What kind of endpoints can be used to settle the switch point? An obvious area in the search for endpoints deals with health and perhaps the most robust endpoint would be the length of life.

The length of human life has undergone a dramatic change during the past centuries. This phenomenon is probably observed worldwide but has been most precisely recorded in developed countries. It is best described as the "squaring off" of the survival curve. The data available from the past 500 years demonstrate a continuous increase in life expectancy. In a shorter perspective, looking at the second half of the previous century, this increase in the human lifespan has continued. Moreover, there is a clear correlation between survival and health. In Gothenburg, Sweden, for example, the general health, activity and well-being of 70-year-old people have continuously improved from one decade to the next.

How can one reconcile these observations with the statement that stress forms an increasing threat to our health? I have not been able to find a good answer to this question. However, it seems clear that the impact of stress has undergone a profound change in the sense of being more and more of psychosocial character than before. The role of infection, malnutrition and poor housing has decreased dramatically. Psychosocial influences during different periods are hard to measure objectively. Possibly their negative impact has also been reduced, but certainly not at all to the same extent as the more material factors. In fact, according to some authorities, psychosocial stress brings an increasing threat to our modern society.

Stress in Health and Disease. Edited by Bengt B. Arnetz and Rolf Ekman
Copyright © 2006 WILEY-VCH Verlag GmbH & Co. KGaA, Weinheim
ISBN: 3-527-31221-8

In any event this threat is severe enough to call for careful attention. Not least, the evolutionary perspective seems to be relevant. Various mechanisms that long ago were essential for survival now have the potential to create serious problems.

The enormous knowledge accumulated in the present volume should provide a useful basis for reaching an integrated view based on further analysis. A careful study of this impressive treatise can thus be strongly recommended.

Nobel Laureate in Medicine 2000   *Arvid Carlsson*

Preface

Groundbreaking research during the first part of the 20th century by researchers such as Pavlov, Cannon, Hess, and Selye has provided us with a better understanding of the physiological consequences of fear and mental stress. In the second part of last century, Mason, McEwan, and Salpolsky, just to mention a few, were able to demonstrate the specificity of the stress response. Researchers also identified structures and mechanisms in the brain coordinating stress response and enhanced our understanding of short- and long-term consequences on health and well-being.

Today, we recognize that stress is of paramount importance both in health and disease. Without a healthy, timely and temporarily defined stress response, we are unlikely to survive, neither on the Savanna thousands of year ago, nor today challenged by microbes, nor in the globalized and increasingly competitive society. However, sustained activation of the stress response will attenuate our ability to stay healthy and increase our likelihood to succumb to environmental challenges and disease.

Some of today's most challenging public health threats, including cardiovascular and Alzheimer's diseases, premature aging, metabolic syndrome, obesity, and diabetes are all linked to stress. Stress might not be the root cause, but a contributing factor in the initiation and progress of diseases. These major public health threats, in addition to malignant conditions, appear to have immunological malfunction in common. Moreover, it is not sufficient to be genetically at risk; environmental factors appear to play an important triggering role. This is apparent in understanding the socioeconomic gradient of many public health disorders, that is, the better off we are as compared to others, the healthier we are.

In order to understand the mechanisms behind stress, our body's response to stress, its relationship to health and disease, and, ultimately, the treatment and prevention of stress, we need to cross scientific silos. No one discipline will have the ultimate answers. Not even one scientific paradigm is likely to come with the ultimate answers. We need to think trans-disciplinarily. We need to consider how we can move knowledge, not only from the lab bench to the clinic and society at large, but also how to reverse this information flow. We truly need a new roadmap, just as has been proposed by the NIH Director Dr. Zerhouni.

Actually, stress might be one of the most fruitful areas in which to apply innovative new thinking and paradigms in order to not only improve mechanistic understanding, but to enhance our ability to implement new knowledge into society and improve overall public health.

Stress in Health and Disease. Edited by Bengt B. Arnetz and Rolf Ekman
Copyright © 2006 WILEY-VCH Verlag GmbH & Co. KGaA, Weinheim
ISBN: 3-527-31221-8

In the current book, *Stress in Health and Disease*, we decided not to take the easy route. It would have been simpler to only invite some of the world's most re-nowned biological and molecular stress researchers, or some of the most recog-nized organizational stress researchers. But we did not think such a format would have added sufficiently to the vast amount of stress literature already published. Rather we decided to take the challenge and invite globally outstanding researchers representing a wide array of scientific disciplines, all relevant to stress, but which rarely meet in today's busy research environment.

We asked experts on history, molecular medicine, endocrinology, brain imaging, sleep, recovery, organizational stress, global health and a range of other disciplines to tell us their view and perspective on stress. We requested a lot from these au-thorities. We asked them to be very specific and focused on their area of expertise. We asked them to challenge the current paradigm. We also asked them to accept sometimes rather harsh editing in order to make sure the book met the mission – understanding stress in health and disease from a multitude of perspectives. Thus, when you read the book, be aware of the active role the editors played. We take full responsibility for this, with the ultimate vision to offer a book that not only presents the state of the art when it comes to stress in health and disease, but also contributes to new and challenging questions that will encourage the coming generation of stress researchers to stretch their experimental design and hypothe-ses. We also hope the book will encourage meetings and collaborations of research-ers and practitioners from a wide array of fields.

This is the first attempt to create a truly trans-disciplinary book on stress – both with regard to the disciplines included as well as its application to real-life settings. The book represents a work in progress. We would be very happy to hear from you how we can improve the book in coming editions and if there are areas you, the reader, think we should have included. Or, are there perhaps superfluous areas that do not belong in a book on stress?

We hope you enjoy this book, that you find some things familiar and universally "true" and other things challenging. We also hope the book generates new ap-proaches in the study and application of stress research.

Finally, we would like to thank all contributing authors. It has been a true joy to work with you all. Without your open minds and timely collaboration, we would not have succeeded. We also would like to thank our publisher, Wiley-VCH, which met the challenge to release a trans-disciplinary book on stress in health and dis-ease. We owe a tremendous amount of thanks to our project editor, Dr. Rainer Muenz, as well as the copy editor, Mrs. Cathy Beesley, and the production manager, Mrs. Dagmar Kleemann, who provided endless professional and social support, en-suring that the editors were optimally challenged and stressed (with sufficient re-covery time).

"Boundaries between disciplines are not barriers, challenges us to find new words and approaches"

Bengt B. Arnetz, MD, PhD
Detroit
April 2006

Rolf Ekman, MD, PhD
Göteborg
April 2006

List of Contributors

Torbjörn Åkerstedt
IPM and Karolinska Institutet
Box 230
17177 Stockholm
Sweden

Ahmad Aljada
Division of Endocrinology, Diabetes
and Metabolism
State University of New York at Buffalo
and Kaleida Health
3 Gates Circle
Buffalo, NY 14209
USA

Susan L. Andersen
Harvard Medical School
Laboratory of Developmental
Neuropharmacology
McLean Hospital
Belmont, MA 02478
USA

Bengt B. Arnetz
Division of Occupational and Environmental
Medicine
Wayne State University
101 E. Alexandrine
Detroit, Michigan 48201-2011, USA and
Division of Social Medicine
Uppsala University
Uppsala Science Park, 751 85 Uppsala,
Sweden

Majed Ashy
Harvard Medical School
Department of Psychiatry
Developmental Biopsychiatry Research Program
McLean Hospital
Belmont, MA 02478
USA

Andreas Backlund
Mälardalen University
Högskoleplan 2
Gåsmyrevreten
721 23 Västerås
Sweden

Christian Berne
Department of Medical Sciences
Uppsala University
751 05 Uppsala
Sweden

Per Björntorp[†]

Ajay Chaudhuri
Division of Endocrinology, Diabetes and
Metabolism
State University of New York at Buffalo and
Kaleida Health
3 Gates Circle
Buffalo, NY 14209
USA

Paresh Dandona
Division of Endocrinology, Diabetes and
Metabolism
State University of New York at Buffalo and
Kaleida Health
3 Gates Circle
Buffalo, NY 14209
USA

Rolf Ekman
Institute of Neuroscience and Physiology
Neurochemical laboratory
Mölndal/SU
43180 Mölndal
Sweden

Hege Randi Eriksen
Director of Research
HALOS/University Research Bergen
Affiliated with the University of Bergen
Christiesgt. 13
5015 Bergen
Norway

Björn Folkow
Sahlgrenska Akademien
Dept. of Physiology
University of Göteborg
Box 432
40530 Göteborg
Sweden

Mats Fredrikson
Department of Psychology
Uppsala University
Box 1225
751 42 Uppsala
Sweden

Perry N. Fuchs
Department of Psychology
College of Science
University of Texas at Arlington
501 S. Nedderman Dr. – Ste. 313
Arlington, TX 76019-0528
USA

Tomas Furmark
Department of Psychology
Uppsala University
Box 1225
751 42 Uppsala
Sweden

Robert J. Gatchel
Department of Psychology
College of Science
University of Texas at Arlington
501 S. Nedderman Dr. – Ste. 313
Arlington, TX 76019-0528
USA

Husam Ghanim
Division of Endocrinology, Diabetes and
Metabolism
State University of New York at Buffalo and
Kaleida Health
3 Gates Circle
Buffalo, NY 14209
USA

Markus Heilig
National Institute on
Alcohol Abuse and Alcoholism (NIAAA)
10 Center Drive, 10/1-5334
Bethesda, MD 20892-1108
USA

Isabella Heuser
Department of Psychiatry
Charité – Campus Benjamin Franklin
Eschenallee 3
14050 Berlin
Germany

Karin Johannisson
Department of History of Science and Ideas
Uppsala University
Box 629
751 26 Uppsala
Sweden

Ulf Johanson
Mälardalen University
Högskoleplan 2
Gåsmyrevreten
721 23 Västerås
Sweden

Rollin McCraty
HeartMath Research Center
Institute of HeartMath
14700 West Park Avenue
Boulder Creek, CA
USA

Bruce S. McEwen
Laboratory of Neuroendocrinology
The Rockefeller University
Box 165
New York 10021, NY
USA

Tommy Olsson
Department of Public Health and Clinical
Medicine
Umeå University Hospital
90185 Umeå
Sweden

Yuan Bo Peng
Department of Psychology
College of Science
University of Texas at Arlington
501 S. Nedderman Dr. – Ste. 313
Arlington, TX 76019-0528
USA

Maria Petersson
Department of Molecular Medicine
Endocrine and Diabetes Unit
Karolinska Institutet/Karolinska University
Hospital
171 77 Stockholm
Sweden

Russell D. Romeo
Laboratory of Neuroendocrinology
Rockefeller University
Box 165 Weiss Research Building
New York 10021, NY
USA

James Rubin
Mobile Phones Research Unit
New Medical School Building
Bessemer Road
London SE5 9PJ
UK

Jacqueline A. Samson
Harvard Medical School
Depression Research Facility
McLean Hospital
Belmont, MA 02478
USA

Robert Sapolsky
Departments of Biological Sciences, Neurology
and Neurological Sciences
Stanford University
MC 5020
Stanford, CA 94305-5020
USA

Nicole C. Schommer
Department of Psychiatry
Charité – Campus Benjamin Franklin
Eschenallee 3
14050 Berlin
Germany

Anna Söderpalm
Institute of Neuroscience and Physiology
Sahlgrenska University Hospital
41345 Göteborg
Sweden

Bo Söderpalm
Institute of Neuroscience and Physiology
Sahlgrenska University Hospital
41345 Göteborg
Sweden

Martin H. Teicher
Developmental Biopsychiatry Research
Program
McLean Hospital
Belmont, MA 02478
USA

Töres Theorell
National Institute for Psychosocial Factors and
Health
Box 230
171 77 Stockholm
Sweden
and
Department of Public Health Sciences
Karolinska Institutet
Box 220
171 77 Stockholm
Sweden

Dana Tomasino
HeartMath Research Center
Institute of HeartMath
14700 West Park Avenue
Boulder Creek, CA
USA

Akemi Tomoda
Harvard Medical School
Developmental Biopsychiatry Research
Program
McLean Hospital
Belmont, MA 02478
USA

Holger Ursin
Institute of Psychology
University of Bergen
5000 Bergen
Norway

Kerstin Uvnäs Moberg
Department of Physiology and Pharmacology
Karolinska Institutet
171 77 Stockholm
Sweden

Lars Weisæth
The University of Oslo
Boks 1072 Blindern
0316 Oslo
Norway

Simon Wessely
Psychological Medicine Division
King's College London
Strand
London WC2R 2LS
UK

A Multifaceted View of Stress

1
Modern Fatigue: A Historical Perspective

Karin Johannisson

"There exists, both within and without the ranks of the medical profession, a widespread belief that the exigencies of modern life are producing an ever-increasing amount of nervous diseases."
– H. C. Wood, *Brain-Work and Overwork* (1896)

1.1
Introduction

At the general meeting of the British Society of Medical Psychology held on 21 November 1900, a dramatic increase in mental disorder cases was discussed. Three major causes were indicated: heredity, internal and external toxins, and *stress*. Laboratory experiments had demonstrated that stress was a triggering factor; rats had been placed in treadmill-cages and subjected to extreme stress. Physiologically, the process of illness could be described as a loss of energy. "If, then, it is a disease in which the danger lies in stress," one doctor pointed out, "we must see many people whose nervous systems will go to pieces unless they can be taken away from the stress in which they are living, whether that be on the stock exchange, or in any other professional occupation where the nineteenth century pressure is very great" [1].

The similarity between the situation at the turn of the 19th century and that of today is striking in regard to an increasing decline in mental health. Both eras define their times as being characterized by major changes, increased information flows, and heavy demands on the urban individual – and all of it happening in a whirling market economy. At both points in time, new diagnoses appear that identify and legitimize the symptoms of stress and internal discomfort in a culture strongly marked by competition, achievement, and a high tempo.

The unifying component in this case, seems to be the perception of an accelerated rate of change, an ever-growing flow of innovations which, on a subjective level, is in danger of creating spontaneous feelings of inadequacy, of not being

Stress in Health and Disease. Edited by Bengt B. Arnetz and Rolf Ekman
Copyright © 2006 WILEY-VCH Verlag GmbH & Co. KGaA, Weinheim
ISBN: 3-527-31221-8

able to keep up mentally, physically, and emotionally. This is what makes up modernity's identity – the expectation that the individual be limitlessly adaptable, flexible and progress-oriented. Modernity means being involved in a world where, "all that is solid melts into air," says modernity researcher Marshall Berman, citing Karl Marx. "To be modern is to find ourselves in an environment that promises us adventure, power, joy, growth, transformation of ourselves and the world – and, at the same time, that threatens to destroy everything we have, everything we know, everything we are" [2].

One concrete way to relate the perception of mental stress at the the last turn of the century to that at the recent one is to compare two medically and culturally legitimized diagnoses that – within their respective contexts – are considered to reflect abnormal fatigue. These diagnoses are neurasthenia and chronic fatigue syndrome.

However, the purpose here is not primarily to find absolute similarities, something that would be based on the concept that illness can be reduced to historically neutral phenomena, but rather to study how the clinical pictures are constructed and which scientific and cultural explanatory models work well together. Ultimately it also involves a new way of approaching the complicated process by which diagnoses are created.

1.2
Overstrain and Modern Society in 1900

During the last half of the 19th century, the Western world underwent a dramatic social change. Industrialization, an expanding capital market, and massive urbanization created new patterns of human contact. New technology represented an altered living environment. Special risk scenarios and pathology myths surrounded electrification and the telegraph. New kinds of transportation – trains, streetcars, and later the automobile – represented new relationships between the individual and time and space. The railway, particularly, was considered to carry special risks. The mental and physical stress was symbolized in the speed itself, in the train's shaking, vibrations, and sudden stops, as well as in the hustle and bustle of the railroad stations. Timetables, crowding, loudspeaker announcements, warning bells; all of this, together with the city's disorder, created an uncontrolled stream of sensory stimulation.

A number of scientific theories on modern society's effects on the vulnerable individual were developed. These included the theory of evolution that, in its social Darwinist formulation, emphasized the battle for survival; the theory of thermodynamics maintaining that the individual's energy was limited; and various civilization theories that saw alienation and fragmentation as the inevitable price of progress.

All of the prominent contemporary sociologists – Georg Simmel, Émile Durkheim, Ferdinand Tönnies, and Max Weber – pointed out the inner conflicts that appeared when old ways of life were replaced by new ones, and the individual, denied his habitual security and value bases, felt lost in a changing world. Many people spoke of growing fatigue. The French psychologist Pierre Janet interpreted this fatigue as symptomatic of a gigantic alienation. Others referred to civilization and evolution as sensibilizing processes. If the individual could not protect his vulnerable self from too-rapid change and the effects of cultural shock, the result was pain.

The situation was described as being serious. Overworked, tortured patients were crowding doctors' consulting rooms. Their case histories could probably be copied into a present-day scenario without any changes [3].

> Merchant, who has been suffering for several years from insomnia, anxiety, and a strong feeling of pressure in his head:
> I work from 8 o'clock in the morning until 10 o'clock at night. I can hardly take any time out to eat; usually I eat on my feet, and then it's cold, tasteless food. By 10 o'clock in the evening I'm so tired that I have trouble finding the strength to close my books. During the night the day's events whirl through my head, so that it isn't until early morning that I can enjoy any rest. When I arise, I'm deathly tired, and find that I must drink a few glasses of brandy in order to be fit for work again.

> Young businessman, who suffers from insomnia and agoraphobia, has been incapable for months of any intellectual work:
> We work from 8 in the morning to 8 in the evening, with barely 15 minutes to eat lunch. In the evening, when work is over, a group of us young men meet at a café, where we eat and drink gleefully until 2 or 3 in the morning. I never get enough sleep … When I travel, I do it at night so that I can work during the day.

Many doctors report similar cases. The problem is overstrain resulting from overwork and too little rest. Life in a modern city puts a great deal of pressure on an individual. Competition and the struggle to be recognized dominate finances, industry, art, and science. Everyone wants to get ahead. They work intensively to be successful, but feel mostly fatigue and dissatisfaction. For distraction they leap on entertainment and hectic travel. This particular combination of overstrain and overstimulation results in illness. Overstrain is mental, primarily intellectual, but it can also be caused by long-term worry, personal unhappiness, and disappointments.

The argument is thus that mental work drains the body. Overstrain is a condition that causes illness, and is directly related to a lifestyle characterized by the overuse of one's mental energy.

1.3
The "Fatigue Problem"

The overstrain theory was central in science, medicine and the media around the turn of the 19th century. Fatigue plays the role of progress' perpetual goddess of revenge. There is a huge literary discussion of the relationship between society, fatigue, and ill-health.

This analysis is constructive. Fatigue is seen as a sign of the body's refusal to bow to the modern industrial society. It is not identified as depression, illness, or unwillingness to work, but rather is perceived as a border, even as a kind of awakening – a sound signal from the body of the need for rest and recuperation. If fatigue can be interpreted as the self's natural resistance to increased demands for productivity, then the same interpretation indicates the necessity of creating a better order for the human being in an industrial society.

Fatigue, thus, represents the limits of the individual's physical and mental capabilities, as well as the limits that society cannot overstep without working against its own interests [4].

The overstrain theory was a purely physiological theory borrowed from the laws of thermodynamics, particularly the law dealing with the constancy of energy and that dealing with heat loss (entropy). Translated from a physical to a physiological plane, they gained status as scientific explanatory models for the fragile relationship between the human being and society. The logic was this: the body has at its disposal a predetermined amount of vital energy. In the healthy body this energy is evenly distributed, with special depots in areas like the brain, the digestive system, and the genitals – which in turn have an internal reflex relationship to each other. Overconsumption of energy in one area means that other areas "starve". According to this economic model, intellectual energy drain thus presents a risk to the individual's sex life and digestion. Every exertion reduces the finite energy capital, and deficits are expressed as ill-health. Continuous external stress threatens to create an irreversible energy drain, a kind of gradual heat-exhaustion of the soul and the body.

This concept of fatigue had a unique ability to translate an external set of problems to inner levels, and to make the body the place where a greater social set of problems could be studied. During the last decades of the 19th century, medical models for a culture in crisis were developed, based on either the degeneration theme or on the overstrain theme. Doctors tried various evaluation methods to translate the individual's response to external stress into a medical science. As concrete physiological conditions, the forms and degrees of fatigue – from tiredness to exhaustion, overstrain, and breakdown – could be identified. At first these conditions were also perceived to be objective, measurable, and possible to deal with. German physiologist Wilhelm Weichardt's sensational announcement in 1904 that he had discovered a vaccine against fatigue turned out, however, to be a disappointment.

Until the 1870s, fatigue had hardly been seen as a medical problem except as a marginal phenomenon in various depressive conditions like melancholy, nostalgia, ennui, spleen, or acedia. At the turn of the century there were hundreds of studies of muscle fatigue, nervous exhaustion, brain fatigue, asthenia and neurasthenia, and nerve fatigue. In most countries overstrain theories appeared in the medical discussions during the 1870s.

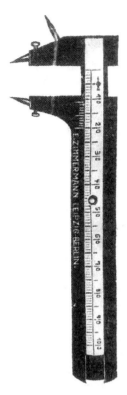

Fig. 1.1. Esthesiometer. Several technical instruments were introduced to measure individual stress levels, e.g., the ergograph, registering muscle fatigue, the algesimeter, estimating pain, and the esthesiometer, measuring stress levels via skin sensitivity. The greater the loss of mental energy, the lower the capacity to state the distance between two points placed upon the skin (so called spatial limen). Even though the esthesiometer measured mental fatigue only indirectly, it became popular for fixing limit values for overstrain, particularly in school children. Foremost, however, it was used to register loss of sensitivity in nerve-lesion or trauma. It was further developed in order to be applied to minute skin areas, registering exceedingly small distinctions. The most advanced versions were using hair of varying diameter.

Two main arenas were identified for fatigue problems; one was connected to industrial work, and the other to intellectual work. The first was based on a well-known 18th century metaphor, the human machine. The human body and the factory machine both represented motors that changed energy into mechanical work; in conditions of imbalance, exhaustion, or overheating their efficiency would be dramatically reduced.

A number of laboratory studies on the working body were initiated. These included attempts with special instruments – the ergograph, which measured muscle fatigue, and the esthesiometer, which measured the skin's sensitivity – to register very small changes in the physical process during a specific task (Fig. 1.1).

Soon scientists had investigated many aspects of exhaustion, including the role of fatigue in accidents, sick leaves, and "blue Monday" syndromes. Using increasingly refined measurement techniques, they hoped to successively expose the principle of the body's energy system, identify the economy of muscular action, and find methods for organizing the consumption of both muscle energy and neural energy. They were particularly interested in determining the critical difference between exhaustion and overstrain. This difference also defined the borderline between the normal and the pathological, or between capacity and incapacity, respectively, after recuperation through rest.

The second arena for investigating the problem of fatigue was connected with groups that represented high consumption of mental energy; these included schoolchildren, students, scientists, and intellectuals, i.e., "brain-workers." All over Europe, even in a small country like Sweden, there was a dramatic increase in ill-health among young people at school. Their symptoms were, among others, eye and sleep problems, anemia, chlorosis, and nosebleeds. In France, people talked about an epidemic of overstrain and intellectual exhaustion triggered by decades of educational reforms in combination with murderous demands ("*l'éducation homicide*"). Researchers tried using the ergograph to demonstrate that the intense mental strain caused by tasks such as solving a mathematical problem or memorizing Latin or poetry also caused muscle fatigue. A stressed brain could likewise produce restlessness and mental hyperactivity that marked an individual's character and personality.

Based on this activity, exhaustion appeared to be a strategic threshold value for the individual's adaptive capacity to modern society. The fatigue problem was a social problem, the responsibility of which therefore had to be shared by the areas of medicine, technology, education, and politics.

There was a hierarchical distinction made between the kinds of fatigue experienced by the manual worker and the intellectual worker. Mental work was determined to be more energy-consuming than heavy industrial work or mechanical office work. The effect of brain stress on the body was thus seen to be greater than direct stress on the body. Distinctions like this confirmed an ancient order between body and soul, as well as between the fatigue of the privileged and that of others. When Karl Marx pointed out that exploitation actually created fatigue, his opinion ended up halfway between the current political discourses. A working-class woman could not, according to the dominant discourse, be overexerted. She might possibly be worn out; a concept associated with the lower class until the middle of the 20th century.

Fatigue – as a measured physical and mental reaction and as a socially constructed concept – thus came to be part of several different explanatory models, including those of labor organizations, social medicine, occupational medicine, and psychiatry. As an indicator of the body's and the soul's conditions at a given point in time, overstrain stands out as a condition of decided social and medical significance. It was a matter of protecting the individual from overwork, as well as from overstimulation. Especially in the feverish tempo of the big city, mental fatigue risked being spontaneously compensated for by an equally energy-consuming appetite for entertainment and consumption. It was characterized by luxurious interior decoration, clothes and food, and by extravagance in bodily, sexual, and sensual pleasures. Some people even claimed that modern society's depleted neural energy could be defined as a special psychophysiological condition, ennui, which explained the artistic peculiarities of the European *fin de siècle* style. According to these interpretations, individual and collective fatigue, not modern esthetics, were the source of the subjectivism, experimentation, and nostalgic retrospectivism – as well as of the drug culture and gender-crossing within the gay, dandy, and Bohemian lifestyles.

1.4
Neurasthenia

One particular kind of ill-health, neurasthenia, appeared among the effects of overstrain. It represented mental fatigue in its pathological form.

The name was coined in 1869 by George Beard, an American doctor, and it referred to "the forms and types of nervous fatigue that originate in the brain and the spinal cord." It was defined as the disappearance of nerve energy [5]. The diagnosis specified the diffuse spectrum of suffering earlier characterized as nervous, e.g., neurosis, spinal complaints, hysteria, or hypochondria. These could be divided up into a number of subtypes, such as the cerebral, the sexual, and the traumatic. They included a large number of symptoms (Beard himself names about 80), from headaches, insomnia, pains, and sensitization of all the sense organs, to anxiety, melancholy, and a long series of phobias. The primary symptom was a feeling of paralyzing fatigue. He claimed that the condition was related to the modern lifestyle, and that it affected mainly the overachieving groups in the forefront of civilization like businessmen, stockbrokers, and intellectuals. Neurasthenia was, he said, a cultural illness nourished by the modernization process itself.

The diagnosis spread rapidly to Europe, where it began a long journey. In Sweden it was introduced in the Board of Health's disease classification in 1890, and soon showed high numbers of sufferers. This is an outstanding example of what can be termed the institutionalization of an illness. When a diagnosis comes into existence – as both name and concept – and is medically and culturally legitimized and exposed in the mass media, it also tends to attract those who exhibit the typical symptoms.

Neurasthenia was generally described as reduced nerve energy expressed as chronic fatigue that shut down or slowed down cerebral, emotional, and bodily activity. The neurasthenic was overcome by powerlessness, emotional instability, and sudden weakness. A reduced ability to concentrate, pay attention, and listen was also noted. In addition to the esthesiometer, an audiometer provided measurements of "the degree of distraction" (actually hearing). Memory problems were also observed to be a general characteristic of the neurasthenic, and even difficulty in remembering his/her own symptoms. Something else that struck many doctors was that the loss of energy seemed to trigger a number of emotional fatigue symptoms in the ability to experience sorrow, involvement, and empathy.

Comparisons of otherwise healthy but mentally exhausted people with neurasthenic patients showed that it was a matter of a difference of degree, and not of any other specific difference. This seemed to explain the fact that neurasthenia was primarily limited to the intellectual professions, i.e., to those social categories consuming large quantities of nerve energy. The neurasthenia diagnosis demonstrates how a number of values of race, sex, and class infiltrate medical science.

Beard considered the idea that neurasthenia could affect "the savage" absurd, but others, such as the well-known neurologist Jean Martin Charcot stated that a person from the working class could also be affected, especially after painful emotional experiences or conflicts with a new, unfamiliar environment. The category of "traumatic neurasthenia" was generally reserved just for the working class. The gender aspect presented problems, as this diagnosis, especially in the Scandinavian countries, tended to be a woman's issue. At the *fin de siècle*, 80–90% of the more serious cases of neurasthenia were reported to be women. Since intellectual over-strain could not be associated with women (most of whom had access to neither higher education nor the professions), it was necessary to take on gender-specific explanation models of neurological, gynecological or psychological type.

Patients were generally divided up into two main types; one was the depressive, hard-to-reach, and nonverbal, and the other the exalted, communicative, and verbal. Patients could also be sorted by two main types of symptoms: primarily psychological or primarily somatic (e.g., persistent headaches, neuralgic backaches, neuromuscular asthenia, mortal fatigue, and increased sensorial sensitivity). The descriptive mania that characterizes the neurasthenia literature is remarkable; it is as though the slightest symptomatic shift and each sign must be registered. The patients themselves are also described as intensely concentrated on the minute details, constantly producing sets of symptoms that became more and more complex.

As far as symptoms were concerned, neurasthenia did not actually appear as a disease in its own right, but rather as an unstable reflecting system of other diseases. This, in turn, seemed to reflect the provocative identity of the illness; it leaves no part of the individual being unaffected. To the doctor, the neurasthenic's symptoms formed a sort of bodily text or image, and his/her task was to interpret and give meaning to the patient's perception of the illness. As it would be for a critic confronted by an abstract modernistic painting, the idea was to discern the structure in a chaos of signs and figures, in which even the absurd and apparently incomprehensible had to be included.

At the beginning of the 20th century, doctors appeared quite desperate about neurasthenia's extremely many-faceted set of symptoms. The name "asthenia" was suggested in order to separate "energy diseases" from the greater concept of neurasthenia. Many of neurasthenia's psychic symptoms ended up inconveniently outside the physiological explanatory model that could clarify physical and mental exhaustion, and fit better under the heading of neuroses. The borderlines between different exhaustion conditions had to be defined; the straightforward physiological causes were won back from the complex neuropathological ones.

Asthenia was thus not defined in relation to a greater sociocultural scenario but rather as the physiological effects of a perceived loss of energy. The classical treatment forms rejected rest and care. Doctors were not to advise their fatigued patients to stay away from work and activities. On the contrary, only by mobilizing their inner energy resources and returning to work could they recapture their energy and health. The primary strategy was to exercise mental powers of resistance, to resist and deflect the unconscious flow of associations and fantasies that took command over one's being when the energy allowance was low.

Studies of fatigue problems thus emphasized the significance of the economy of energy, i.e., of the equilibrium between the individual's inner energy capital and the social requirement. The various degrees or categories of tiredness are structured in steps. Fatigue meant a condition that was reparable by rest. Exhaustion was defined as the "accumulation of fatigue with a gradual capability of recuperation," and overstrain as a condition where the option of recuperation by rest was no longer possible. These conditions functioned as a kind of regulator for work capacity. The machine metaphor was used frequently. Running a machine beyond its adjusted rhythm and capacity was neither effective nor rational. It was more a matter of increasing effectiveness by identifying the optimal equilibrium between inflow and outflow of energy.

When the criticism of modernity had lost ground, and the modern welfare society could be glimpsed behind the industrial expansion, fatigue was released from its role in political cultural analysis. The issue was moved from a greater social stage into the closed rooms of science. As a problem related to production and labor organization, it was assigned to occupational medicine or environmental medicine. As a symptom of pathology processes within the body, it was assigned to virology and immunology. As an expression of depression and inadequacy, it disappeared into psychiatry.

1.5
Between Nervous Fatigue and Chronic Fatigue: Stress

After World War I, the fatigue problem was transformed from an issue of high political and scientific concern into a technical topic, which in the occupational area was connected particularly to industrial rationalization. During the 1940s and 1950s interest was defined primarily by military needs, increased airplane traffic, the beginnings of space research, and later by various security issues related to air travel, traffic, and accidents.

As mental fatigue was related to exterior pressure, the problem was relegated to psychiatry, where it was also given a certain amount of attention. During the 1920s and 1930s it was still possible to use neurasthenia as an umbrella diagnosis. A differentiation was generally made between constitutional neurasthenia, characterized by chronic dejection, and abnormal susceptibility to fatigue with concentration problems and memory blackouts, acquired neurasthenia also affecting the mentally well-balanced as a result of overstrain, and study neurasthenia, energy drain connected with intellectual fatigue. Feminine neurasthenia was defined in its own special category as being "characterized by its exterior intensity of dejection ... and by weakness. Patients literally lack energy and fortitude, and are unable to go about their usual tasks ... They are unable to walk; some have great difficulty in keeping themselves upright ... some of them are completely confined to their beds" [6]. There was a general element of complex passivity and powerlessness combined with muscular asthenia noted in women's neurasthenia, which was otherwise seldom seen.

In the realm of psychiatry, fatigue could also be interpreted in various models. "Neurasthenic fatigue has nothing to do with overstrain," wrote the well-known Swedish psychoanalyst Poul Bjerre in 1924. Work performance and the exterior work situation play small roles in comparison with the "interior complex job," i.e., the battle to control inner impulses, setbacks, and complexes. The most significant and most disastrous feature of neurasthenic fatigue is its mechanization, that is, an individual's "tendency to ... continuously seek corroboration of one's own weakness, which in turn is lodged in a physical complaint that then legitimizes the illness role." Thus the proper treatment is not rest; instead the fatigued person must be fed "new impulses, new obligations, indeed, why not new conflicts?"

However, the fatigue problem had no status in the public arena. It is as though it was relegated into the shadow of the 20th century's huge modernity and welfare projects. My general thesis, that certain illness syndromes are mirrors of society (or to put it differently, that a subjective feeling of ill-health is translated into the symptoms that society, culture, and social affiliation legitimize), can also be applied in a scenario of nonaffirmation. When fatigue, alienation, and nostalgia are no longer supported by current discourses, they risk being rejected or even stigmatized.

A concept that at this microlevel seems to be better adapted to a society characterized by rationalization, effectivization, and auspiciously pounding machines within the framework of a collective welfare utopia, is that of stress.

This word existed, thus, as early as the turn of the 19th century with the same meaning that it has today, but without defined physiological components. It had no real impact then, and was out-contested by the concept of nervous tension, which fit within the established neuropathological interpretive model. Nervous tension indicated, like stress, a general condition of worry, irritability, and strain. Similarly, it was also described as a condition that was negatively associated with demands of external performance and adaptation. Both concepts mesh to a great degree with the diagnoses that each particular period names and legitimizes: neurasthenia and nervous fatigue or, respectively, chronic fatigue syndrome and burnout.

1.6
Chronic Fatigue Syndrome

Since neurasthenia had lost ground as a diagnosis during the 1940s and 1950s, the medical fatigue problem waited several decades for new legitimizing names. Associated primarily with a neurotic, asthenic, or depressive personality – or to a female identity – it had a total lack of social status. Similarly, overstrain and the nervous breakdown were framed in a half-scientific, half-mythologized dimension as names of antiquated reactions outside of the expected normality.

Not until the late 20th century were fatigue and overstrain brought to the fore with new medically legitimizing names, chronic fatigue syndrome and burnout.

The breakthrough was in the 1980s. In the mid 1980s a remarkable new disease was reported; it was popularly called the yuppie disease, but was soon given a more dignified name, chronic fatigue syndrome. After what seems to have been an acute outbreak in the Lake Tahoe district in Nevada, the illness came to be associated with well-educated young career people (the word yuppie comes from "young urban professional"). The illness mobilized major mass media and scientific interest, and spread quickly – as neurasthenia once had – to Europe [7].

The explanation was linked primarily to two scientific models that were of great interest then, the virological and the immunological models. Both of them could be combined with the lifestyle factor as the triggering cause. The virological model suggested infection with the Epstein–Barr virus, or, alternatively, another microorganism like herpes, borrelia (which causes Lyme disease) or some other that had not yet been isolated. The immunological model, saying that it was a matter of weakened immunity, pointed first in the direction of similarities with the great nightmare of the 1980s, HIV/AIDS, but thereafter towards various external and internal toxins. Both of the interpretive models mirrored the dramatically increased risk awareness prevalent in the late 20th century associated with contagion and toxemia from the external environment. Clinical ecologists and a number of ideological groups had a huge media impact with theses about risks to the health from the modern lifestyle and consumer culture. Suspected culprits included overuse of antibiotics, chemical additives, insecticides, genetically modified food, toxins from the air, earth, and water, metal excretions, and threatening radiation from electrical equipment, display screens and cell phones.

It has been maintained that chronic fatigue syndrome is nothing more than the old neurasthenia in a new guise. It is true that they both center on great fatigue. While the neurasthenic was considered to suffer from reduced neural energy resulting from external tension, the chronically fatigued individual was believed to suffer from a virus attack or weakened immunity resulting from an external threat. A systematic comparison of the syndromes also shows that there are definite overlaps [8].

The main issue is simply fatigue; a feeling of exhaustion so extreme that it makes any kind of work, exertion, or activity impossible, even distractions like conversation, music, or literature are unthinkable. Other symptoms in common are pains in the muscles and joints or even all over the body, feverishness, persistent headache, a feeling of pressure, sleep problems, a series of neurological symptoms like oversensitivity to sound and light, and memory and concentration problems. In fact the only symptom characteristic of chronic fatigue syndrome that George Beard *didn't* name was sore lymph glands.

We are thus confronted with two sets of symptoms that are almost identical, but which appear at different times, under different names, and are analyzed by different interpretive models. Every such interpretation, in turn, mirrors both a scientific position and the culturally acceptable codes of its time. It can be claimed that in the same way that neurasthenia was a compilation of the concepts (especially of fatigue as a standard of value of modernity) that caught the interest of both the public in general and the scientific world of the time, chronic fatigue syndrome is built on the very timely conception of the biologically vulnerable individual in a threatening, highly rationalized living environment.

Neurasthenia and chronic fatigue syndrome share the basic theme of overburdening the body's own reserves. In both cases the overburdening is explained by the demanding lifestyle of the times. Much of the past's connection between neurasthenia and the hectic pace of city living is also true of today's connection between illness and stress. To the 19th-century doctor the stressors caused reduced nerve energy, while to today's doctor it is a series of complex neural, immune, and endocrine processes. Neurasthenia offered the individual, in the same way as chronic fatigue syndrome, the right to be ill with something that was both medically verified and legitimate in relation to culture and social position. Both were – initially – associated with society's well-educated, overachieving groups. Neurasthenia was an acceptable and even honorable diagnosis for professional men. Beard reported that at least 10% of his patients were male doctors, and others were businessmen, bankers, lawyers, and government officials. The diagnosis therefore appeared to be an emblem of a select group (those with ambition, success, intellect, cultivation, sensibility), while it rescued the patient from negative labels like neurosis, hypochondria, or depression. Chronic fatigue syndrome initially had the same status, associated with a risk group characterized as well-educated, young career men and women. The strength lay here, also, in a biomedical interpretive model that allowed the patients to be spared stigmatizing psychiatric diagnoses.

Parallels between neurasthenia and chronic fatigue syndrome are also striking. The question is really how lessons learned from the earlier diagnosis can be used to help in understanding the later one.

One lesson is that when a diagnosis undergoes a change in class (from high to low) and gender (from male to female) there is a risk that it will lose status. As neurasthenia decreased greatly after World War I (without disappearing entirely), it had undergone precisely this change of class and gender. As a syndrome it was no longer associated with class-conscious refinement or with intellectual achievements. A number of symptoms could be separated out and assigned to other medical or psychiatric diagnoses. What remained was a mixture of unspecified functional symptom and expressions for mental suffering that seemed increasingly antiquated, especially the fatigue. As time went on the diagnosis disappeared from the public mind.

We can speculate similarly about what will happen to chronic fatigue syndrome. If the parallel with neurasthenia continues, it would mean that this diagnosis will eventually disappear, and for the same reasons: the syndrome is too unspecific, scientific medicine is not able to identify a biological sign, it is no longer culturally acceptable, or it is swallowed up in new illness names.

It can also be claimed, however, that the diagnosis has already been replaced by another one that is better adapted to the acute social set of problems – burnout.

1.7
Burnout and Modern Society in 2000

The concept of burnout has, interestingly, never been associated with a primary biological cause. It has instead been analyzed as a syndrome produced by society, labor organization, or the vulnerable relationships between people, mainly those in the professional spheres.

The rise of this diagnosis has been dizzyingly rapid. During a period of a very few years around the turn of the century in 2000 it appeared from relative anonymity to reach epidemic levels, primarily as a threat to whole labor markets. In Sweden, it was reported that every other teacher was at risk of burnout. Business people, stockbrokers, doctors, and high achievers linked to the expanding field of information technology (IT) were other groups affected. Never has an illness been so openly connected with society itself.

One approach is also to interpret the phenomenon via a greater social diagnosis, that of an achievement-, control-, and tempo-incited culture characterized by labor organizations that are increasingly anorexic, in which fewer and fewer must do more and more. Old structures distinguished by stability, security, and inertia seemed to be replaced by neurotic cults of change, manic corporate cultures ("funky business") and short project jobs. Individual performances were pressured. Employers demanded not just competence, involvement, and independence of their employees, but also flexibility and accessibility. The individual expected, in turn, quick and visible rewards. No one had time anymore for the old coffee breaks and socializing. New technology required new knowledge as well as uninterrupted accessibility; it was necessary to adapt oneself to a continuous flow of information and communication, even a new time-and-space conception.

A second approach is the medical one. Burnout is defined as a condition of illness, and not as a feeling, a rebellion, a cultural criticism, or a healthy reaction. Feelings of inadequacy and the body's spontaneous resistance are assigned to the only dimension that lends legitimacy – the field of medicine. Of course there is also a concrete medical aspect to this. Physical and mental stress as well as exhaustion beyond the possibility of recovery create not just fatigue but also weakened immunity, vulnerability, and sleep problems; these in turn open the doors for negative events in the body. We concentrate for a major part of each day – whether intellectually or as consumers of media information, with health and exercise activities, or with entertainment and adventure. The demands on us are many; they include knowledge, skills, and enthusiasm, as well as good health, charisma, creativity, and success. Our work, marriages, children, homes, bodies, and our own beings – all these can be made into projects in eternal motion toward change, refinement, and perfection.

In this connection we might ask ourselves whether burnout isn't just a name for a problem that doesn't have anything at all to do with illness. "People aren't angels," wrote a well-known Swedish political economist in a 1980s article that attracted widespread attention, referring to that decade's increasing frequency of sick leaves. They are, instead, rationally calculating beings who take advantage of the welfare system when they can to optimize their own life projects. Interpreted this way, the epidemic burnout would actually be about the dream of a work-free income, of a narcissistic culture that seeks pleasure – not overwork – and views the illness label as a way to avoid the demands [9].

But we can also examine more constructive explanations. One is to search in the syndrome's own history. Keying in the word "burnout" in a bibliographic search program gives rapid results: the entire first wave of literature was produced in the

USA around the mid-1980s. Christina Maslach's pioneering work *Burnout* was published in 1982, and was quickly followed by others. It gives the definition and the clinical criteria, including physical, mental, and emotional exhaustion, uneasiness, and lack of empathy. The diagnosis was initially created for people in the caring professions, e.g., social workers, nurses, and therapists, who in dealing constantly on a personal basis with others' weaknesses, were drained of their own energy.

Their reactions were to burn out; the simile was that of a burning match as it blackens, turns to ash, and then to nothing. Some people also claimed that the burnout syndrome could be divided into three stages that corresponded to the three degrees of burn injuries. The first-degree burn is characterized by short-lived, reparable damage. The second-degree burn is more painful, causes tissue damage, and takes time to heal. The third-degree burn causes very great pain, serious tissue damage, and deep scarring, and requires an extended healing process.

Burnout was thus already a well-defined diagnosis in the 1980s, but it never caught on outside the USA. One explanation lies in the personality type with which it was identified – individuals who were adaptable, had low self-reliance, and were sensitive and subject to feelings of guilt. Burnout was thus hardly a diagnosis suited to the financial achievers, the hungry market people, or the sophisticated IT people who were then just starting out. There was instead another diagnosis with similar symptoms that was popular during the 1980s, one that was indeed associated with the high achievers: chronic fatigue syndrome.

It is no great exaggeration to say that the status of an illness is determined by the status of those who have the illness. Some typical such candidates have been elite males with type A behavior (overstrain, neurasthenia, myocardial infarction), as well as the outcasts of society such as homosexuals or drug addicts (venereal disease, tuberculosis, AIDS). The victims of burnout in the 1980s belonged to neither of these groups. They were feverish workers in the caring professions. And they were mainly women.

Once again we see an illustration of how a diagnosis must mesh with contemporary cultural codes to attain real success. It was as though the spectacular 1980s demanded spectacular illnesses. The mass media devoted intense interest to a new kind of illness that was connected with the period's atmosphere of crisis, catastrophe, and threats. These included mercury poisoning, electricity and display screen sensitivities, and pain syndromes. There was talk of sick buildings and sick water, of killer streptococci and aggressive viruses, and of course of AIDS. The world appeared to be ill, and so did we.

It was as though the gray, unglamorous burnout didn't fit into the pattern. The diagnosis wasn't taken seriously until the front lines of society – the high-achieving intellectual workers like teachers, doctors, and IT consultants – appeared to be victims. But this, in turn, was not possible as long as burnout was classed as an illness affecting those with low self-reliance and depressive personality types, primarily of the female gender, i.e., in an interpretive model that laid the blame on the inadequate individual. What was needed was a redistribution of the blame. It was not until this blame was placed on the actual labor organization and a social dimension, or in other words, on a cause external to the individual, that burnout became more popular.

1.8
Conclusion

From a historical perspective, fatigue related to stress was intensely discussed around the year 1900 as well as around the year 2000. As a symptom it has been given different diagnostic names, first of all neurasthenia, then chronic fatigue syndrome and burnout. The diagnoses all have fatigue and weakness at the centers of their clinical pictures. This fatigue can be specified on several levels, from stress-related fatigue to exhaustion and long-term chronic fatigue feelings, to a more serious level as in overstrain and burnout. One key factor is that the fatigue is not primarily related to physical exertion, but rather is described as mental, emotional, or existential, and is associated with feelings of inadequacy and an imbalance between demand and ability. In all cases there is thus a relationship with stress.

A comparison between the key medical concepts formulated in 1900 and in 2000, to describe the delicate interaction between the individual and the demanding, unstable world, also shows clear parallels. Nervous tension corresponds to stress. Neurasthenia and overstrain correspond to chronic fatigue syndrome and burnout. In the same way that nervous tension could lead to overstrain with neurasthenia as the clinical manifestation, stress can lead to chronic fatigue or burnout. The depersonalization and emotional exhaustion that is seen as typical for burnout syndrome is also discussed in connection with the typical neurasthenia patient.

Diagnoses thus mirror more than physiological and biochemical events in the body. They project the contemporary cultural values and social codes, class and gender structures, and expected relations between individual and society. This is true on both the individual and collective levels. Certain conditions of social anxiety seem, for example, to be inseparable parts of the actual endeavor to be modern. These include stress, restlessness, fatigue, alienation, fragmentation, and nostalgia (and this last may be the reason for the wave of nostalgia sweeping through society today just as it did at the last turn of the century).

The high status of fatigue in the Western world's self-image around 1900 highlighted a deep cultural anxiety related to the rapid changes due to industrialism and the market economy. Combined with fatigue's actual meaning in industry's definition of efficient manpower, the fatigue problem was incorporated into various medical interpretive models. It also entered into other scientific theses, for example the one concerning the constancy of vital energy or the one on modernity as an energy-draining process. Medically legitimized and reformulated into a diagnostic name (neurasthenia), the overstrain image was brought back to the culture (the accepted set of norms and conceptions), where it was exposed by the mass media to offer the individual interpretive models, meaning, and context for subjective illness.

The question is whether an equally sweeping analysis can be attempted for the relationship between perceived fatigue and the society of today. During the 20th century the individual was encompassed gradually by a dramatic process of welfare development. After World War II, a state of social and economic depression, unemployment, and decreasing birthrates was turned around in most Western countries. In Sweden the Social Democratic drive and a series of central social policy changes built the "People's Home," a Swedish model of stability, equality, and optimism about progress. When the stress concept was redefined in the 1940s, it was primarily a scientific issue, though one with a broad impact. It was not yet of immediate interest as an instrument of social analysis, although during the 1960s quite a bit of attention was paid to the unhealthy effects of haste.

It is no great exaggeration to maintain that stress first enters the public consciousness when a new social situation lends the concept a new, well-defined role.

This point was reached in the 1980s, when an older welfare model was dismantled and the industrial society's stable structures were replaced by a market-controlled economic model with mobility, globalization, and freedom of choice as its standards. A vacuum of values occurred as new information technology and rapid communications confronted the individual with great demands. Speed, adaptability, and flexibility became expected qualities within the increasingly rationalized labor organizations. The rise of welfare, a favorable insurance policy (though marked by large national differences), and a new work ethic had simultaneously increased the possibility of expressing inner reluctance as illness. Sick leaves and consumption of medications showed dramatically increased frequencies. A spectrum of new syndromes arose, reinforced by the brutal reminder of AIDS of a loss of biological control. Medicine met the raised illness frequency with increased resources and great openness, and also with increased medicalization in the form of new disease names connected to viruses, toxins, radiation, and stressors. Pain, depression, and fatigue could be placed in meaningful patterns.

A second question is how this process looks when new syndromes appear, and are given names and definitions. Historical and contemporary case studies of individual diagnoses (neurasthenia and chronic fatigue syndrome) indicate that consensus on an illness is reached by negotiation between different players. The doctor's knowledge and laboratory tests create options for a new category of illness or a new significance for a new category of illness, but do not decide the social part of its progress and spread [10].

Thus, there is an aspect of every diagnosis that can be called the social construction of disease. This also doesn't mean that anything can be called a disease or that the disease doesn't, in fact, exist. It indicates rather that the identity an illness possesses – from its traditional medical identity (cause, diagnosis, prognosis, and treatment) to its meaning for patients, doctors, and the surroundings – is never a neutral consequence of biological factors. It functions instead as a social process with several participants, including doctors, patients, the health insurance system, the pharmaceutical industry, the media, and the cultural codes that constantly redefine what will be permitted to be called sick.

This means that illness always exists in a medical dimension, but that its sociology and epidemiology must be analyzed on a greater social stage. It is here that the images and myths are created, and here that the legitimized, opinion-forming processes are acted out. Seen from this perspective, we can assert that the concept of stress has been transformed from a psychophysiological condition to a simultaneously explanatory, forgiving, and challenging social diagnosis.

A final question is whether the historical perspective offers any useful knowledge. At the turn of the 19th century collective and individual fatigue was interpreted as an immediate, physiologically measurable effect of external stress. Fatigue was defined as the limit beyond which an individual in the industrial society could not be forced, and therefore also as the limit beyond which social demands on the individual became counterproductive. The machine metaphor was important; if the person/machine was run so hard that it broke down, then the effectiveness that was the specific goal of production was counteracted. This association inspired very intensive research on both the fatigue that was directly caused by labor organizations and working conditions, and that caused by the contemporary cultural codes, including competition, performance demands, superficialized human relations, and narcissistic individualism.

If the same conclusions were to be drawn today it would mean that fatigue, under its time-adapted name of chronic fatigue syndrome, burnout, exhaustion syndrome, or any other, could be interpreted as a limit for the individual's physical and mental adaptability. An action program aimed at negative labor structures could be formulated. It could also be aimed at negative cultural values, loss of collective identity, and the cult of the young, invulnerable body.

Modern fatigue science focuses specifically on the sophisticated interactions between, on the one hand, the body's neural, hormonal, and immunity systems, and on the other hand the individual's life-conditions, and social and gendered structures. This means that the problem is not just a medical concern, but ultimately a political and humanistic responsibility.

References

1 *J. Mental Sci.* **1901** 47, 226–244.
2 M. BERMAN **1983** *All that is solid melts into air. The experience of modernity.* Verso, London, p. 15.
3 A. MATHIEU **1893** *Neurasthénie.* Paris.
4 A. RABINBACH **1992** *The human motor. Energy, fatigue, and the origins of modernity,* University of California Press, Berkeley, p. 23.
5 G. BEARD **1869** *A practical treatise on nervous exhaustion.* New York. See also: F. G. GOSLING **1988** *Before Freud. Neurasthenia and the medical community 1870–1910,* Urbana University Press, Urbana; G. F. DRINKA **1984** *The birth of neurosis: myth, malady, and the Victorians,* Simon and Schuster, New York; M. GIJSWIJT-HOFSTRA, R. PORTER (eds.)

2001 *Cultures of neurasthenia. From Beard to the First World War,* Rodopi, Amsterdam.
6 H. BERG **1903** *Läkarebok,* Göteborg, p. 1330.
7 R. A. ARONOWITZ **1998** *Making sense of illness. Science, society and disease.* Cambridge University Press, New York.
8 S. E. ABBEY, P. E. GARFINKEL **1991** Neurasthenia and chronic fatigue syndrome: the role of culture in the making of a diagnosis. *Am. J. Psychiatry,* December, 1638–1646.
9 B. SÖDERSTEN *Dagens Nyheter,* October 27, 1990.
10 C. E. ROSENBERG, J. GOLDEN (eds.) **1992** *Framing disease: studies in cultural history.* Rutgers University Press, New Brunswick, xiii–xxvi.

2
Evolutionary Aspects of Stress

Björn Folkow

2.1
Introduction

The very existence of this book illustrates how human health depends not only on our physicochemical–microbiological environment but also on our psychosocial one. They differ fundamentally both in nature and in the routes by which they can impose threats to health, as schematically illustrated in Fig. 2.1, which depicts not only the various "levels of control" (I–VII) that are common to all mammals, but also via which of these levels these two types of environmental challenges initiate their effects.

In these respects man and other mammals are remarkably alike, and this includes the mechanisms utilized in coping with the two types of threats. Thus, noxious physicochemical–microbiological factors invade the organism by means of airways, gastrointestinal tract and/or skin, i.e., at the organ–system level (III). From there, they can reach all organ systems via the circulatory and lymphatic systems, or sometimes via nerve tracts, and harm their cellular–biochemical processes. For millennia, these types of health threats and disorders have been the major target for medical interventions, from the era of "witch doctors" to present-day organ–system specialists. One reason is the often obvious links between cause and disorder, and particularly so as the time-lag between cause and effect usually is fairly short.

Fig. 2.1. Schematic diagram, illustrating the seven (*I–VII*) main levels of organization and control in higher organisms. To the *left* is shown how psychosocial stimuli reach the brain via the "telereceptor" senses (vision, hearing, olfaction). If judged as harmful, the brain can via "triads" of responses, involving (a) behavior, (b) autonomic nervous system and (c) hormonal system, adjust all lower levels of organization (including genetic expressions via some hormones) so as best to cope with the situation. To the *right* is shown how noxious influences in the physicochemical–microbiological environment invade the organism at the organ–system level (*III*), i.e., via airways, the gastrointestinal tract and/or skin. From here on they can spread via the blood stream, lymph, or sometimes nerve tracts to all cells and disturb their processes.

Stress in Health and Disease. Edited by Bengt B. Arnetz and Rolf Ekman
Copyright © 2006 WILEY-VCH Verlag GmbH & Co. KGaA, Weinheim
ISBN: 3-527-31221-8

HUMAN ORGANISM

(I) CNS level (mental functions)

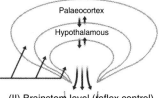

Psychosocial environment:

Harmful influences invade via:
Highest CNS levels which, by means of neurohormonal links influence all other levels.

Telereceptor information

Physicochemical environment:

Harmful influences invade via:
Respiratory system
Gastrointestinal system
Skin and mucous membrane

(II) Brainstem level (reflex control)

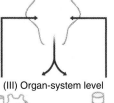

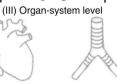

(III) Organ-system level

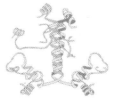

(IV) Cellular level

(V) Sub-cellular level

(VI) Macromolecular level

(VII) Genetic code

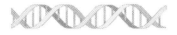

In contrast, psychosocial challenges present a vastly more complex situation, as their initial target is the central nervous system (CNS). The brain receives information about the environmental situation via signals from the "telereceptor" senses – vision, hearing, olfaction – that more or less continuously scan what is going on in the surroundings. Whenever these signals by the brain are interpreted as potentially harmful – or alternatively as appealing – the cerebral supercomputer can in anticipatory, and often "emotionally charged" fashions respond to the new situation. This is accomplished by combining all three efferent control links – (A) the somatomotor system, (B) the autonomic (visceromotor) system and (C) the hormonal system – into suitable and properly graded "triads" of coping behaviors for the situation, described in Section 2.4. In principle, B and C are then so adjusted as to make A as efficient as possible. Particularly in primitive life this is all-important, as the gain of a split second can mean the difference between life and death, e.g., when a cheetah hunts an antelope.

When, however, oft-repeated or chronically involved, these psychosocially induced neurohormonal expressions can result in considerable disturbances to health, and also cause serious disorders or even death. As links between cause and effects here are immensely complex, it may take years before true diseases ensue. This explains why disorders caused by mental stress have long been neglected – and often still are in an era where reductionism and molecular events dominate biomedical thinking.

As the literature relevant to this topic is enormous, reference is mainly given to review articles or books that cover various aspects of the field, and provide access to more important studies of experimental, epidemiological or other nature.

2.2
Man's Situation in a Phylogenetic Perspective

The mentioned triads of coping patterns that serve to protect self and species in a merciless environment are physiologically organized at the paleocortical (limbic) and hypothalamic levels of the brain. Here man and other mammals are, as mentioned, remarkably alike in neuronal architecture, circuit couplings, transmitters etc., implying that these brain regions were in general fully developed already some 100 million years ago – and parts of it even earlier in lower animals and birds. Thus, the human brain differs from those of other mammals, mainly because in our species the superimposed neocortical level has shown, in, biological terms, an unusually rapid growth and differentiation during the last few million years. However, even this difference is quantitative rather than qualitative in nature, though its consequences are remarkable indeed, in terms of present-day cultural–technical achievements. Nevertheless, man should perhaps remain humble concerning neocortical organization, because dolphins seem to more or less match *Homo sapiens* in the size of the hemispheres, when related to lean body mass. Accordingly, dolphins exhibit such remarkable mental performances that they have sometimes been called "people of the oceans", although their medium of existence no doubt imposes restrictions on what they may accomplish.

There are also other reasons for humility when it comes to man's neocortical accomplishments, namely if they are related to the very long time it has taken for our species to reach what we call civilization. This has been outlined and documented by the physiologist J. Diamond in a fascinating way in two recent books [1, 2]. Further, to paraphrase my colleague in exercise physiology, P.O. Åstrand, the situation is memorably illustrated if one compares man's evolutionary history with a 42-km-long marathon run. It may then be appropriate to start the run some 2 million years ago, when our African ancestors seem to have produced the first few primitive tools to help them in their struggle for survival. However, it was perhaps 300 000–400 000 years ago our species first began to spread from tropical Africa to other parts of the globe, i.e., when only 6–8 km of our run remained. This relatively late exodus toward cooler global regions was probably mainly due to the fact that man is, indeed, a tropical species. Thus, at naked rest our ideal thermoequilibrium is at 27–28 °C environmental temperature, which is why our thermoregulatory sweating system has a capacity of 8–10 L a day. For such reasons any migration required easy access to fresh water, and thus would follow streams, or coastlines where streams end, after which came protective coverings when chilly regions were reached, as well as the use of fire.

In these long and slow migrations, the Australian continent seems to have been reached some 40 000–50 000 years ago, i.e., when only about a kilometer of the run remained. It occurred across Torres Strait, which at this time was far narrower due to the enormous amounts of water that were bound in the massive ice cover to northern global regions during the last Ice Period. It was probably the same Ice Period that delayed man's access from northern Asia to the American continents until some 15 000–20 000 years ago, i.e., when only 300–400 m of the run was left. It must have occurred along the ice border in the Bering Sound region, which certainly demanded protective clothing. Arrival in the Pacific Islands occurred far later, and mainly from southeast Asia, as it called for ocean-going canoes or timber rafts, when first some 1000 years ago the Hawaiian Islands were reached from the Tahiti region. To some extent, migration to the Pacific Islands may also have occurred from South America; Heyerdahl and colleagues proved this possible in 1947, simply by doing it.

The start of agriculture – and hence chances for domilication instead of a hunter–gatherer's or shepherd's migratory life – goes back about 7000–8000 years in time. It seems to have started along the Euphrates and Tigris rivers in present-day Iraq, where wild wheat was growing and gradually cultivated, and probably around the same time in southeast Asia on the basis of wild rice. Thus, this fundamentally important prerequisite for stable cultural development occurred when only some 150 m of our species' marathon run remained – or a mere 350–400 generations ago. Finally, the "Machine Age" started 200–250 years ago, when only 4–5 m of the run remained while the modern industrial–postindustrial era is like the last few decimeters of man's marathon run [3].

In general, therefore, during more than 99.5% of the 2-million-year period, or over some 100 000 generations, our species has survived as small groups of hunter–gatherers, bound together by emotional links and roaming around in search of food and fresh water, a type of life demanding light equipment and a minimum of requisita, and which only a generation or two ago was still the case in remote corners of the globe. (An example: when the gold-rush started in Western Australia the roaming Aborigines thought that the gold diggers were silly and stupid, collecting these immensely heavy and useless golden stones ...) Considering this enormous time span, human beings must already have been fairly like people of today when it comes to intellectual potential thousands of generations ago. Thus, the long-sluggish, and regionally highly variable pace of material–cultural development has probably mainly been determined by such factors as local access to – or lack of – environmental resources.

For example, in his fascinating book *Guns, Germs and Steel* [2], the physiologist J. Diamond illustrates how differences in material culture closely relate to regional differences in natural resources. He became interested in such problems, when he – being also an outstanding ornithologist – visited the New Guinea remote highlands for bird-watching. He then noted how his stone-age aboriginal friends were – as he states – about as clever as his faculty colleagues home in Los Angeles, and nevertheless they led a stone-age lifestyle. He then made a heroic attempt to find out why. Thus, though always fairly rare, high intelligence must have been man's creative cotraveler for thousands of generations, and been fairly evenly spread among the groups of humans, migrating along coastlines and into continents in search of food, water and protection. After all, to survive as a hunter–gatherer in harsher global regions certainly demands respectable mental qualities gradually chiseled out by the tough principle of survival of the fittest. By means of such selection processes concerning neocortical abilities – as combined with age-old behaviors of protection, imprinted at the paleocortical–hypothalamic levels of the brain – present-day *Homo sapiens* faces an entirely different, and biologically artificial "Brave New World." It is created by the very same neocortical qualities that for thousands of generations have helped skilled hunter–gatherers along the road.

Paul McLean, former director of psychophysiological research at the National Institutes of Health (NIH) in the USA, has used a colorful metaphor to illustrate man's situation in today's psychosocial environment: he compares the interactions between our neocortical and paleocortical–hypothalamic brain levels with that of a more or less competent rider of an inherently restive horse. As long as the rider is in full command of the horse, they represent an efficient combination of skills and force, but when the horse is driven against its instincts by a foreign situation, its emotional responses tends to take over, and it may even throw the rider.

In other words, there is a inherent potential conflict between the neocortical and paleocortical facets of the human mind, which are particularly obvious when new challenges are met with. For example, when an ever-avalanching stream of stimuli are experienced as mentally stressful, it may disturb the balance between the two brain regions, leading to mental strain – to use the terms stress and strain appropriately (see Section 2.3). Then the same emotionally colored triads of expression that were designed eons ago for coping with overt physical threats and challenges are elicited, but they are not always as purposeful in present-day life.

After all, in a biological perspective the psychosocial climate of the modern hectic–competitive society is entirely artificial and seen from such an angle it is, in a way, natural that the brain responds with neurohormonal expressions associated with emotional displays. Neither is it strange that these reactions, when repeated or chronic, can cause disturbances and disorders, but it has taken a very long time to understand what is going on, simply because highly complex psychophysiological mechanisms and neurohormonal expressions are involved. In this context, it is therefore worthwhile to mention a few milestones in the biomedical search for a truly physiological and biochemical understanding of what is going on between mind and body, when man can become physically sick from mental challenges.

2.3
From Intuitive Insight to Experimental Documentation

Since the dawn of culture, observant people have noted how strong emotions can profoundly affect bodily functions, and even lead to death; this is not infrequently reflected in ancient scripts like the Old Testament. Furthermore, as long as arts have existed, these expressions of mind–body interactions have fascinated poets, writers, sculptors and painters, long before scientists tried to find out what was going on. An example from a millennium ago: The Icelandic Tales visualize the immense wrath and frustration of young Glum, when he had lost a dispute at the Iceland Thing, by the following low-key, though chilling, description of his reactions: "Then Glum turned homewards, and a huge laugh came over him. It took him so that his face became white while tears poured from his eyes. It was commonly so when bloodshed was in his mind." Better than pages of modern psychological–analytical prose, this laconic text reflects a mental turmoil of magnificent and scaring dimensions.

But doctors early intuitively understood that important events were going on. Thus, as long as 1500 years before young Glum's display, Hippocrates, the "Father of Medicine," somehow understood how important interactions between mind and body could be to health, and how they are affected by both the physical and social environments of a patient. Though the number of useful drugs at that time could be counted on the fingers of one hand, clever physicians could be quite successful. For example, in ancient Alexandria the Hippocratian school taught students that if doctors met their patients in such a way as to gain their full confidence and trust from the start, "then half the cure was won" – from which the term placebo ("I will please") stems.

It would, however, take nearly two-and-a-half millennia – in fact, it was only a few decades ago – before it was experimentally shown how placebo effects are actually due to strictly physiological processes in the brain. It implies an engagement of cerebral endorphin neurons, and for that reason placebo effects can be more or less eliminated by the endorphin-blocker narloxon. Moreover, such mentally induced activations of cerebral endorphin mechanisms result not only in mental sedation and pain relief, but also damp sympathetic activity, enhance parasympathetic activity and even stimulate the immune system and its defenses against infections, tumor cells etc. Hippocrates and colleagues probably smiled in their esculapian heaven when their "fancy" placebo effects were thus shown to reflect strictly physiological brain mechanisms that mobilize the "inner forces of healing." Still more important things are bound to be detected in this fascinating field.

These early, though mainly intuitive, insights by early doctors concerning mind–body interactions, and their importance for health and disease, were to some extent obscured in the 1630s–1640s, when the brilliant French mathematician and philosopher René Descartes (Cartesius) presented his philosophical work. The reason was that it contained also the concept that only man has a soul, considered to be a spiritual entity separate from the body, though perhaps residing in the epiphysis. In contrast, animals were thought to be mere complex machineries, and unfortunately often treated accordingly. Church authorities were, of course, delighted by this "Cartesian dichotomy", but it hardly promoted holistic views in medicine, which had its remarkable experimental start around the same time. Thus, in 1628 William Harvey in London published his classic experimental analysis of the circulation of blood in *De Motu Cordis*, whereby a new approach to biomedical problems began.

Nevertheless, the Cartesian dichotomy may to a great extent be responsible for the fact that the brain remained *terra incognita* in experimental research for another 250–300 years. Thus, it was not until the 1910s–1930s that experimental studies suggested that the brain also directs the autonomic–nervous and hormonal systems, much of which is outlined in a Physiological Reviews volume [4]. In a way, indications in this direction had already appeared in Charles Darwin's 1872 book *The Expressions of the Emotions in Man and Animals*. In his thorough observations of birds and mammals he had been struck by the close similarities between man and other mammals when facing, e.g., danger and how this indicated the involvement of basal parts of the brain.

However, real breakthroughs in this field came first during the 1930s–1950s, thanks to scientists like Ivan Pavlov in St Petersburg, Walter Bradford Cannon in Boston, Walter Rudolf Hess in Zürich and Hans Selye in Montreal [4, 5]. For example, in his classic studies of conditioned reflexes in dogs, Pavlov noticed how these CNS-dependent mechanisms became profoundly disturbed after trained dogs had accidentally been exposed to severe mental stress, as they nearly drowned in their cellar during a Neva flood. Studies of (and unfortunately also deliberate induction of) traumatic mental strain, thereby had their start.

Cannon analyzed the extensive sympathohormonal activations in dogs and cats in fear or rage, calling adrenaline the "catastrophe hormone." Further, with Bard he showed how these mechanisms are organized in the paleocortical–hypothalamic regions of the brain, while the neocortex has in this respect important inhibitory influences [4].

Hess mapped out these brain sections by means of precise topical stimulations in conscious cats, showing how separate activations of small neuron groups could largely induce all types of natural emotional patterns. It also became evident that all the three efferent links were engaged in various "triad constellations", though few details were known. For this Hess was awarded the Nobel Prize in Physiology or Medicine in 1949, and had not Cannon died a few years earlier he might well have shared the prize with Hess.

Selye – Hungarian-born, and educated in Prague, though working in Montreal from the 1930s – exposed rodents to severe physical, and hence also mental insults, and thoroughly analyzed the results. He showed how they all led to activations of the hypothalamic–hypophyseal–ACTH–glucocorticoid axis, resulting in characteristic changes in metabolism, organ functions and in the immune system [6]. Fluent in several European languages – though perhaps least so in English – Selye called this state of profound bodily and mental disturbances "stress", a word which has since become one of the most commonly used, and misused, in biomedicine, and in daily jargon as well. The proper word should have been "strain" as stress causes strain (compare Hooke's law of elasticity: the elasticity modulus equals stress/strain). Actually, later in life Selye jokingly said to his co-worker Paul Rosch, now director of the American Institute of Stress, that had his English been better in younger years, he would have been world-reknowned as the "Father of Strain" instead of being called the "Father of Stress" [7].

Anyway, these pioneer findings during the 1930s–1950s made it clear that the sympatho–adrenomedullary axis and the hypophyseal–ACTH–glucocorticoid axis are the main efferent links used by the brain when mental challenges are at hand – and then closely linked to somatomotor-determined behaviors. Extensive studies during subsequent decades have vastly increased both knowledge and interest in this difficult though highly important field. Among other things, it had the result that the WHO in 1960 sponsored an international conference in Prague, where the involvement of stress-related mechanisms in primary (essential) hypertension was intensely debated between the "CNS" and "kidney" schools. The WHO then asked the endocrinologist–clinician Joseph Charvat in Prague, the French neurophysiologist Paul Dell in Paris and the present author to try to outline to what an extent – if any – that mental stress may contribute to cardiovascular disorders in general, and this was published in 1964 [8]. However, at the time the Cartesian dichotomy seemed to still influence thoughts concerning bodily disorders, because the WHO added a cautious footnote to the article, stating "… it does not necessarily reflect the opinions of the World Health Organisation."

Among the important experimental studies in animals during later decades, the work by Henry, with coworkers like Stephens and Ely and using group-living rodents as models of human society, should be noted particularly [9, 10]. They will for this reason be dealt with further in subsequent sections, as will related group studies in primate monkeys by Clarkson, Kaplan, Manuck et al. [10]. Of studies in man, Roger Sperry's Nobel-Prize-awarded discovery concerning hemispheric functional differentiation deserves mention in this context, as it also revealed how the neocortical control of emotions and emotional expressions are organized. To grossly simplify: the left hemisphere has a preference for analytical approaches to situations and problems and for detached matter-of-fact attitudes; usually well expressed as it also commands speech. In contrast, the "silent" – though by other means expressive – right hemisphere is characterized by holistic evaluations and intuition–emotion-valued approaches to problems.

Important consequences of the mentioned animal studies, and of the hemispheric specialization concerning emotions and their expressions, are surveyed in the Acta Physiologica Scandinavica volume [10] honoring James P. Henry's pioneer work. For example, surveys by Wittling, by Shapiro, Jamner and Spence and by Wang discuss various aspects of right-hemispheric dominance with respect to emotions and emotional displays, as does Henry himself in this mini-review volume. It has important implications concerning man's situation in today's society, as becomes further evident in Sections 2.5 and 2.6. In a way, modern society is increasingly dominated by "left-hemispheric rationality", from how children are educated in schools to how society and production are run. As a result, for mental health – and hence health in general – important right-hemispheric qualities tend to be set aside, as they are less concerned with materialistic affairs. Is it perhaps these biological fundaments of the human brain's design that partly explain why stress-related disturbances and disorders are increasing in the midst of abounding material affluence which, in turn, is the result of a dominance of "left-hemispheric activities"?

2.4
Organization of Stress-Induced Response Patterns

2.4.1
General Aspects

Since the mentioned pioneer studies, knowledge has greatly increased concerning the functional organizations of the cerebral control of actual triads of neurohormonal responses. They represent the decisive mechanisms by which higher organisms cope with the positive and negative challenges met with in a primitive existence [9, 10]. In a way, these centrally controlled response patterns have much in common with how nations nowadays organize their military and civil preparations for coping with, e.g., international threats: here, any conceivable challenge is planned for, both concerning military engagements (i.e., somatomotor-linked behaviors), and concerning adjustments on the "inner front", such as industrial mobilizations, production and distribution of nutritional supplies, and so on (i.e., the visceromotor and hormonal adjustments) – all in order to ensure top efficiency in danger [5]. And all can be put into full action by a signal from the command center.

In the present context four of these preformed triads of response will be described in more detail, simply because they are particularly important and common whenever mammalian organisms meet situations experienced as potentially threatening. The very same patterns thus occur in human beings, facing instead the often symbolic–artificial challenges typical of modern life: here "mice and men" are equals, with the same ancient repertoire of responses, though they are of course often activated by widely different environmental stimuli [9, 10].

However, on two points *Homo sapiens* differs from other mammals, again mainly quantitatively, but with important consequences. First, thanks to a more sophisticated neocortical superstructure, man can better learn to distinguish between types and grades of mental stimuli, and hence to better select between important and trivial ones, which latter are then neglected. Had this not been possible, life in modern society may well have been intolerable, a type of coping ability that may fail in some mental disorders, whereby the mind is overwhelmed by environmental stimuli. Second, once an emotion is elicited, man can learn, though within limits, to suppress the somatomotor component of the triad in situations where this is socially appropriate. For example, it is hardly proper to start fist fights in parliamentary debates (though in hot-tempered societies it happens), or to jump for joy if one gets four aces in a hand of poker. Small children only gradually learn this type of coping, and choleric people perhaps never do. Animals are in these respects more 'honest,' in the sense that their emotions always show up in behaviors. This is illustrated by one out of many American shaggy dog stories, i.e., about the poker-playing dog who unfortunately always lost to his master because he wagged his tail whenever he had a strong hand of cards.

Anyway – and this is important in man's situation – once an emotion is evoked, the corresponding autonomic–nervous and hormonal parts of the triads cannot be suppressed and will therefore be fully induced – though perhaps only showing up to others as a blanched face (compare to young Glum in immense wrath). Though socially cohesive, such voluntary suppressions of somatomotor displays imply that preformed biological response patterns are broken up: the inner neurohormonal adjustments – meant to support behavioral exertions by increasing blood supply, mobilizing nutritional stores, and so on – then occur in vain. Animals are not able to distort their emotional expressions in such ways. When angry, dogs wholeheartedly enter into furious fights, but when it ends, so does the mental engagement; they relax and lick their wounds.

Man's ability to dissociate emotional responses in this way may, however, have serious biological consequences. First, the emotional state *per se* tends to become more long-lasting, because physical activity stimulates muscle ergo-afferents which, in turn, activate cerebral endorphin neurons, damping the emotional engagement (see, e.g., survey by Jonsdottir, Hoffman, Thorén in [10]). Second, the inner neurohormonal effects are correspondingly prolonged, so that mobilizations of fatty acids and glucose from nutritional depots are not used as intended, and will therefore remain longer in blood and tissue fluids.

Thus, modern life *per se* is characterized by decreasing physical activity in combination with increasing mental engagements in a hectic–competitive environment. In all these respects modern life is fundamentally different from the type of existence that our species has known for 99.5% of its existence – and for which we were biologically designed – from brain function down to cellular biochemistry. With such a background it is perhaps not so difficult to understand that nowadays, when we have never been so well-off, psychosomatic disturbances and diseases are a rapidly increasing threat to health. One may paradoxically perhaps say that it is a biological health sign that we so react to a biologically artificial life style. In any case, where the situation is acute, it invites mental tension and discomfort after a hectic workday, often inducing an urge for physical activities. This probably explains things like the jogging fad, whereby the triads' dissociation is at least in part compensated for and mental balance reestablished.

2.4.2
The Four Triads of Response

Among the many ways in which the brain can respond to environmental stimuli, four of them are of special interest here, and their general character is fairly well-known from both animal and human studies [5, 10]. Various names have been used, but they will below be denoted as follows: A, the vigilance ("freezing") reaction (VR); B, the playing dead ("inhibitory") reaction (PR); C, the defense ("alarm") reaction (DeR) and D, the defeat ("surrender") reaction (DfR). Their differences concerning neurohormonal effects on inner organs and metabolism are schematically illustrated in Fig. 2.2, and further described below.

VR and PR are in general episodic events, usually over within a minute or so,

	Vigilance reaction (VR)	Playing-dead reaction (PR)	Defence reaction (DeR)	Defeat reaction (DfR)
Sympathetic system	↑	↓	↑	↑↓
Parasympathetic system	↑↓	↑	↓	↑
ACTH-glucocorticoid axis	0 ?	0 ?	↑	↑
Heart	↑↓	↓	↑	↑↓
Blood pressure	↑	↓	↑	↑
Gastrointestinal system	↓	↓ ?	↓	↑
Kidney function	↓	↓ ?	↓	?
Immune system	↑ ?	0 ?	↑	↓

Fig. 2.2. A highly simplified illustration of the, in many respects drastically different, neurohormonal adjustments in the vigilance reaction (*VR*), the playing dead reaction (*PR*), the defense reaction (*DeR*) and the defeat reaction (*DfR*). The *arrows* indicate increase or decrease; their size extent. Two *arrows* in opposite directions indicate differentiated nervous discharge. "*Zero*" indicates no or insignificant change; a *question mark* that the effect is not fully known.

though VR can occur often in daily life, whether among antelopes on African savannas or among people living a hectic big-city life. However, their usually short duration implies that associated neurohormonal effects on inner organs are brief too, though in the acute situation important parts of the display.

By contrast, DeR and DfR can be quite prolonged when the situation is experienced as more or less continuously challenging or threatening, and DfR can even end in chronic states of frustration and despair. For such reasons, they are particularly important in the modern hectic–competitive life, as their visceromotor–hormonal influences on inner organs and metabolism often result in disturbances and disorders in the long run. Moreover, due to widespread effects on inner organ systems, as on skeletal muscle tone, heart rate, intestinal motility, and so on, afferent signals from these sites are induced, which may be experienced as alarming. This is reflected in old expressions like "heartfelt" or "it hurts my stomach", etc. Particularly where a "sore point" is at hand somewhere in the body, like tender neck muscles, a sensitive stomach or a "nervous" heart, the associated increases in afferent signals may so dominate in a stressful situation as to border on stigmatization: a "flight into disorder" from a mentally pressed situation, where the involved links are schematically illustrated in Fig. 2.3.

DeR and DfR will therefore be described in much detail below, and it will also be illustrated how they can decisively contribute to now-common "disorders of regulation", when often or chronically involved. It is, in a way, a paradox that age-old psychobiological response patterns, that for millions of years have served to protect self and species in primitive life, can today socially backfire and, in the long run, more seriously threaten health than most disorders with a physicochemical–microbiological background [11, 12].

2.4.2.1 The Vigilance (Freezing) Reaction (VR)

VR is induced whenever sudden stimuli reach the brain: an unexpected noise, the sight of a predator or the like. Ongoing activities are abruptly stopped and, in a tense and immobile position (freezing), all attention is directed toward the source, ready for fight or flight. Respiration is transiently interrupted in inspiratory position and, on the inner front, a combined sympathetic–parasympathetic pattern is induced, which is only known in part. Anyway, blood pressure increases, where systemic vasoconstriction is combined with vagal bradycardia. VR has been analyzed both in conscious birds (ptarmigans) by Steen and coworkers [5], and in awake cats by Mancia et al. [5], via topical brain stimulations by McCabe et al. [13] and, in human beings exposed to sudden stimuli, by Anderson et al. [14]. Thus, when intensely involved in man it may substantially increase blood pressure.

If, however, the initiating stimulus proves to be harmless, VR usually fades away, but if danger really is at hand, VR can within seconds shift over to DeR, PR or, sometimes, to DfR. Which of these patterns that the cerebral computer chooses after an initial VR depends on the nature of the situation, but to some extent also on species. For example, an opossum rat often prefers PR (in the southern USA, often called playing possum), while lions may prefer DeR and all-out attack. Again, subordinate members of group-living animals, when suddenly facing the aggres-

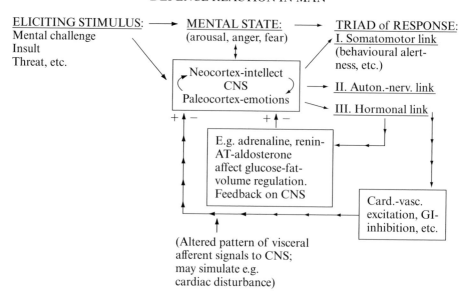

DEFENCE REACTION IN MAN

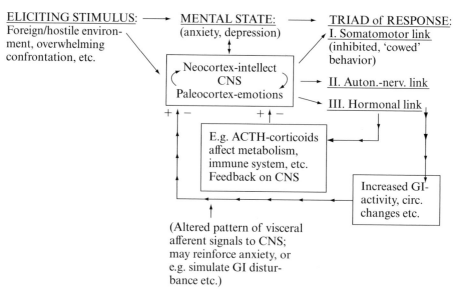

DEFEAT REACTION IN MAN

Fig. 2.3. Schematic illustration of how, e.g., the defense and defeat reactions may become involved in daily human life, in terms of types of eliciting stimuli, induced mental state and ensuing "triads" of expression, i.e., change of behavior, autonomic–nervous and hormonal functions. It is also indicated how some of involved hormones, as well as afferent nerves from inner organs, have feedback effects on the brain, often reinforcing emotions and experiences of changed inner organ functions – sometimes to the extent that these effects, rather than the eliciting mental challenge, dominate the experience – perhaps even resulting in an "escape into disorder" from intolerable psychosocial situations.

sive dominant, may prefer DfR – but all four types of reaction are available in all mammals, including man.

In well-camouflaged species in particular, VR has an additional protective value, as they are very difficult to detect in freezing. The author once experienced how a nesting ptarmigan bird, instrumented for telemetric ECG recordings by Steen et al. at the Institute of Arctic Biology in Tromsö, Norway, was impossible to detect even at a distance of only 5 m, though revealed telemetrically by the bradycardia, typical for VR. On approaching further VR suddenly shifted to DeR, with intense tachycardia, and the bird escaped in flight. Further, on a moose hunt in Norway we heard an animal approaching in dense bushes. I then noticed how respiration stopped in inspiration position and heart rate slowed down, but when the huge moose bull suddenly showed up, DeR and tachycardia occurred – presumably both in moose and hunters. Over to ordinary daily life: there are probably many occupations where rapid and frequent shifts of environmental stimuli quite frequently induce VR, and with that pressure peaks and transient respiratory interruptions, to the extent that, according to Anderson's group, blood CO_2 values are enhanced [14].

2.4.2.2 The Playing Dead (Inhibitory) Reaction (PR)

When animals are in acute danger, and chances for flight or attack seem excluded (being cornered), a dramatic inhibitory response can occur: motility and muscle tone, as well as respiratory movements, are suddenly and completely inhibited, and the animal hangs slack if lifted by tail (sometimes experienced by opossum hunters believing that they shot the animal dead, but it got scared by the missed shot and went into PR).

On the inner front, a transient but immediate loss of consciousness seems to occur, suggesting a centrally induced suppression of locus caeruleus activity at brain stem level, whereby its catecholamine-dependent actions on brain activity ceases [5, 13]. In the cardiovascular system such a profound vagal bradycardia can occur that the heart almost stops. At the same time generalized sympathetic inhibition leads to vasodilatation, further accentuating the marked blood pressure fall. Thus, such animals appear to be dead, which may protect them from such predators that only eat prey that they have themselves killed.

The opossum is, as mentioned, the perfect model of PR displays, but PR seems to be used for protection by many species, particularly when well-camouflaged in colors, and then alternating with VR. For example, when people find "sick" deer calves abandoned by their mother in the woods, it most likely is a healthy newborn calf displaying PR, while its mother waits anxiously behind bushes that stupid foreigners should have the sense to leave. Further, the old fable about the cunning fox, surprised by the farmer in the chicken house and "pretending" to be dead and would then escape, in all likelihood stems from such a situation: the fox was not at all cunning, but deadly scared and went into a full-fledged PR.

Man's emotional fainting is in all likelihood our version of PR, and exactly the same neurohormonal adjustments then occur. Further, it is typically elicited by sudden fear or by intensely embarrassing situations, but can sometimes be elicited by unexpected great joy. Shakespeare, with his magnificent command of words, somewhere described man's emotional fainting as follows: "... an inward flight from the slings and arrows of outrageous fortune ..."

PR is, however, not necessarily an all-or-none inhibitory response. At milder stimuli of the same character, it may merely be experienced as a sudden mental and physical weakness, where the legs give out and one feels inclined to slump down in a chair (being "entirely shocked"). The author vividly experienced this as a schoolboy, with some friends when we ran into a moose cow with newborn calves on a stroll in the woods. With raised fur and lowered ears she charged us and we started to run, but our legs would not work and we fell, laughing hysterically but in great fear. She, however, with mission accomplished, turned away and vanished with her youngsters to our immense relief. Thus, milder variants of the inhibitory PR are probably common in all mammals, with the full-fledged playing dead as the most extreme variant of an age-old protective mechanism.

2.4.2.3 The Defense (Alarm) Reaction (DeR)

DeR is by far the best studied and known among the emotional response patterns, not only because it is particularly important, but also because it is that most easily induced in conscious experimental animals. Thus, even when animals are, for example, in a chronic DfR situation, they tend to promptly shift over to DeR when confronted by people, making it difficult to trace the initial DfR-related neurohormonal pattern. Another example: years ago we tried to induce PR in opossum rats in the laboratory environment, but they all responded with DeR. Evidently we could not mimic the typical situation for PR displays for opossums, which, in a way, also illustrates how – even in primitive opossums – it is a matter of highly sophisticated brain mechanisms that can alternate at the slightest change in situation.

This is, incidentally, the reason why it can be very difficult to analyze emotional responses in man under laboratory conditions. A memorable example: we were interested in whether emotional blushing is part of DeR, and by which mechanism it is then induced. The hospital had a nurse, known by all to blush at the slightest provocation, and we asked whether she could volunteer as an experimental subject. Courageously she did, and by local anaesthesia we blocked sympathetic nerves to one-half of the face, recording blood flow in the two cheeks by various means. Then we tried increasingly drastic stimuli to induce a blush – but she remained quite undisturbed and did not blush at all in the unanaesthetized side of the face. Finally, the local anaesthesia faded away and we had to stop the study. When she was ready to leave, I thanked her profusely for her kindness and courage – and she got warmly red all over her face ... This exemplifies how neocortical interferences can dramatically interfere with paleocortical–hypothalamic mechanisms, which makes man quite a difficult experimental model when it comes to mechanisms of this kind.

Anyhow, the term defense reaction – once chosen to denote how this pattern shows up, e.g., in experimentally threatened cats or dogs – may give the erroneous impression that DeR only occurs when real danger is at hand. However, like the other response patterns, DeR is a well-graded one, being only marginally induced at weak arousal stimuli, though no doubt with maximal displays when situations are experienced as life-threatening. The well-graded engagements of DeR in man is perhaps best illustrated by the fact that it is mildly induced experimentally by such trivial and harmless stimuli as playing electronic ping-pong, or by exposing people to forced mental arithmetic (i.e., subtracting, say 47, from 5000 every time a metronome signals: within short most people display a beautiful DeR – but the example above also illustrates how neocortical interventions may distort responses) [3, 5, 11, 13].

The somatomotor component of DeR is characterized in animals by attack or flight, where the choice depends on situation and species.

However, in man this component is often, though within limits as exemplified earlier, more or less suppressed or diverted, though electromyographic recordings are likely to reveal increased tension in several muscle groups, e.g., shoulder and back. On the inner front, a widespread though differentiated neurohormonal pattern is induced, which down to the last detail is the same in animals and man.

The limbically–hypothalamically directed discharge overrules bulbar and local control mechanisms and intensely engages the sympathetic nervous system, though in a differentiated fashion and combined with inhibition of parasympathetic activity [5, 13]. Thus, in the cardiovascular system DeR superimposes an anticipatory adjustment that is highly suited for supporting an all-out muscle exertion in attack or flight. For example, the systemic vasculature is neurogenically adjusted to increase blood supply to skeletal muscles, myocardium and brain, while blood flow to the kidneys, gastrointestinal tract, most skin regions, etc., is reduced, at the same time as ongoing activities are here suppressed by sympathetic neurohormonal influences. Concomitantly, blood depots, like the voluminous venous side, is adjusted by sympathetic nerves so as to enhance venous return to the heart, where both rate and contractility are stimulated, all serving to increase cardiac output.

Further, via sympathetic nerves and adrenaline, nutritional depots are mobilized, glucose being released from the liver and free fatty acids from adipose tissue. On the fluid–electrolyte side, sympathetic activation includes a β-receptor-mediated engagement of the renin–angiotensin–aldosteron axis, serving to reduce salt–water excretion, while the suppressed gastrointestinal secretion, if anything, improves intestinal salt–water uptake, contributing to enhanced plasma volume. Even mild engagements of DeR increases salt appetite, an adjustment also serving to enhance plasma–extracellular fluid volumes – first shown by Denton et al., in stressed rabbits and confirmed in other species [10, 11]. The essential elements of DeR are illustrated in the left part of Fig. 2.4, modified from Henry and Grim [15] and their excellent 1990 survey. As a result of these neurohormonal adjustments, DeR is usually characterized by substantial increases in blood pressure, though the key element is to elevate cardiac output enough so as to secure a maximal blood supply to skeletal muscles, myocardium and brain at all costs, for an optimal flight/fight exertion. When this follows, the metabolically induced accentuation of muscle vasodilatation so modifies the balance between cardiac output and systemic resistance that the net increase in blood pressure is fairly modest.

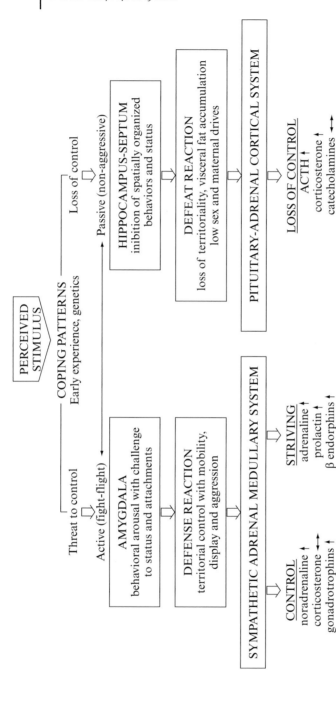

Fig. 2.4. Schematic illustration of the defense reaction and defeat reactions, as analyzed and perceived by Henry et al. [15], on the basis of experimental studies of group-living rodents. Shifts between the two reactions are common in striving for control. The defense reaction prevails when organisms are challenged but manage to maintain control, while if control is lost the defeat reaction dominates concerning both behavior and neurohormonal expressions. Modified from Henry and Grim [15].

As, however, the somatomotor component of DeR is more or less suppressed in human civilized life, the net results of even mild DeR engagements in man often end up in substantial blood pressure increases. Occasionally this can precipitate catastrophe in elderly persons if coronary or cerebral arteries are past their best, because an intense DeR can easily increase the work load for the myocardium five- to sixfold, and mean arterial pressure 50–60%. This is colorfully illustrated by what happened to the eminent British surgeon and scientist John Hunter about two centuries ago. Of choleric temperament – and with coronaries narrow enough to give him frequent angina pectoris attacks – Hunter once said: "My life is at the mercy of any rascal who chooses to annoy me." And when he once exploded with anger at some fool, this was his predicted and sudden end.

At the other end of the spectrum, marginal DeR activations, which often occur in modern life, perhaps mixed with VR episodes, whenever attention is raised, usually imply that the heart rate increases, say, 20% and blood pressure 10–15% but, even so, all the other mentioned changes occur in the background, correspondingly balanced. In, for example, daily office work today, blood pressure is at its highest level during work hours, reflecting mild DeR engagements, while the by far the lowest values occur during sleep. This has become evident from several ambulant blood pressure recordings, like that by Omae et al. in Japan [11, 13]. They also showed how genetic profiles were expressed, because in subjects predisposed to primary (essential) hypertension the work–time blood pressure elevations were (percentage-wise) three times higher than in ordinary normotensive subjects. It is via these milder, though more long-lasting, or/and frequent, DeR activations over years that modern life's psychosocial climate can, in the long run, decisively contribute to the perhaps most common among civilization disorders, primary (essential) hypertension [11, 12, 15, 16]) – and then often more or less combined with DfR and the metabolic syndrome (MS) [17, 18], as discussed in Sections 2.4.3 and 2.5 below.

2.4.2.4 The Defeat Reaction (DfR)

Intense variants of this neurohormonal reaction occur when organisms experience stressful situations as so overwhelming that coping attempts, by, e.g., DeR, end in mental exhaustion and despair. This is illustrated in Fig. 2.3, and in the right part of Fig. 2.4 from the classic work of Henry and coworkers [9, 10, 15]. Again, the inner neurohormonal expressions of DfR are, as in DeR, VR and PR, the same down to the last detail, from mouse to man. However, while sympatho–adrenal activation dominates in DeR, the hypothalamic–pituitary–adrenocortisol axis forms the dominant element in DfR, as combined with e.g., central suppressions of growth hormone and sex hormones. As a result, profound behavioral and metabolic changes ensue, further resulting in a corticoid-related suppression of the immune system.

Autonomic nervous changes in DfR are less well-known than those in DeR, but the two certainly differ considerably (Fig. 2.4): in DfR a mixed sympathetic–parasympathetic engagement is at hand, as systemic resistance and blood pressure increase modestly as combined with vagal bradycardia. Further, parasympathetic activation to the gastrointestinal tract seems to occur, as, e.g., gastric mucosal blood flow and secretion increase. Thus, rats exposed to situations that lead to DfR engagement often respond with gastric mucosal ulcerations; this is sometimes used as an experimental model to test antiulceration drugs. Likewise, in their well-known experimental subject – and senior laboratory assistant – "Tom", Wolff and Wolf could observe, via his gastrostomy fistula, that gastric secretion and blood flow increased markedly when Tom was in a state of frustration–resentment or depressed. However, when scared, i.e., in a bout of DeR, Tom responded with intense blanching of the gastric mucosa and secretion stopped.

With respect to the somatomotor link, and hence behaviors, intense DfRs lead to general inhibition and withdrawal, with neglect of food intake, grooming, protection etc. It is not then so surprising that such consequences of intense DfR, in combination with the mentioned metabolic effects, and immune system suppression, can end in death. For example, in overpopulated animal colonies where migration is impossible, dominants secure survival by means of DeR and aggression, while weaker group members display DfR, general withdrawal and neglect, and ultimately often die [5, 9, 10] – nature's tough stamping-out method in situations where species survival has priority over individual welfare.

Concerning man, old scripts like the Bible mention situations where deep sorrow and despair lead to death. Further, outstanding biomedical scientists, like Walter Bradford Cannon and Stewart Wolf, were deeply interested in exploring what could be the biological events behind so-called voodoo deaths, known to occur e.g., in primitive tribal societies, when violators of some taboo were, at ceremonial rites, excluded from society to become nonpersons. In such situations it is hardly surprising that profound DfRs can be elicited: left alone in the jungle or desert, in a state of severe depression with associated metabolic and immunological disturbances, it is not so strange that death may ensure without any physical punishments being inflicted. One may wonder how often similar events occur in modern society when merciless news media run amok against a social or political sinner against some of today's taboos. We are, after all, only few generations apart from what we used to call primitive society. And there is certainly no lack of superstition.

Such striking expressions of intense DfR aside, marginal or mild forms are – as in DeR – common in daily life. Anyone can wake up one morning, facing a tough agenda that makes one inclined to stay in bed and vegetate – until a bout of DeR may reverse the mental balance. Thus, mild expressions of DfR are not only common but are presumably fairly harmless and part of ordinary life. Some examples: Frankenhauser et al. [3], experimentally exposed students to problem-solving tests, either relatively easy and confidence-inducing ones, or tougher and tending to cause anxiety and feelings of pending failure. They used changes of catecholamine and glucocorticoid levels in blood as markers for engagements of DeR and DfR respectively. When tests induced feelings of pending failure, an increased catecholamine release became associated with raised glucocorticoid levels, suggesting a combination of mild DeR and DfR activations.

Likewise, among group-living animals like rodents, wolves or some monkeys – and certainly in *Homo sapiens* as well – subordinate group members are kept in a state of mild DfR by dominants. This serves to maintain group stability, not least because the associated suppression of sex hormones reduces aggressiveness, and thereby ranking fights and other forms of intragroup disturbances.

2.4.3
DeR and DfR Involvements in Animal Models of Human Society

In Henry's classic studies of mouse "societies" [9, 10, 15], long-term consequences of psychosocial turmoil were followed in detail. With a life span of only 2.5–3 years these tiny rodents could be followed from cradle to grave in a strictly controlled way. Further, genetically linked differences in, e.g., stress sensitivity could also be explored by using various inbred strains.

In these miniature and time-compressed models of human society, persistent mental stress could be induced by such simple means as by repeatedly and randomly shifting individual animals between colonies. This led to frequent ranking confrontations with displays of varying intensity, not only of DeR, but also of DfR when group members experienced a loss of control and social support. The differences between the two patterns are seen in Fig. 2.4, modified from Henry's own illustrations.

These studies illustrate well how prolonged states of DeR and DfR, or frequent shifts between the two, can end in bodily disturbances and, in the cardiovascular system, closely mimicking man's primary hypertension and the MS. Further, it was shown how this was not only dependent on extent, type, and duration of stress exposure but also on genetic profile and sex. By applying the same principle of group studies to primates (cynomolgus monkeys, with over 95% genetic commonality with man), Kaplan, Clarkson, Manuck and colleagues [10, 19] have particularly explored the long-term consequences of DfR, i.e., in group members who in social controversies tend to loose control and social support – though this no doubt contains elements of shifts between DeR and DfR with time.

Here the monkeys end up with metabolic profiles that closely resemble those seen in man's MS, and after 1–2 years in such a defeat situation they also exhibit one of the MS's most serious sequelae in man, i.e., coronary atherosclerosis [17–19]. Mice and rats are less inclined to present this complication, but in other respects changes are closely similar among species. Such atherosclerosis also developed in the DfR-exposed monkeys when they were on diets natural for their species, but was, as expected, further aggravated when atherogenic foods were given. The influence of sexual profiles could also be followed, because male monkeys were worse off than females, If, however, females were ovarectomized, they not only became social outcasts, but also showed more severe coronary atherosclerosis.

These animal models of man in man's society are, of course, immensely important, as one can explore the key role that psychosocial stress and its neuroendocrine consequences *per se* has; in man these are such common civilization disorders as primary (essential) hypertension (PH) and the MS. At the same time, they also illustrate the importance of genetic profiles, of diet and of other living conditions – i.e., the multifactorial nature of such disorders.

But they also provide highly important information about other aspects of psychosocial contacts, like the influence of perinatal and early life experiences for emotional displays in adult society life. For example, in one facet of Henry's mice studies, juvenile mice were kept completely isolated from mother and siblings from the day they no longer needed their mother's milk, but still needed her nursing as well as contacts with siblings. When such mice, having grown up in social isolation but with their other needs for successful development met, were introduced into well-established mice societies on reaching adulthood, "all hell broke loose", to quote Henry. They proved unable to handle social contacts, reacted with intense DeR and aggressiveness at the slightest confrontation and caused endless turmoil, with fights and deaths where, depending on physical strength, either the intruder or his mates succumbed.

The parallels to human juvenile delinquency and related problems in modern society are obvious, and frightening, and should invite further studies concerning both preventive and handling principles. Thus, animal studies have not only been of the profoundest importance for studies of various bodily disorders in man, but are perhaps even more important concerning how mind and body interact, and how psychosocial disturbances of various kinds are key elements in some of modern society's most common disorders and mental deviations. And the reason is simply that the all-important paleocortical and hypothalamic regions of the mammalian brain are down to the finest details organized and functioning in the same way throughout the mammalian kingdom. As this, however, is to a considerable extent masked by superimposed neocortical adjustments in man, it has been poorly understood for too long, and hence neglected.

2.5
Implications Concerning Man in Modern Society

We are thus now in the last few decimeters of our species' marathon run, but with brains and bodies designed for handling the 42 km of the run already accomplished. In the preceding Sections, an outline in general principle of the physiological design of the central and peripheral mechanisms involved here has been attempted. Much of the interest, and examples, have been focussed on cardiovascular consequences of prolonged psychosocial challenges leading to mental strain and thereby elicited neuroendocrine expressions. This is not without reason, because about two-thirds of deaths today, and a striking portion of care and costs for disorders, are directly related to cardiovascular disorder, in which stress-related elements are increasingly common.

Despite the unparalleled material affluence in postindustrial society, populations nevertheless often experience their life situation as insecure, with lack of continuity, of control and of social support. The animal models mentioned illustrate what this can mean, and it is also reflected in such aspects as average lifespans in modern society, according to the epidemiological analyses discussed in Wilkinson's book *Unhealthy Societies – The Afflictions of Inequality* [20].

Because cardiovascular stress-related disturbances are, as mentioned, not only common but also often serious, they have been the focus of much medical attention. However, thanks to the widespread neurohormonal influences of DeR and DfR, virtually any tissue or organ system can be affected. Thus, stress-related disturbances may be experienced almost anywhere in the body, and particularly so when some region – in one way or another – has a weak spot; be it shoulders, back muscles, stomach or/and colon, or the heart itself. Then inductions of DeR or/and DfR will especially activate afferents from such a region, whereby a tense mental situation in, e.g., work life may be experienced mainly as stomach troubles, extrasystoles or aching shoulders. This may so dominate attention that the underlying psychosocial conflict is neglected, and therefore not mentioned when the subject contacts a doctor for his/her heart troubles, or wherever the troubles are experienced.

Other chapters will certainly discuss such and related problems, but it should be remembered that DeR- and DfR-related effects very often lurk in the background. As, however, the present author has been particularly involved in problems related to cerebral influences on cardiovascular control, some examples of stress-related contributions to cardiovascular disorders will be briefly summarized here, but are discussed at length in other survey articles [11, 12, 15, 16, 18, 19].

Of particular relevance here are primary (essential) hypertension (PH) and the metabolic syndrome (MS), briefly mentioned above in Sections 2.4.2 and 2.4.3. The reason is that PH encompasses almost half of populations above age 40–50 years, and so does MS, and often they are more or less mixed, though DeR engagements often dominate in PH and DfR in MS. Both being multifactorial where, besides actual stress-related neurohormonal influences, genetic predisposition and lifestyle factors such as diet, lack of exercise etc. come in, together they impose an increasing threat to health today.

In PH, the long-term engagements of the mentioned neurohormonal influences gradually induce a *per se* normal, and locally induced "structural upward resetting" of left-heart and systemic proximal resistance arteries. This adaptive resetting, induced by intermittent functional increases in wall load, as reinforced by trophic influences from catecholamines, angiotensin, etc, acts as a structural amplifier, to use Korner's expressive term [11]. As a result, the cardiovascular system will also operate at a raised pressure level when superimposed functional drive mechanisms are at ordinary levels. Moreover, it introduces a potential positive feedback interaction between functional excitatory influences and the structural amplifier [11, 12, 16], tending to aggravate the situation with time.

Actually, modern antihypertensive drugs mainly act by hindering this built-in positive feedback interaction by damping the neurohormonal functional drive mechanisms whereby, when treatment really is efficient (which it unfortunately only is in roughly one out of six to eight PH cases), the adaptive structural upward resetting of left heart and systemic arteries tends to show regression with time. It deserves mention here that the use of regular exercise, presumably by engaging central endorphin mechanisms that damp sympathohormonal tonic activity and cause mental relaxation, by Korner et al., has been shown to be about as efficient as most drugs used when it comes to early phases of PH – apart from the many other health-improving effects that regular physical exercise has [11].

MS provides another example of multifactorial civilization disorder, where psychosocially induced, particularly DfR-related neurohormonal disturbances prove to be of key importance; the work by Björntorp et al. [17, 18] is notable here. For example, in a survey of 51-year-old men in the city of Göteborg, Sweden, they found that no less than 35% exhibited the typical metabolic changes for MS, and DfR, such as increased or disturbed ACTH–glucocorticoid secretion combined with depressed release of growth and sex hormones, abdominal adiposity, disturbed glucose balance, etc, etc. On the mental side, frustration and depressive moods were common, and similar situations were subsequently traced in women. This should be compared with what has been observed in group-living monkeys and rodents, where prolonged DfR engagements had been induced by psychosocial turmoil as described in Section 2.4.3.

In a way, material affluence is increasingly associated with mental disturbances and the civilization disorders outlined here, to such an extent that they impose greater threats to health than disorders related to physicochemically–microbiologically induced ones. As was outlined in Section 2.3, one major reason seems to be that left-hemispheric talents have so dominated in an unparalleled technical–economical progress that too little room has been left for the – in the long run – perhaps even more important right-hemispheric qualities of the human brain – and "the horse tends to throw the rider off the saddle", to use McLean's colorful metaphor (see Section 2.3).

2.6
Concluding Remarks

From a vast number of studies, performed both in various animal species and in man, and dealing with how higher organisms react to psychosocial challenges, a number of now well-documented conclusions may be drawn:

- The brain regions responsible for such reactions, i.e., paleocortex (limbic system) and hypothalamus, are down to the fine details similarly organized in all mammals, mouse and man being in these respects equals.
- These brain regions contain a number of neuron groups from which, almost like from a keyboard, a variety of response patterns can be induced, serving to protect self and species in a primitive existence. They are all so organized as to efficiently cope with environmental stimuli of virtually any type – positive or negative: Via (A) the somatomotor link behavior is so changed as to best handle the new situation, while (B) the autonomic nervous system and (C) the hormonal system so adjust inner organ systems, metabolism, fluid–electrolyte balance as to best support the behavioral response.
- These vitally important triads of response, designed some 100 million years ago to cope with almost any type of challenge, are all of great interest, but two of

them are of particular relevance in this context, i.e., the defense reaction (DeR) and the defeat reaction (DfR).

- While DeR and DfR are in general most appropriate in primitive life's acute situations, where attack/flight and submission–withdrawal respectively are the solutions, they can – when often involved over longer periods – induce organ–system and metabolic disturbances via their extensive neurohormonal influences. Here man is, in a way, especially exposed, as the behavioral–somatomotor link of DeR–DfR is usually suppressed for social reasons, so that the inner mobilizations of circulation, metabolism, etc. occur more or less in vain, with a number of consequences.

- Because of the widespread neurohormonal influences of DeR and/or DfR, almost any tissue, or function, can be afflicted, and particularly so, if they are for other reasons sensitized–stigmatized. When this is the case, whether it is a matter of heart, stomach, back muscles or whatever, regional afferent nerves will be more easily activated in psychosocial situations where any or both of these patterns are engaged. Not infrequently, such local signs are experienced as more troublesome than the underlying mental reaction *per se*.

- Such increasingly common civilization disorders, as PH and the MS are almost absent in hunter–gatherer or small-group herding–agriculture societies. When, however, such populations, like the Australian Aborigines, are confronted with the mixed blessings and left-hemispheric evaluations of modern society, the mentioned multifactorial disorders have often devastating consequences. Then their admirable skills to thrive in desert-like bushland appear useless, resulting in loss of dignity and of sense of control and social support. It is hardly strange that frustration, depression and DfR-related disorders abound.

- Such psychosocially provoked disorders have also been experimentally induced in group-living mice, rats and monkeys, if their social order is repeatedly disturbed – perhaps by merely shifting members between established groups. Experienced as threats to, or loss of, control and social support, DeR and/or DfR engagements gradually lead to PH and/or MS-like disorders.

- Both in man and animals genetic profiles are important cofactors here, as are factors such as imbalance between food intake and physical activity, which reflects the multifactorial background of both PH and MS. Beyond doubt, however, long-term psychosocial challenges, causing DeR- and/or DfR-related neurohormonal activations are the key elements here. Thus, in more or less stress-protected population enclaves in modern society, as in semiisolated nuns, as shown by Timio et al. [10, 11], PH is virtually absent.

- When it comes to genetic profiles predisposing to PH and MS, expressions like genetic 'defects' are not seldom used in this macromolecular era of research. However, between the ages of 35 and 65 years, no less than 45% of the population in, e.g., Spain have blood pressures at or beyond the level that should be treated according to the World Health Organisation, and the high occurrence of MS was also mentioned in Section 2.5. It is hardly likely that up to half or more of present-day populations are in these respects genetically defective. Actually the inherent tendency to be more easily aroused and exhibit DeR, a common sign in human PH (and a cardinal element in e.g., the SHR* model of human PH), must have been of survival value during over 99% of our species' existence. If such biological characteristics now backfire by predisposing to PH and other civilization disorders, it should rather be taken as a sign of an unhealthy psychosocial environment [20].

- From points 1–9, it follows that it is an increasingly hectic, competitive and rapidly changing society that needs to be adapted to fit man's genetically linked mental constitutions, because the reverse is not only impossible, but biologically an unethical approach. Undoubtedly the use of various drugs to combat civilization disorders are of great value, but in reality they represent a delaying defense concerning disorders that should be handled by preventive means.

- Preventive means are nowadays the first line and self-evident way by which physicochemical–microbiological threats are met with. With the knowledge now available about how man responds to psychosocial pollution and threats, it should be equally self-evident that large-scale preventive measures in the psychosocial environment are required. Among other things, such talent profiles that are related to right-hemispheric functions (see Sections 2.3 and 2.4) should be stimulated far more, and form an integral part of education and in how work life and society life should be organized.

- Considering the gigantic total costs for stress-related disturbances and disorders, the long-term gains of a biologically based improvement of the psychosocial climate will be even more enormous economically and, what matters much more, concerning general well-being and health.

- A major hindrance for this is, paradoxically, the dominance of the technical and economical forces behind the material welfare created, simply because this dominance has been coupled with lack of knowledge, and hence disregard for the basic psychobiological characteristics of mankind. Again one traces an imbalance between left- and right-hemispheric profiles and talents, and a lack of understanding of the consequences, as the left-hemispherics have so far been so successful, technically and economically.

- A major problem here is that economic–technical forces in their planning usually do not encompass, for example, the expenses that ensue from psychosocial disturbances of mental and physical health: they are, so far, supposed to be accounted for by other means, or they are deliberately "swept under other(s) carpets." However, the rapidly mounting costs resulting from unemployment due to "rationalizations", premature pensions and stress-related ill-health and disorders, are all in the final end taken from the taxpayers' pockets. Thus, a major responsibility of society is to achieve full insight and control over such complex, though increasingly important problems.

References

1 DIAMOND, J. The rise and fall of the third chimpanzee. London, Vintage, 1997.

2 DIAMOND, J. Guns, germs and steel. London, Vintage, 1998.

3 FOLKOW, B. Mental stress and its

* The Okanoto-Aoki spontaneously hypertensive rat (SHR)

importance for cardiovascular disorders; physiological aspects, "from-mice-to-man." Scand. Cardiovasc. J. 35:163–172, 2001.

4 EICHNA, L.W., McQUARRIE, D.G. (eds). Central nervous system control of circulation. An NIH-supported symposium. Physiol. Rev. 40, Suppl. 4:1–311, 1960.

5 FOLKOW, B. Physiological organisation of neurohormonal responses to psychosocial stimuli: Implication for health and disease. Ann. Behav. Med. 15:236–244, 1993.

6 SELYE, H. Stress of life. New York, McGraw Hill, 1956.

7 ROSCH, P. Reminiscences of Hans Selye and the birth of 'stress'. Health Stress: Newsl. Am. Inst. Stress 9:1–8, 1997.

8 CHARVAT, J., DELL, P., FOLKOW, B. Mental factors and cardiovascular diseases. Cardiologica 44:124–141, 1964.

9 HENRY, J.P., STEPHENS, P.M. Stress, health and the psychosocial environment. A sociobiolgical approach to medicine. New York, Springer Verlag, 1977.

10 FOLKOW, B., SCHMIDT, T., UVNÄS-MOBERG, K. (eds). Stress, health and the social environment. James P. Henry's ethological approach to medicine, reflected by recent research in animals and man. Acta Physiol. Scand. 61, Suppl. 640:1–179, 1997.

11 FOLKOW, B. Considering "the mind" as a primary cause. Handbook of hypertension, vol. 22. Hypertension in the twentieth century, chapter 3, eds.

W. H. BIRKENBAGER, J. T. S. ROBERTSON, A. ZANCHETTI, Amsterdam, London, New York, pp 59–79. Elsevier, 2004.

12 FOLKOW, B. Man's two environments and disorders of civilisation. Aspects on prevention. Blood Pressure 9:182–191, 2000.

13 FOLKOW, B. Perspectives on the integrative functions of the sympato-adenomedullary system. Auton. Neurosci., 83:101–115, 2000.

14 ANDERSON, D.E., CHESNEY, M.A. Emotional inhibition, breathholding and sodium-sensitive hypertension in women. Primary Psychiatry 8:66–70, 2001.

15 HENRY, J.P., GRIM, C. Psychosocial mechanisms of primary hypertension. Editorial. Hypertension 8:783–793, 1990.

16 FOLKOW, B. Physiological aspects of primary hypertension. Physiol. Rev. 62:348–504, 1982.

17 BJÖRNTORP, P. Behavior and metabolic disease. Int. J. Behav. Med. 3:285–302, 1997.

18 BJÖRNTORP, P., HOLM, G., ROSMOND, R., FOLKOW, B. Hypertension and the metabolic syndrome: Closely related central origin? Blood Pressure 9:71–82, 2000.

19 KAPLAN, J.R., MANUCK, S.B., CLARKSON, T.B., LUSSO, F.M., TAUBE, D.M. Social status, environment and atherosclerosis in cynomolgus monkeys. Arteriosclerosis 2:359–368, 1982.

20 WILKINSON, R.G. Unhealthy Societies, the afflications of inequality. Routledge, London, New York, 1996.

3

Stress – It Is All in the Brain

Hege R Eriksen and Holger Ursin

3.1
Background

This chapter presents the reasons for the unpredictable and individual responses to stress. This chapter differs from many other presentations of stress by assuming that stress is an adaptive and necessary response, which explains why it is found in all species with a brain, in all human cultures, in all ages, and both genders. If stress was not adaptive and necessary, it would not have survived the test of evolution. Only under very specific circumstances may the response overshoot and become a potential source of disease.

Evolution brings two main sources of variance between individuals, securing species survival even if the surroundings shift. One source is genetic variance due to sexual reproduction; the other is the development of a brain storing information specific for that brain. The reason for the complex and sometimes unpredictable relationships between stress and health is this individually stored information. There is a brain in between the challenge and the responses. Cognitive processes in the brain determine the outcome. The vast individual differences in reactivity to stressors, and the health consequences, are determined by the expectancies this particular brain has acquired. This is handled by a cognitive activation theory of stress (CATS), offering formal definitions which may be operationalized and measured.

In this chapter the stress response is a general alarm in a homeostatic system, producing general and unspecific neurophysiological activation from one level of arousal to more arousal. The alarm occurs whenever something is missing. Formally, the alarm occurs when there is a discrepancy between what should be and what is: between the value a variable should have, the set value (SV), and the real, or actual value (AV) of the same variable. The alarm drives the organism to solve the problem, and increases performance. The stress response, therefore, is an essential and necessary physiological response.

3.2
Introduction

About the only utilization of stress we know where no brain is involved, is in mechanics and in plant ecology. Stress produces strain in elastic materials, in a reasonable and linear fashion. Stress is also used for plants that wither away when exposed to environmental conditions beyond their adaptive resources. For the vertebrates there is a brain between the external events and the internal events. A fish, a bird, a rat, a human, and even a zebra evaluate the events and respond according to previous experience and prewiring of the nervous system.

The analogous use of a term with strict definitions in mechanics is a source of endless confusion and erroneous attributions on the relations between external loads and health consequences. A main source of this situation is a hedonistic position that everything that feels uncomfortable should be avoided, and probably leads to disease and disaster. This is assumed to happen even if there is a human brain between the event and the expected consequences. Another source of confusion is that the term stress is used for the stimuli (stressors, load), the experience of stress, the stress response (alarm: increased arousal, behavioral responses, efferent impulses to muscles, hormones, internal organs, the "Cannon–Bard effect"), and the feedback to the brain from the alarm (the afferent component, the "James–Lange principle"). We will treat these separately as the load, the experience, the alarm response, and the feedback from the body. Please note that this organization represents a feedback loop that may be a positive feedback loop, i.e., the response facilitates itself, and also note that there is an information handling device in the loop, the brain. This represents the cognitive element, which we define simply as handling information. Based on present and previous information the brain decides whether the activity in the loop is to be sustained, increased, or ignored. Finally, this fact makes it possible to intervene with cognitive interventions and information, or simply previous experience, in man and animals.

Thus, the stress concepts are:

- the input (stimulus, load, challenge)
- the experience, the cognitive evaluation in the brain
- the response (activation: increased arousal, behavioral responses, efferent impulses to muscles, hormones, internal organs) (Cannon–Bard effect)
- the experience of the changes in the body (afferent impulses and signal molecules to the brain) (James–Lange effect).

3.3
The Starting Point: Consensus Statements

Even if the use of the term stress is inconsistent, confused, and used as an attribution for almost any illness, there are some points that appear to be accepted by all or most behavioral scientists that have contributed to the literature. There are exceptions in the physiological literature, where stress may mean anything that elicits activity in one or several brain–endocrine axes. If this is then used for claiming relationships to health or disease this may be too much of a leap.

In a review of the literature up to 1990, Levine and Ursin [1] stated that there were three statements that appeared to represent consensus:

- There are no common physical characteristics of stress stimuli.
- All stimuli are evaluated or filtered by the brain before gaining access to any response system.
- Psychological (emotional) loads are the most frequently reported stress stimuli.

In a review of the psychological aspects of psychoneuroendocrinology Ursin [2] found that the statements were unchallenged, and pointed out that Mason formulated most of these principles as early as 1968. To the best of our knowledge of the literature, these statements are still valid in 2004.

3.4
The Alarm: When and Why Does this Alarm Occur?

Brains regulate a high number of processes simultaneously. Humans are aware of some of them, and may pay attention to some they normally ignore or are unaware of. Animals may be conditioned to use information from autonomic processes previously believed to be autonomic; vegetative responses may be controlled instrumentally by biofeedback processes. We will return to the "paying attention to" factor in the discussion of sustained alarms, potential ill effects from this, and the potential use of attention in cognitive treatment of illness believed to be related to stress.

Since the brain qualifies as a simultaneous and parallel information processor there has to be a system for giving priority to systems that are out of control. As a self-regulating system the brain operates following a rather simple general formula. A general, unspecific alarm response occurs whenever there is a discrepancy between what is expected or the normal situation i.e., the set value (SV) and what is happening in reality, i.e., the actual value (AV). In general, the alarm occurs in all situations where expectancies are not met. It occurs as a response to novel stimuli, in situations where there is something missing, or where there is a homeostatic imbalance, or when there is a threat to the organism [1]. This follows simple and basic principles from general control theory, and represents a cognitive reformulation of homeostatic theory. All brains have many such SVs, with corresponding AVs, one for each variable the brain controls, or attempts to control. This ranges from osmotic pressure to the social climate. The basic principles are the same.

Therefore, we regard the general and unspecific stress response as a nonspecific alarm response, eliciting a general increase in wakefulness and brain arousal, and specific responses to deal with the reasons for the alarm. We refer to this increase in arousal as activation in line with traditional neurophysiological thinking since Moruzzi and Magoun [3].

The alarm continues until the discrepancy is eliminated, by changing the AV, or the SV, when this is possible. The alarm is uncomfortable; the alarm is the "drive" component that is required to make drive reduction theory work, since it drives the individual to the proper solutions. Therefore, the alarm is a safety system, which guarantees priority to serious and sudden discrepancies. On the other hand, the brain must also be able to turn the alarm off, if there are no possibilities to correct the situation. A hungry rat does not run around in his or her cage searching for food if there is no food available [4].

Since we find this pattern of response in all vertebrates, at all ages, and in all cultures, it is biologically difficult to accept that this response is all bad. If it was a prewired suicidal bomb ticking every time the organism is subjected to a challenge we would probably not be around to ponder these questions. The response is there because it is a necessary response for survival.

The alternative view is to regard alarm or – more common – fight or flight as an archaic part of our biological heritage. Even if our ancestors needed the response, we are no longer in need of it. This view is found in many different versions; the most influential paper being perhaps Charvat et al. [5]. The common element is that arousal is costly, and leaves scars in civilized man. Some of the theories assume that energy mobilized must be used, for instance in overt aggressive acts. If it is not used or released, some kind of pressure builds up, and may even give increased blood pressure or other horrors. This appears to be a remnant from old psychodynamic and psychosomatic theories, what has been referred to as "the hydrodynamic pressure cooker position." More recently, it is assumed that the alarm may only be used conservatively; too frequent a use may damage your health. We will return to this "allostatic load" position under the discussion of potential harmful effects from sustained alarm.

3.5
CATS: From Words to Formal Logics and Theory

One reason for some of the confusion that appears to exist in the stress literature is a lack of stringent definitions and inconsistent use of words. Even when defined the same word may cover different concepts (stress), or the same concept may be covered by different words (coping, strategies, plans, mastery, and efficacy). For those of us for whom English is a second language, translation and back-translation are another source of confusion.

The cognitive activation theory of stress (CATS) offers definitions formulated in symbolic logic [6]. We believe this is the only way to formulate concepts if they are to qualify as components of a theory. Formal definitions make it possible to operationalize and quantify the concepts for empirical research in man, as well as in other species. There is one major disadvantage; it appears to be extremely difficult to communicate the system. In this text we use the system with caution, and it should be possible to read this text without referring to the symbols. Perhaps it is some solace in just knowing that there is such a consistent system somewhere, something like an instruction booklet you check only when everything else fails?

3.6
Expectancies: What Do Brains Really Do?

The easiest way of handling stress is to refer to any stimulus as stress or stressor that results in a physiological stress response, for instance an increase in plasma levels of cortisol. It is also relatively easy to use the term for whatever acts on the body via the hypothalamus and its releasing factors, or through the autonomic nervous system. However, this leaves us with a major problem: there is such an immense variance in the response to the stressor. This is what the brain is all about.

Basically, the brain stores expectancies. To perform complex acts like catching an insect a frog must direct its movements to where the prey is expected to be in the next time interval. When the brain has established that one event precedes another, the brain expects the second event after the first event has been presented or the response has been performed.

All brains store the relations between stimuli, and between responses and stimuli. This stored (learned) information is what we refer to as expectancy. Formally, expectancy is the particular brain function of registering, storing and using the particular information that one stimulus (event) precedes a second stimulus, or that one response leads to a particular outcome. Less formally, brains learn (store) that certain stimuli precede other stimuli. This is classical (or Pavlovian) conditioning. Brains also learn (store) that certain responses precede stimuli, or consequences. This is instrumental (or Skinnerian) conditioning. These reformulations of learning theory are often referred to as cognitive reformulations. The main advantage is that this offers a frame of reference for the information processes in the brain which makes it unnecessary to distinguish between higher and lower forms, conditioning versus insight and planning, and other anthropocentric notions which we hold to be confusing and confounding.

To sum up then:

- stimulus (S) expectancy: S1 precedes S2 (S1 $\Rightarrow$ S2)
- response (R) expectancy: R1 precedes S2 (R1 $\Rightarrow$ S2)

Expectancy is an essential element in many reformulations of learning theory from the last decades. Edward Tolman (1886–1959) used the concept, systematized to a Hull-like set of postulates by MacCorquodale and Meehl [7]. The CATS formulations rest heavily on Bolles' cognitive formulations, which follow closely those of Tolman. When a rat learns an instrumental response for food, it typically first learns that certain cues predict food, and then learns that certain responses produce food, for instance pressing a bar in the Skinner operant box. In an avoidance situation it first learns the stimulus contingencies predicting shock, and then learns that it is possible to avoid the shock.

The CATS formulations are developed from the "two-process" theory of learning. Briefly, there are two stages in any learning situation. The first stage, stimulus–stimulus learning, is to be regarded as classical conditioning. The second stage, response learning, represents instrumental conditioning. This position is developed further to regard phase one (classical conditioning) as acquisition of stimulus expectancies, phase two (instrumental conditioning) as acquisition of response expectancies. These cognitive reformulations are necessary to explain how the brain determines the health consequences of stress.

3.7
Expectancies: Priorities, Probabilities, and Values

The alarm response gives priority to unexpected events and to events where the reason for the alarm is not eliminated. Since the brain is above all an organ designed for multiple, simultaneous tasks there must be a system for giving priorities beyond simple novelty. Again, we attribute these processes to expectancies, and to a system for ranking priorities. This requires quantification, and we quantify expectancies in three dimensions: acquisition strength, perceived probability, and affective value.

The acquisition strength, H, or habit value (the strength of learning) of an expectancy expresses the strength on a scale of 0–1 according to the general principles of learning theory. This depends on properties of the events ("salience"), the contiguity in the presentation, the number of presentations, and how often the events are occurring together (the predictive value).

The perceived probability (PP) of an expectancy expresses the probability of the expected event, again on a scale of 0–1, as it is perceived by the individual. This is a subjective evaluation of the probability based on learning (the H value). It may differ considerably from the true or objective probability. For the stimulus expectancies, a high level of PP is often referred to as predictability, while high levels of PP for response outcomes may be referred to as control.

The affective value (A) of an expectancy covers the hedonic value of the expected outcome, i.e., whether the expected outcome is attractive, aversive, or neutral on a scale of -1 to $+1$. This decides the reinforcing properties of the expected event.

3.8
Variance in Stress Responses: Stimulus Expectancy

The easiest way to reduce or even eliminate an alarm response is simply to deny that there is any danger. This is psychological defense, a cognitive mechanism which we only measure in humans, since it requires verbal communication. Theoretically, CATS defines psychological defense as a distortion of stimulus expectancies. Within traditional ego psychology or psychodynamic theory, defense used to encompass all strategies, including response expectancies, and coping. This is still influential in literature on stress, and in many animal studies. Toates defined stress as a "chronic state that arises only when defense mechanisms are either being chronically stretched or are actually failing." To Folkman and Lazarus [8], defense was a coping strategy.

The CATS position linking cognitive defense strategies only to stimulus expectancies is an essential and central element in the theory. Within ego psychology, the first systematic distinctions between defense and coping seem to have occurred in 1963 [9]. Norma Haan [9] saw all strategies used to handle threats as having two poles, one related to defense, one to coping. Defense involved distortions of reality; coping was used for strategies associated with accepting the true nature of the situation ("Cope if you can, defend if you must").

Defense is a filtering mechanism encompassing cognitive mechanisms that distort, deny or explain away threatening stimuli. Reducing fear by distortion of true relations between stimuli may be dangerous, particularly in situations where the stimulus really is signaling physical danger. Accordingly, there are controversial claims that perceptual defense measured with a tachistoscopic technique predicts inadequate behavior in many different types of dangerous tasks requiring split second decisions. The potentially life threatening aspect of high levels of perceptual defense may be due to information processing requiring 100–200 ms longer in these individuals.

3.9
Variance in the Stress Responses. Coping: Positive Response Outcome Expectancies

The most elegant way of handling a threatening or challenging situation is actually to handle it, and to know that you are handling it. CATS refer to this as coping, which is defined as a positive response outcome expectancy. In simpler language, the individual has learned (acquired an expectancy) that in this situation there is a response that gives a good result. An additional feature relevant for health issues is that this positive response outcome expectancy tends to generalize: most or all responses lead to positive results.

In English, and in the stress literature, coping is sometimes used for the act, and sometimes for the result. This double meaning in the common language has, in our opinion, unfortunate effects on the scientific and the clinical literature. It is only when defined as positive outcome expectancy that the term coping has any predictive value for stress, arousal, and health.

Weiss was the first to use coping in the animal literature, but not in our meaning. He claimed that numerous coping attempts, in the absence of feedback, would result in stomach ulcers and a depletion of noradrenaline in the brain. Coover et al. used coping specifically for rats in avoidance learning. When given shocks for the first time, rats showed a high level of arousal, both behaviorally and measured by a rise in plasma corticosterone. However, when the avoidance response had been well-established, there was a clearcut reduction in the corticosterone level, and in overt expressions of the behavior. The authors concluded that the animals had learned not only a correct response, but also that this response eliminated the shocks, and used the term coping for this type of learning. They described the animal as "a minimally aroused, behaviorally relaxed, coping rat."

Many previous authors had commented upon the relaxed nature of the animals in late stages of avoidance. When the performance is approaching a level of perfection, the performance becomes stereotyped ("asymptotic", "mastery") with a decrease in overt emotional reactions. Within traditional learning theory, the reduction in overt fear is due to the avoidance responses, removing the animal from the fear stimulus. However, this reduction is so fast and efficient that it terminates the anxiety reaction before "it is more than minimally elicited". In CATS we suggest that this low level of arousal is due to an expectancy of future events, tied to the expectancy of a positive outcome of the avoidance act.

Ursin et al. tested this position in an experiment with parachutists. They assumed that when the trainees had acquired the proper response, arousal would be reduced. It turned out that the coping, the trust in ones own abilities to perform jumps, came very early in a learning phase. Actually, in a training tower situation, the subjectively reported fear, and the vegetative and endocrine responses to the jump were reduced after the first training sessions, long before their performance had reached any acceptable level. It was not the performance, or the feedback from evaluation of the performance, that mattered, it was the subjective feeling of being able to perform that reduced the stress responses.

3.10
Variance in the Stress Responses. Lacking or Negative Response Outcome Expectancies: Helplessness and Hopelessness

While coping is related to health, optimism and high quality of life, lack of coping is what most people associate with stress, illness, and disease. In CATS it is essential to relate negative health outcomes with negative or lacking outcome expectancies. It is not the task at hand which determines the health status; it is whether or not the individual expects to be able to cope that really matters.

There are two possible outcome expectancies that both relate to depression, anxiety, and even to illness. Helplessness is the acquired expectancy that there are no relationships between responses and reinforcement. Hopelessness is the acquired expectancy that most or all responses lead to a negative result.

Helplessness occurs in experimental situations with uncontrollable and unpredictable negative events, or unpleasant life events beyond their control. The expectancy is that there is no relationship between anything the individual can do and the outcome. The classical experimental situation is the experimental neurosis occurring after unpredictable negative events. Mowrer and Viek introduced the term "sense of helplessness" for the condition arising from nonescape situations. Two of R.L. Solomon's students, Overmier and Seligman [10], found that dogs with previous experience with inescapable shocks did not learn avoidance tasks. They found that this state of helplessness generalized to situations where control is possible. Translated to CATS, the *PP* of avoiding the aversive stimulus with a response is the same as for no response. In other words, the response is without any perceived consequence for the occurrence of the aversive event. The organism has no control.

As for coping, helplessness tends to become a generalized response expectancy, for all possible responses, in man as well as in animals. Seligman offered helplessness as a cognitive model for depression. The changes in hormones, immune variables, and brain biochemistry during prolonged states of helplessness support the validity of this model. However, when the helplessness expectancy is truly approaching zero, and the individual accepts that there is no solution, the arousal may be reduced. Arousal may also be reduced if the helplessness leads to secondary gain and support from society. In such cases helplessness may function as a coping strategy, and the secondary gain may reinforce and sustain the helplessness condition.

Hopelessness is more directly opposite of coping than helplessness, since it is a negative response outcome expectancy. There is control, responses have effects, but they are all negative. This is an even better model for depression, since it introduces the element of guilt. The negative outcome is his or her fault since the individual has control. The "hopelessness theory of depression" is now an important part of the cognitive tradition in depression research and treatment.

To summarize, the outcome expectancies here are:

- Coping: all my responses lead to a good result.
- Helplessness: my responses have no effect on anything.
- Hopelessness: all my responses lead to bad results

3.11
The Variance in Coping Concepts

Coping is often defined as the acts or strategies chosen (see *Ways Of Coping*, a very important questionnaire). However, the strategy chosen does not predict the result or the internal state, and, therefore, it does not predict health effects. More relevant for the CATS position (coping as positive response expectancy) is the Lazarus differentiation between active and passive coping. Passive coping may cover withdrawal strategies; if they also involve perceptual distortion CATS covers this by the defense term.

Another term frequently found in this literature is the concept of control. The term control is frequently used to cover the ability to handle stress and work, i.e., in many ways for the phenomena we refer to as coping. In humans, the term control is used in the most influential model in analyses of potential psychosocial work factors for health: the demand–control model [11]. High demands, low control, and low social support carry the highest risk of illness and disease [11]. However, for the internal state, it is the results that count. When control is combined with positive outcome expectancy, the predictive power may increase. This may be because hopelessness also involves control; the difference is that the result is unacceptable and unpleasant. CATS defines control as an acquired, perceived high probability of a given response outcome, regardless of the value of the outcome. The term control, therefore, is not identical to coping.

The essential aspect is the subjective or perceived feeling of being able to control the situation. This may or may not develop into positive response outcome expectancy, or indeed negative outcome expectancy. The generalization of the expectancy from one situation to all situations is the important aspect. Individuals feeling that they have control over their situation are said to have an internal locus of control. Self-efficacy is another related concept, defined as the belief that an individual can act in a way that leads to a particular goal. When this expectancy is generalized it becomes identical with the CATS coping concept. However, most often the term is related to one particular strategy or treatment. The generalized self-efficacy concept also relates to self-esteem, neuroticism, and locus of control, as measured with standardized questionnaires. There are also other related, or perhaps identical, terms. Toughness, an increased ability to deal with the stressor, develops through repeated exposures to a variety of stressors. Other related concepts are hardiness, high self-esteem, affective stability, mastery, sense of coherence, and older concepts like the "instinct of mastery" of Hendrick, and the effectance concept of White.

When defence mechanisms are accepted as coping strategies, the nomenclature becomes more complex. In the Ways of Coping scoring system, and derivatives of this form (for instance CODE, as used in The Netherlands and in Norway [12]) two consistent factors are identified, instrumental and emotional coping. In the CODE form, defence appears as two independent factors, one related to hostility and one to withdrawal strategies.

3.12
Covert Coping

Even if the brain has established hopelessness or helplessness as its response outcome expectancy, it will still keep trying new strategies. One likely set of strategies is avoidance, passive or active. If the avoidance behavior is successful, the behavior may be instrumental, the brain then establishes more positive expectancies. In truly serious situations where no such solutions are available, inactivity, depression, and social isolation may be the only way to handle the situation. This is a characteristic of many chronic pain patients, interpreting the pain as a catastrophe, and entering into avoidance and inactivity.

In muscle-pain patients this is often referred to as fear avoidance, implying that the patient is avoiding movements because they are afraid of movements inducing pain, and damaging their muscles further. In other words, this inactivity is a passive avoidance, following the Mowrer nomenclature, motivated by fear and by pain.

Another strategy is to establish success in other fields of life. One particularly unfortunate strategy available to humans is to take it out on family members when the job situation is intolerable. This is similar to displacement strategies in animals, frustrating important behavior patterns may lead to strange or inadequate responses like meaningless pecking on the cage. These response patterns are picked up by Theorell's covert coping items, with items covering depression, passive avoidance, and defensive behaviors [13]. These behaviors are related to illness and disease risks (see later).

3.13
Outcome Evaluations, Fear, Anxiety and Alarm

The expectancies stored by the brain are a way to prepare for the future. Acts are determined by the expected outcome. It may be an unfamiliar way of thinking, but when the frog aims at a fly, it sticks the tongue out to a place in space where the fly most probably is when the tongue reaches this point. The frog's brain does not aim at the fly, but at the location where the fly probably will be when the tongue gets there along an abstract trajectory.

Brains, therefore, act very much on probabilities and predictability. Predictability is used both for the true relationships between events, and the subjective or learned (perceived) relationship. Only the acquired (learned) relationship is related to internal state of the organism. In addition to the alarm, there are also emotions attached to these expectancies. To a large extent, fear, anxiety and the general well-being are all determined by what is probably going to happen. Perceived predictability offers formal definitions of fear and anxiety.

A highly probable as well as a highly improbable event are both predictable, and are concurrent with low arousal. Uncertainty produces high arousal. However, predictability in itself is not enough to predict the internal state, or the behavioral consequences. In situations where the affective value of the expected event is highly unattractive, high PP leads to high arousal rather than low. This is a reasonable definition of fear. When the PP of the unattractive event is low, the arousal is low, this is safety. If the PP of an unattractive event is at chance level, that is, the PP is close to 0.5, the arousal is high, this is uncertainty, or simply anxiety. Fear and anxiety are also often different in their time perspectives; fear is of a specified event in time and space, anxiety is uncertain for the time dimension as well.

So we have:

- Fear: high PP of unpleasant event.
- Safety: low PP of unpleasant event.
- Anxiety (uncertainty): PP of an unpleasant event at chance level (PP close to 0.5].

A very extensive literature from humans and nonhumans show that predictability, a sense of control, and feedback all permit the organism to reduce its levels of arousal. This requires information about the relationship between responses and their results. This is referred to as feedback. Without feedback rats develop stomach ulcerations. Low feedback affects the level of corticosterone. Predictability is an even stronger factor. In rats it was sufficient to shift from a fixed ratio of reinforcement to the same, but variable ratio to produce significant increases in plasma corticosterone.

3.14
Access to the Alarm System

The Sokolov [14] model for orienting responses and habituation was important for the development of cognitive theory and control theory in neuroscience. Sokolov ascribed orienting responses – and neurophysiological activation – as responses to mismatches between what was expected (SV) and what really happened (AV). Orienting responses, in man and animals, occurred to events that did not correspond to any templates in the brain. When such templates had been acquired, there was no longer a response to the stimulus; the orienting reflex was extinguished (habituation).

Sokolov based his theory on sudden, brief events. CATS expands this to include all events with mismatch between SVs and AVs. Sokolov demonstrated that orienting occurs also when an expected stimulus does not appear, or when response expectancy is not met. Rats trained to barpress for water on continuous reinforcement (CRF) have higher values if shifted to a variable interval (VI) schedule; while VI-trained rats have lower values if shifted to a CRF schedule. Predictability, therefore, is important for arousal.

The affective value of the expected event also counts. Cues signaling positive events (e.g., food to hungry rats) produce a decline in the corticosterone response. Thirsty or hungry rats have high levels of plasma corticosterone when there is uncertainty about whether food (or water) is coming or not, and low levels when there is a very high or very low probability that food (or water) is coming [4]. The *PP* of success, therefore, has a decisive influence on the arousal level. Increased arousal, or stress, is not a direct function of deprivation unless there is some probability that the missing item may be available. From a biological point of view it would be inadequate if, for instance, the food or water-deprived animal kept running around in its cage when food or water is not available. Instead, they are quiet until some cue signals that the deprivation period may be over.

3.15
Stress as an Alarm System: Adaptive or Maladaptive?

The ability to respond to changes and challenges in the environment with a general alarm response should be regarded as an essential element in the total adaptive and self-regulating system of the organism [1]. Since arousal and stress are essential elements in all complex brains – in fish, birds, and mammals – the activation response must be assumed to be adaptive. A maladaptive system would not survive the test of evolution.

The stress response is dynamic and develops over time. When coping has been established, there is still a short lasting phasic arousal when individuals handle a difficult task. It has been known for more than 25 years that parachutists and pilots have a brief heart rate increase, and a sympathetic drive (adrenaline rise in plasma) when they perform at their highest level. In men, this arousal may be accompanied by an increase in plasma testosterone levels. This type of phasic arousal, referred to as anabolic arousal, is related to health and improved performance in the elderly. Any training session involving loads on the skeletal muscles and the cardiovascular system lead to similar stress effects. This is the training effect of stress, as illustrated in the CATS diagram (Fig. 3.1).

Still stress is held to be a major source of all types of illness and disease. Used in this way stress is a nondescript and ill defined attribution concept. One reason for these assumptions is that the response is uncomfortable, therefore assumed to be incompatible with health and happiness. The feedback from normal arousal responses (increased heart rate, increased sympathetic tone) may be felt as uncomfortable, in particular if the feedback is interpreted as dangerous: stress is bad for you. The arousal is there to drive the organism to provide specific solutions to abolish the source of the alarm, as well as the alarm itself. Within CATS, the arousal will be sustained until the reason for the arousal is eliminated. In other words,

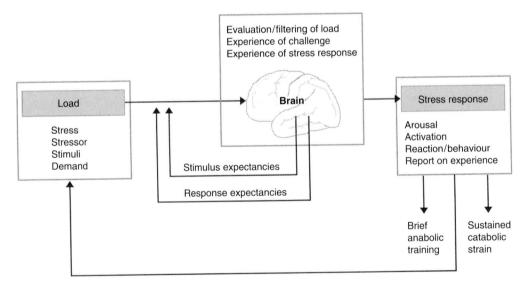

Fig. 3.1. The four main aspects of stress. The load (*1*; stressor, stress stimuli) is evaluated by the brain (*2*) and may result in a stress response (*3*; alarm) that is fed back (*4*) to the brain. The physiological stress response may lead to training or straining, dependent on the type of activation. Phasic arousal is seen in individual with a positive expectancy. Sustained arousal may lead to pathology (strain). The brain may alter the stimulus (*5*) or the perception of the stimulus, by acts or expectancies.

arousal turns off arousal by initiating and driving the system to produce the proper actions.

A weakened organism may not tolerate the alarm response, but then it is not the alarm that is to blame. Avoiding all situations that produce arousal is impossible, even if we attempt this in the care of the seriously ill person or animal. However, this strategy is not optimal for preventing disease and illness.

The stress response, therefore, is an optimal, positive and desirable alarm response, where physiological resources are mobilized to initiate and improve performance. It provides the necessary tool for an immediate resetting of priorities; and for sustained alarm if the correcting devices are insufficient. Under what circumstances may this adaptive, necessary alarm response lead to disease and illness? The brief version is that this occurs when there is no way to turn the alarm off. The long version should explain how this is possible. There are two main hypotheses in the literature, the allostasis theory [15], and the sustained activation theory [1, 6].

3.16
Allostatic Load – Repeated Strong Arousals – Training or Straining?

Weiss claimed that numerous coping attempts would result in stomach ulcers and a depletion of noradrenaline in the brain. The essential element in his finding was that this happened only in the absence of feedback, which is compatible with the CATS position on what produces sustained activation. The more recent position of McEwen [15] is that repeated arousals may have a cumulative straining effect. Rather than a training effect he assumes that there is an accumulation of "wear and tear of daily experiences and major life stressors" [15]. The pathophysiological model assumes that changes in the vegetative, neuroendocrine and immune systems that are adaptive in the short run somehow become damaging if they are not shut off when no longer needed. This statement is close but not identical to the sustained activation position of CATS. The main difference between the two positions is the assumption of cumulative effect of repeated arousals (or adaptive responses).

McEwen refers to the term allostasis from Sterling and Eyer, which represents a reformulation of the homeostasis principle, "stability through change." It is common knowledge that physiological processes are regulated by feedback loops. Any deviation from the SVs of any system sets up corrective processes, sometimes even as a preparatory response. If the organism expects, for instance, a decrease in body temperature as a drug effect, the opposite processes are initiated (opponent process theory). The term allostatic load implies that there is a price for homeostasis; the organism pays for repeated overactive or inefficient adaptive or allostatic responses. This is stored or accumulated in the organism as receptor desensitization and tissue damage.

The concept is carried even further to postulates of development of a failure to adapt, as a loss of allostasis [16]. In their analyses of the MacArthur studies of aging they have constructed a cumulative biological risk index based on known and established risk factors (blood pressure, waist–hip ratio, blood lipids, indicators of glucose metabolism, endocrine activity, etc), and they use this as their operationalization of their allostatic load concept. Then, but probably only then, they find significant relations between allostasis and future morbidity and mortality. However, in these reports there is still a substantial missing link between the results and their interpretation. There is no doubt that their cumulative biological index represents significant risk factors for health. The issue is to what extent this index is a meaningful operationalization of allostatic load, or, simply, whether there is any real cost of adaptation. What they do find is that there is a cost in lack of adaptation.

3.17
Sustained Activation

According to CATS, there are no ill effects of shortlasting arousal in the healthy organism; it is a healthy and necessary response. Challenge and loads are necessary for training, the systems must be taxed in order to stay healthy, and get stronger. Use it or lose it. It is when the brain does not find any solutions, and is unable to shift to other motivational systems, that problems may occur. In those cases, and only in those cases, the alarm may become damaging. This appears to us to be more precise than the cautious formulation of the McEwen model, where adaptive changes in the short term may become damaging if they are not shut off. McEwen assumes that the damage occurs when the adaptive responses are no longer needed. We assume that the alarm itself makes sense, but may be more than a nuisance when it does not lead to any solution.

The problem with the sustained activation hypothesis, as with the allostatic load, is that even if both are convenient models, it is very hard to measure sustained activity. Homeostatic mechanisms dampen the endocrine changes we try to identify. There is no reason to doubt that at least animals left in noncoping situations develop serious tissue damage. Rats in situations beyond their control may develop gastric ulcerations, hypertension, cardiac failure, immunological deficits, or changes in the brain biochemistry similar to those occurring during depression and psychoses. In humans, it is generally assumed that similar situations may produce disease, illness, somatization and sensitization [6]. The missing link is the endocrine, immune and vegetative evidence for sustained activation as the mediator.

There is accumulating evidence that the solution may be in the circadian rhythm, in the shifts between activity and restitution. Recent data point to the importance of recovery for resetting the basic levels after the challenges of the day, building up the energy used [17]. Any efficient training session for muscles and the cardiovascular system consists not only of load using energy, but also sufficient rest to build up the energy to a higher level than before the session. We assume, but cannot prove, that this also is the case for the rest of the organism. For plasma cortisol, in exposed groups, basal values may be increased, while stress values are lower than in coping control subjects. We interpret that as an indication of a lack of restoration of the system. The cortisol system has not returned back to normal basal levels after a night's sleep, and has lost some of its power to respond to the challenges of the day. This interpretation is reasonably close to the McEwen and Seeman positions on lack of adaptation. However, within CATS this occurs in individuals that are faced with challenges they do not expect to be able to handle.

If this thinking is right, there should also be relationships to sleep and sleep quality. Insomnia may be characterized as a state of hyperarousal from a clinical point of view. It is also associated with changes in the control of heart rate, which again is affected by coping. Short periods of sleep deprivation elevate evening cortisol levels, and insulin levels and insulin resistance.

3.18
Stress and Disease: Coping and Health

Weiss claimed that numerous coping attempts, in the absence of feedback, would result in stomach ulcers and a depletion of noradrenaline in the brain. We have regarded this as sufficiently analogous to the situation in humans, as described by Karasek and Theorell [11], to produce a composite figure comprising both sets of data (see Fig. 3.2). The model predicts disease, especially related to cardiovascular disease.

Sustained activation or allostatic load represent the attempts to find a pathophysiologically acceptable pathway from stress to somatic pathology. The final pathology (organ selection) depends on genetics and environmental factors interacting with the sustained arousal.

Sustained activation, therefore, is one of the three known routes to disease and illness: genetic disposition, environmental factors, and sustained activation. However, there is also another route which may be even more important from the point of view of behavioral medicine, and is highly related to the expectancies, coping, helplessness and hopelessness. This is the effect these variables have on the choice of lifestyle. Lifestyle (smoking, diet, inactivity) is by far the most important killer, and the most important source of illness. This raises two more questions for the relationship between CATS and health.

The first is the potential role for sustained activation giving rise to sustained attention to signals from the body. This may give rise to sensitization to afferent signals from processes that may or may not be abnormal, but may eventually develop into permanent disability. Subjective and unexplained health complaints (muscle pain, fatigue, gastrointestinal problems) are the most important sources of sickness absence and encounters with medical care. These conditions have a strong relationship with lifestyle, to the choice of activities, and to the interpretation of their condition.

Second, we will also discuss the CATS position on the unequal social distribution of illness and disease may be related to motivation for choice of lifestyle,

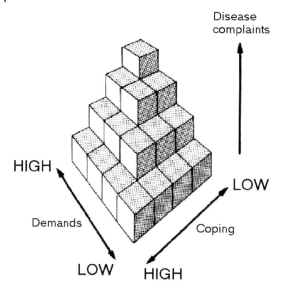

Fig. 3.2. Composite figure, based on relations described in animals and in humans. Disease, illness, and subjective health complaints are highest in individuals with high demands and low control in humans [11]. In animals, high levels of coping attempts (*demands*) combined with low levels of feedback (*control*) produced ulcers. In our own studies we get the best predictions for subjective health complaints when the *axes* are labeled demand and coping. Modified from Ursin and Murison.

which may represent unequal reinforcement schedules for the development of coping.

3.19
Sustained Activation, Sustained Attention and Sensitization

Muscle pain, tiredness, fatigue and mood changes are often attributed to stress. Common for this set of complaints is the lack of objective signs, or that the complaints go beyond what is regarded as reasonable. The absence of objective criteria makes this an area ridden with controversy and inconsistent health policies. We refer to these conditions as subjective health complaints, and have developed a scale for scoring these complaints, regardless of whether they lead to sickness behavior or not [12]. The complaints are also referred to as unexplained medical symptoms, and an international collaboration has been developed to cover these conditions (www.uib.no/insuhc).

The complaints cluster in three main categories, muscle pain, gastrointestinal problems, and a composite fatigue/mood factor [12]. The same cluster of com-

plaints is found in the somatization syndrome of the DSM IV, and is also characteristic of a multitude of conditions like hysteria, epidemic fatigue, burnout, sick
buildings, and amalgam and food toxicity. The complaints show a high prevalence
in the ordinary population. At the same time, they are also the source of the majority of encounters with the general medical practitioner, and a major source of sickness leave. We have, therefore, suggested that one possible mechanism for the clinical manifestations is based on the subjective tolerance of normal sensations from
the body. Some of us get sensitized to these afferent impulses, and the pain from
muscles or the sensations from the gut become intolerable through a sensitization
mechanism.

Sensitization is an increased efficiency in a neural circuit, due to a change in the
synapses from repeated use. This feedforward mechanism increases the response
to a stimulus. Sensitization is a typical feature of pain pathways; pain produces
pain. This basic neurobiological process may be assumed to have a cognitive analogue, or be regarded as a possible substrate for cognitive and emotional processes,
as is indeed the case for pain pathways. The cognitive correlate may be attentional
bias, or cognitive bias, as suggested by Brosschot [18].

Brosschot [18] proposed that cognitive bias, a well-established and well-
documented phenomenon in experimental psychopathology, is a higher form of
sensitization. Anxious persons give priority to thoughts and information that are
related to their fears. They detect fear-related stimuli at a lower threshold than controls. Selective attention to the fear stimuli may sustain or cause anxiety disorders.
Brosschot [18] found at least some evidence to support the notion that patients
with subjective health complaints (unexplained medical complaints) show sensitization and extensive activation of cognitive networks related to illness and pain.
Members of a family biased by illness in one of their members are likely to interpret somatic arousal as somatic symptoms. Cognitive bias for these stimuli constitute a perseverative negative cognition [18], which manifests itself as worry and rumination. Patients developing these complaints ruminate over the complaints and
the interpretation of the meaning and importance of the afferent impulses. Brosschot [18] refers to this as the "night-and-day watch" of the sensitized organism.

3.20
Rumination and Sustained Activation

Rumination may be defined as "behavior and thoughts that focus on one's attention and one's depressive symptoms and on the implications of these symptoms".
Rumination is linked to depression and depressive symptoms. It may also be used
to describe sustained attention towards other problems such as somatic diseases
and subjective health complaints, and sustained thoughts about stress factors like
health issues, economy, job factors, life events or any other type of worry. Worry
itself is defined as chains of thoughts and images that are negatively affect-laden
and relatively uncontrollable. In the sensitized brain, therefore, constant rumina-

tion and worry – the night-and-day watch of Brosschot – gives rise to sustained activation and becomes a threat to psychological and somatic health.

Rumination and worry are difficult to control, and may become a form of perseverative thinking. Normally, worry – as stress – has an alarm function interrupting and directing awareness towards solving a problem. Worry functions as a preparation making the organism ready for a situation where increased activation is needed. Perseverative thinking and rumination may therefore leave the individual in a prolonged state of psychophysiological action preparation, or – within CATS – in sustained activation [6]. In this context, worry and perseverative thinking are mediators from stressors to pathophysiology through the mechanism of sustained activation.

Perseverative thinking sustains the physiological response to a stressor by prolonging the uncertain state in the coping process, the state in which low control over the stressor is perceived. It may also sustain activation of specific pain and illness-related cognitive networks. Activated illness networks might guide information processing towards overabundant illness perception. This may again result in a higher detection of illness-related internal and external cues, more ambiguous internal and external information will be interpreted in terms of illness, more misattribution of harmless signals to illness will occur, and more and stronger memory traces for illness-related information will be produced. This, again, may be regarded as sensitization, but now at a higher cognitive level, with an assumed sensitization of the neural networks involved [18].

3.21
Too Much Coping – Being Too Good: the Dangers of Narcissism

An essential feature of response outcome expectancies is that the expectancy generalizes; success in one task leads to expectancy of success in other tasks. It is the same with failures, lack of success in one task leads to expectancy of failures in other tasks. For copers as well as for individuals with helplessness and hopelessness, the expectancies may be unrealistic. For the losers it may lead to anxiety and depression. For the copers the expectancy may lead to unrealistic risk evaluations. It may lead to sensation-seeking behavior; if combined with high defense mechanism this may lead to exposure to life-threatening situations.

Highly successful individuals may display personality traits revealing their high levels of self-confidence and high level of positive outcome expectancy. It may reach levels that may qualify as narcissistic. This personality trait is receiving more attention, since it relates to important issues in leadership and social organizations. According to DSM IV, the trait is characterized by grandiose sense of self-importance, fantasies of unlimited success, power and beauty, being unique, requires excessive admiration, expects special treatment, takes advantage of others, lacks empathy, is envious and arrogant. This reads like a list of excessive positive outcome expectancies, except there is also often an uncertainty and anxiety of being wrong, explaining the need for constant reassurance. It also reads like a description of many successful leaders. It should be noted that only when these traits are inflexible, maladaptive, and cause significant impairment or distress do they constitute narcissistic personality disorder (301.81 in DSM IV).

3.22
Social Inequality in Health and in Response Outcome Expectancies

Socioeconomic status is related to health. The socioeconomic differences in health seem to be increasing in Europe, in spite of a general political will to eliminate these differences, and in spite of a significant improvement in health, in lifestyle, and in longevity. We believe that at least part of this variance is to be found in socioeconomic differences in lifestyle which, again, relate to expectancies and coping [19]. Helplessness and hopelessness are not equally distributed over socioeconomic strata, and the compliance and motivation for lifestyle change is easier to obtain in individuals that have experienced that their own efforts matters and give success.

Three mains sources for the socioeconomic gradients in health, within most or all societies, have been suggested. General fitness (biological and psychological) determines your status (survival of the fittest), illness may reduce your status (the "drift" hypothesis), and the lower you are on the social gradient, the more stress you encounter. Within CATS, the gradient in health is related to a gradient in general positive response outcome expectancy. There are social differences in the reinforcement contingencies for the development of coping. Success breeds success, higher social classes have a higher chance of developing coping, and, therefore, may have more motivation, information, and trust in lifestyle changes.

There are also possible endocrine and physiological explanations related to hypotheses on sustained activation. In animals and human societies, social order reduces hostility and conflict. Breakdown of order may be a factor in the increase in cardiovascular pathology reported from Eastern Europe. Some support for this may be found in the animal literature. Ptarmigans (willow grouse), an arctic bird, establish order during winter. The dominating male has low cortisol, high testosterone, high secondary sexual features, and lower body temperature than subordinate males. Once order has been established, fighting decreases. The catabolic stress responses decreases in the whole flock, most in the dominating male, but also in the subordinate birds. Energy is conserved, which is a condition for survival. Similar findings have been reported from other species, including primates.

These psychoendocrine findings are readily explained within the CATS framework. The dominating male has a higher level of positive response outcome expectancy, hence lower arousal. Social order is also established in children, with consequences for the psychoendocrine status.

3.23
Brain Mechanisms

A prerequisite for the CATS position on stress is a general, nonspecific brain stem activation concept. The concept of arousal entered psychology from neurophysiology, with the documentation of a mesencephalic brain stem system for evoking and maintenance of wakefulness [3]. The concept has been controversial, but seems to us to be necessary in physiological, psychological, and clinical science, in man and animals. In a *Science* commentary, Steriade [20] stated that it was "encouraging that the concept of brainstem activation of the cortical processes has been rescued from oblivion and substantiated." Corticocortical and corticothalamic neuronal loops are controlled by activating systems in the brainstem and in forebrain structures. Our position is that this modulation and control depends on the cognitive activity analyzing available information, in this particular situation with the acquired expectancies for this situation. This is the substrate for rumination and sustained attention. We have, however, only a rudimentary understanding of the neural mechanisms of these circuits.

There is a reasonable level of consensus that the activity depends on limbic structures and the frontal lobes, even if there is no general acceptance of specific circuits. In particular, the amygdala and related structures, often referred to as the extended amygdala are involved in pain and fear. Sustained arousal leads to changes in the brain itself. Helplessness and hopelessness in animals produce the same biochemical changes in the brain as those counteracted with antidepressive and antipsychotic drugs. Exposure to inescapable but not escapable shock increases extracellular levels of 5-HT in the dorsal raphe nucleus of the rat. Uncontrolled pain, or stress, bias the brain towards helplessness and depression, whether you look at it from a biochemical or cognitive point of view. There are also morphological changes, connected to the plastic changes that normally happen in the brain. Neurons in amygdala and hippocampus are prone to morphological changes during prolonged and repeated exposures to situations rodents cannot escape or control, for instance restraint. This will affect the normal remodeling and neurogenesis in the hippocampus cells [15].

Some of these changes are attributed to the endocrine effects of the sustained arousal (or allostatic load). However, this is a feedback mechanism; the origin of the endocrine changes is the cognitive activity in the brain itself. It is the controllability of the situation which determines the biochemistry and pharmacology of hippocampus neurons. Social stress in primates produces receptor changes and morphological changes in the hippocampal pyramidal cells. These effects have been related to the feedback effect from the high levels of cortisol ("cortisol intoxication"). Since this constitutes a feedback loop, similar problems exist for the findings on the brain–cortisol relations in humans. Cortisol reactivity and regulation have been related to the long-lasting effects of trauma {posttraumatic stress disorder (PTSD)}, to negative or inconsistent expectancies, and to depression [19]. The intensity of PTSD depends not only on the traumatic event; factors like lack of control and predictability also matter. Feedback loops are hard to analyze; however, they do exist.

3.24
Conclusions

This chapter differs from many other approaches to stress in the emphasis on the positive health consequences of the normal alarm response, occurring whenever the organism is lacking an essential factor. The CATS theory is an expansion of general arousal and activation theory from neurophysiology. The stress responses are normal activation responses leading to an increase in arousal, and corresponding changes in behavior as well as in most or all parts of the body. These somatic changes are mediated through well-described and well-understood mechanisms in psychophysiology, psychoendocrinology, and psychoimmunology. CATS offers a systematic insight in the psychological mechanisms explaining when the alarm occurs, and when it may become maladaptive.

The alarm produces nonspecific changes as part of a general preparation to face any form of challenge or danger. The alarm produces coping behavior. When these are expected to bring positive results the alarm is reduced or eliminated. CATS differs from common stress concepts in emphasizing the difference between the responses, and the expectancies attached to the responses. When these expectancies are positive, there is no health risk in a healthy organism. Ill effects occur only when there is a lack of coping. CATS offers strict definitions of two different expectancies occurring when there is no coping: helplessness and hopelessness. Both states may lead to somatic disease through sustained arousal. Both states may also lead to somatic disease and illness through a lack of motivation to engage in positive lifestyles. CATS, therefore, offers a new and alternative explanation for social differences in health, based on social differences in the reinforcement contingencies for the development of coping.

CATS offers formal definitions that may be expressed in symbolic terms which makes it possible to arrive at clear definitions and consistent use of language. The stress field offers an abundance of terms, which may or may not cover the same or similar phenomena. Through the use of formal symbolic logic the amount of terms may be reduced, or at least translated into a common language. The formal definitions also permit comparisons across species, without referring to nonverifiable assumptions of mental activities beyond the assumption that brains handle information according to basic logic principles.

The adaptive functions of the stress or alarm response do not represent an unfortunate phylogenetic residue. Stress is reported from all complex brains, from fish to birds to mammals. The systematic approach to the expectancies attached to stress stimuli and related responses explains when arousal is sustained and may become a health risk. A better understanding of the relationships between loads, experience of loads, alarm responses, and the subjective experience of these somatic and psychological changes may in itself lead to better understanding, better prevention, better therapy, and healthier lifestyle. Erroneous attributions to normal and adaptive responses are not only wrong. They may actually become true, not because they are true, but because they are held to be true, and give rise to unnecessary concern and worry.

References

1 S. LEVINE, H. URSIN. 1991. What is stress? In: Stress: Neurobiology and Neuroendocrinology. M.R. BROWN, G.F. KOOB, C. RIVIER (eds.) Dekker, New York, pp 3–21.

2 H. URSIN. 1998. The psychology in psychoneuroendocrinology. *Psychoneuroendocrinology* 23:555–570.

3 G. MORUZZI, H.W. MAGOUN. 1949. Brain stem reticular formation and activation of the EEG. *Electroencephal Clin Neurophysiol* 1:455–473.

4 G.D. COOVER, R. MURISON, H. SUNDBERG, F. JELLESTAD, H. URSIN. 1984. Plasma corticosterone and meal expectancy in rats: effects of low probability cues. *Physiol Behav* 33:179–184.

5 J. CHARVAT, P. DELL, B. FOLKOW. 1964. Mental factors and cardiovascular diseases. *Cardiologia* 44:124–141.

6 H. URSIN, H.R. ERIKSEN. 2004. The cognitive activation theory of stress. *Psychoneuroendocrinology* 29:567–592.

7 K. MACCORQUODALE, P.E. MEEHL. 1953. Preliminary suggestions as to a formalization of expectancy theory. *Psychol Rev* 60:55–63.

8 S. FOLKMAN, R.S. LAZARUS. 1990. Coping and emotion. In: Psychological and Biological Approaches to Emotion. N.L. STEIN, B. LEVENTHAL, T. TRABASSO (eds.) Erlbaum, Hillsdale, NJ, pp 313–332.

9 N. HAAN. 1977. Coping and Defending. Academic, New York.

10 J.B. OVERMIER, M.E. SELIGMAN. 1967. Effects of inescapable shock upon subsequent escape and avoidance responding. *J Comp Physiol Psychol* 63:28–33.

11 R.A. KARASEK, T. THEORELL. 1990. Healthy work, stress, productivity, the reconstruction of working life. Basic Books, New York.

12 H.R. ERIKSEN, M. OLFF, H. URSIN. 1997. The CODE: a revised battery for coping and defense and its relations to subjective health. *Scand J Psychol* 38:175–182.

13 T. THEORELL, L. ALFREDSSON, P. WESTERHOLM, B. FALCK. 2000. Coping with unfair treatment at work – what is the relationship between coping and hypertension in middle-aged men and women? An epidemiological study of working men and women in Stockholm (the WOLF study). *Psychother Psychosom* 69:86–94.

14 E.N. SOKOLOV. 1963. Perception and the Conditioned Reflex. Pergamon, Oxford.

15 B.S. MCEWEN. 2003. Mood disorders and allostatic load. *Biol Psychiatry* 54:200–207.

16 A.S. KARLAMANGA, B.H. SINGER, B.S. MCEWEN, J.W. ROWE, T.E. SEEMAN. 2002. Allostatic load as a predictor of functional decline. McArthur studies of successful aging. *J Clin Epidemiol* 55:696–710.

17 J.K. SLUITER, A.J. VAN DER BEEK, M.H. FRINGS-DRESEN. 1999. The influence of work characteristics on the need for recovery and experienced health: a study on coach drivers. *Ergonomics* 42:573–583.

18 J.F. BROSSCHOT. 2002. Cognitive-emotional sensitization and somatic health complaints. *Scand J Psychol* 43:113–121.

19 M. KRISTENSON, H.R. ERIKSEN, J.K. SLUITER, D. STARKE, H. URSIN. 2004. Psychobiological mechanisms of socio-economic differences in health. *Soc Sci Med* 58:1511–1522.

20 M. STERIADE. 1996. Arousal: revisiting the reticular activating system. *Science* 272:225–226.

Stress at the Societal and Organizational Level

4
Collective Traumatic Stress:
Crisis and Catastrophes

Lars Weisæth

4.1
Introduction: The Individual as a Citizen

According to Plato, Socrates left Athens only twice during his entire life. On both occasions it was to take part in a war as a soldier, a citizen in uniform. Both instances testify to his loyalty to his city state.

Aeschylus, founding father of classical drama, did not want that accomplishment inscribed on his tombstone; rather "was at Marathon" was his preferred epitaph.

During this era of Greek democracy, for the first time in human history, the free and independent individual entered onto the world scene. However, when society, his city state or his nation was threatened, the male Greek citizen subordinated himself to the needs of the collective. The individual, even a prominent philosopher and writer, had to be prepared to risk his life to defend society's freedom and independence. The values at stake were thus more important than the existence of the individual.

Until recently, only diplomats could be expected to sacrifice their lives to society in peacetime, in political terror/hostage situation where their nation could not yield to their demands. Suicidal hijackings of passenger planes have, however, created situations in which national leaders must be prepared to make decisions about sacrificing innocent passengers' lives by shooting down the plane if the flight appears to be being used as a bomb that might cause greater loss of life. Thus, terror is a form of psychological warfare in peacetime which makes new demands on citizens' risk acceptance.

The individual's level of commitment to his group and society has been documented to be a most important protective factor during stress exposures, as well as a crucial factor in early therapeutic interventions. One example of this and perhaps the most important finding from research on soldiers' stress tolerance during military operations is the decisive importance of the sociopsychological and sociological factors: Variables that relate to the whole unit, in particular group cohesion and so-called military morale (*esprit de corps*, regimental spirit) and discipline are the best predictors of combat effectiveness and combat stress resiliency. Whereas individual data on vulnerability and degree of exposure to combat are somewhat

Stress in Health and Disease. Edited by Bengt B. Arnetz and Rolf Ekman
Copyright © 2006 WILEY-VCH Verlag GmbH & Co. KGaA, Weinheim
ISBN: 3-527-31221-8

predictive, the mentioned collective factors are the best predictors. After participation in the same combat the majority of soldiers in need of help therefore usually come from the military units characterized by lack of such protective factors. Thus, it is mainly sociopsychological factors that decide the risk of developing a combat stress reaction. Whether psychological injury is to progress to psychiatric illness is again dependent upon sociopsychological factors: The essential preventive and therapeutic elements in correctly applied "forward psychiatry" are proximity, immediacy and expectancy (the PIE principles). Early interventions applied to the soldier without removing him from his unit with an expectation of return to duty maintains his group identity, his pride and his commitment to his comrades. The 10–20% who do not rapidly recover their combat fitness after such interventions turn out to have personality problems.

4.2
Society's Denial of Psychic Trauma and its Consequences to Health

Seen in a historical perspective there is a striking pattern in the knowledge base in the field of psychotraumatology. The insights have been of an episodic kind, i.e., the knowledge that has been won seems to have been lost again. This is true both with regard to the willingness to recognize the existence of potentially psychotraumatizing events, the psychological effects of these events and the employment of interventions that may prevent or cure the harmful effects. It is, for example, remarkable that the knowledge about frontline psychiatry which was developed during World War I, and the efficacious intervention forms that were as decisive for the maintenance of individual health as for the combat strength of the whole unit, were forgotten and had to be rediscovered both during the World War II and the Korean War. The accumulation of knowledge over time which is the common pattern in the world of science seems to have been absent. Rather, there has been a dangerous lack of institutional awareness of the important insights that have been won, which has led to a repetitive circle: First denial, then exaggerations, followed by a true understanding of the problem, only to be forgotten again. Amnesia, as is well-known, is not unusual among persons who have been exposed to traumatic stress, and the same phenomenon seems to occur within society.

Awareness and recognition of psychic trauma might on the one hand threaten our sense of personal invulnerability ("It can't happen here"), and on the other hand implies a shared responsibility for helping. Denial of psychic trauma and blaming the victim both for the event and its mental health consequences are consistent phenomena that needs to be challenged.

This chapter deals with severe stress exposures that threaten or hit large groups of people. We will focus on collective stressors that endanger life or cause loss of life. Firstly, we describe the aspects of stressors that increase the risk of traumatic effects. Secondly, we describe the various forms of stress reactions, the protective factors and forms of therapeutic intervention.

4.3
Central Concepts and Models

4.3.1
Disasters: Incidents and Types

More than one billion people have been affected by disasters during the last 25 years. The smallest and poorest countries are affected most severely by natural disasters, and the poorest and most disadvantaged members of a disaster-affected community are likely to experience the most serious consequences. Therefore, in the majority of developing countries, disasters, because of their severity and frequency, represent a real public health priority. The devastation in Indonesia where the majority of the 300 000 lived who perished in the 2004 tsunami is a good illustration of this fact.

Disaster preparedness was an important part of the strategy for the World Health Organisation (WHO) program health for the year 2000. The goal for the program was that at least 70% of all nations should develop plans for handling the health aspects related to disasters. The plan even included mental health.

Disasters are often divided into two categories: natural disasters and human-induced or man-made disasters. Natural disasters are increasing in frequency and in terms of the number of people affected, while the number of deaths are declining. While on the one hand, modern technology increases safety, on the other, when things really go wrong the consequences tend to become more severe than previously. Since the invasion of Iraq the number of international wars and conflicts have been significantly reduced.

The differences between the categories are of great importance for the psychological reactions that follow. This will be described below. In the future, however, the differences may be reduced for the following two reasons: The enormous difference between industrial countries and the third world in terms of number of killed people in the same type of natural disaster demonstrates the possibility of controlling the consequences of the harmful event: "Earthquakes do not kill people, poor house constructions do." Secondly, the view that the global climate crisis has been caused by human disturbance of the environment may lead many to question whether storm disasters are really natural events.

Natural disasters are perceived as unavoidable, they often develop slowly and in modern society it is often possible to detect the danger at an early stage. The type of disaster is familiar if it is endemic, and the losses met with a fatalistic attitude.

Human-induced disasters differ in important aspects from natural disasters: the event is unnatural, caused by a failure in control systems and did not need to happen, it strikes suddenly, without forewarning and there is someone who is responsible and may be blamed.

Disasters imply a confrontation with danger, loss and grotesque experiences. Total disasters are disasters in which both homes and workplaces are destroyed, as in the areas where the 2004 tsunami destroyed all infrastructure. Partial disasters are those where only parts of the infrastructure have been destroyed. The degree of severity of exposure in various types of disasters may be measured by combining the intensity of the threat, the number of victims and material losses:

- Extensive loss of lives/severe threat/moderate material losses result from industrial disasters, transport disasters, and terrorist attacks.
- Extensive material losses/intense threat/moderate loss of lives result from forest fires, earthquakes, storms, and volcano eruptions.
- Extensive material losses/low threat/small losses of lives result from floods, and drought/crop failure.
- Intense threat/small material losses/low losses of lives result from nuclear power plant accidents and poison spills.

Major accidents/disasters usually strike or affect the following groups:

- deceased, bereaved families
- survivors with physical injuries and their families
- survivors without physical injuries and their families
- witnesses to the event
- rescue personnel (professionals and volunteers)
- health personnel
- body search-and-recovery personnel
- evacuees
- colleagues (in occupational accidents)
- people seen as responsible for causation or mitigation.

The destructive effect of a disaster may be limited to a community, a region, a nation or the event may be truly international, even global in scope. The 2004 tsunami affected much of southeast Asia, but because some affected regions were tourist areas the tsunami became a global case.

From a psychosocial point of view, a classification of disasters based on the geographical distance between the victims and their most important social networks has practical merit. Such a classification comprises communication, community and company disasters. Accidents in the local community and in the work place differ from transport accidents in that there is a geographical nearness between those affected and their families, so that social support is readily available from their networks. This access to human support from family, neighbors, friends and work mates is a great asset which is used in models for psychosocial support in community and company disasters. On the other hand, the geographical concentration of social networks may result in extreme human losses. A high number of deceased within a limited social system might contribute to a disintegration of the system. The sociologist Kai Erikson described loss of communality in Buffalo Creek after at a dam break that killed a high proportion of the village people and destroyed much of the community.

Disasters such as the 2004 tsunami illustrate that a destructive event which is regional can have a truly international and global character because of international tourism.

4.3.2
Communication Disasters

As illustrated by the 2004 tsunami, problems become enormous when the location and the identity of the victims are unknown, which is often the case for travelers, but is less likely in community and company disasters.

Uncertainty about who has perished may be high when there are no passenger lists, as in cases of disasters striking public transport systems or tourist areas.

The immediate and worldwide spreasd of information about the destructive event and the uncertainty of thousands of loved ones create an intense need to get reliable information among families of the victims. The presence of cell phones which allows survivors to inform the next-of-kin of the situation may reduce the otherwise massive search for information. It is impossible completely to avoid this convergence towards the call centers that try to cope with the need for information. Several governments failed in this respect during the 2004 tsunami. Only preselected and trained personnel at call centers can handle the tens of thousands requests per hour which can actualize in the acute timephase in such disaster situations.

When transport accidents occur far from home, the social network is at a distance from the victim. In such cases it has proven to be useful to create an information support center to provide the available, reliable information directly to the next-of-kin about the event and ongoing search-and-rescue, and the presence and conditions of survivors, etc. Families with missing or deceased members may receive crucial information from survivors or rescuers about the fate of their close ones. Victims, survivors and bereaved families in such a center tend to perceive the situation as a shared destiny and this allows for mutual support. Self-help support organizations tend to be organized in such environments. The presence of many of the next-of-kin and survivors is helpful for police identification work and provides the opportunity for clergy to carry out their role in the grief support, and for health personnel to carry out emotional first aid, crisis interventions and other early preventive interventions.

4.3.3
Confrontational Support

Sudden and violent death is accompanied by an increased risk of psychological injuries in bereaved families. The suddenness of death, the often terrifying aspects of the death situation, the geographical proximity, or rather distance, of next-of-kin, the physical condition of the corpse, which may be missing or never found, account for some of the risk. Sudden death implies that no last farewell was bid and that the bereaved had no opportunity to do something for the dying person. The goal for supportive interventions in the acute phase is twofold: to help the bereaved families to grasp the reality of the loss and to facilitate an acceptance of the loss, both necessary elements in the early phase of working through grief. Obtaining information about what happened, the way the message of death is conveyed, visits to the scene of the death, viewing the body, and commemoration have proven helpful. A visit to the disaster areas 4 months after the tsunami struck illustrates some of this: 97.5% of the bereaved family members visited the site of death, 92% reported that they got new information that made it more clear to them what happened to those close to them that had died and more than 60% stated at the end of the trip that these experiences made it easier to accept the fate of their lost ones. This combination of encountering the brutal reality and shoulder-to-shoulder solidarity and support during the encounter, we label confrontational support. It runs counter to the common tendency to overprotect bereaved families, and research findings have indicated that it facilitates the grieving process.

4.3.4
Myths

Since ancient times, people have ascribed supernatural meaning to the sudden, violent natural event. In modern societies, the natural disaster are scientifically explained and as such, generally, the cause is understood by the public.

Nonetheless, when it comes to the expected effects of a disaster, myth often overwhelms reality. For example group panic is wrongly believed to be a frequent response to disasters. Stereotypes of the victim and helper roles may distortedly view the victims as only weak and helpless, the helper as all-powerful and effective. Neither scenario is supported by research findings. In few areas does a full understanding of the psychology of helping have such importance as in disaster relief work. Relief activities based on misconceptions may be wasteful, useless and often counterproductive; the actual recovery of the population may be hampered rather than hastened, so a "second disaster" or "second trauma" is produced.

Why are relief measures sent to disaster stricken areas so often useless? Because it may be the needs of the donor that decides the content, not what the needs of the disaster victims actually are. The ability to distinguish between the need of the victim and the need of the helper is always important in helping professions – and as the urge to help is particularly strong in disaster situations, there is a risk that irrationality might get the upper hand.

Tenacious beliefs widely held by the affected population are also part of the problem: "Dead bodies will lead to catastrophic outbreaks of communicable diseases." This fear-driven belief, which leads to rapid mass burials of unidentified bodies, causes many families great uncertainty about the fate of their missing members and deprives them of a grave to mourn at.

4.3.5
Disaster Stressors

Disaster trauma usually consists of multiple stressors. It often includes both an acute and a chronic event, the primary and the secondary disaster stressors. The severity of the primary stressors are dependent on factors such as suddenness, forewarning and level of preparedness, coping possibility, geographical and numerical magnitude, duration of exposure, number of deaths and other losses, the degree of control and predictability, leadership, competence and social cohesion in the affected population. These factors largely determine the level of traumatic helplessness, anxiety, emotional storm, hopelessness, inhibition, paralysis, confusion and conflict. These immediate reactions are of great importance for subsequent psychiatric morbidity after disaster.

Within medicine and the rescue service, a disaster is defined as an event where the destructions are so extensive that the acute need for help by far exceeds the resources, i.e., the need for rescue efforts and emergency medical interventions are much greater than the immediately available resources.

In contrast to much stress research which mainly has focused on the individual, disaster and war studies focus on the primary group, the family and the military unit respectively.

In individual studies of traumatic stress a frequent finding is the strong relationship between the degree of exposure, for example, danger to life, and the risk of developing a later mental health problem (the dose–response relationship). When it comes to prediction of human response patterns in collective situations, knowledge about relational aspects of the exposure needs to be considered:

- If members of the primary group are together and simultaneously exposed to the same danger, the disaster response is likely to be characterized by reciprocal attachment. For example, individual evacuation is rarely found. If not all can be saved, there is a considerable risk that all will die. In the disastrous fire on the ferry Scandinavian Star in 1989 as many as seven family members died together. Recognizing the imminent danger of the tsunami at Christmas 2004, many parents and grandparents who had dependents on the beach closer to the water than themselves ran towards the danger to rescue their children.
- If members of the primary group are in danger but separated from each other, intensive search-and-rescue behaviors are usually seen. Parents may resist evacuation and insist on searching for their children. Children will be looking for their parents rather than searching for a safe place.
- If members of the primary group are separated from each other during the danger in such a way that some are severely exposed while other are outside the danger area, the same type of intensive search behavior is seen. This contributes to the convergence phenomenon (see below).
- The degree of uncertainty and the person's possibility of control in the disaster situation are important aspects of the stress exposure. If a next-of-kin is centrally exposed in a disaster situation, for example an earthquake, while another family

member is in the periphery, the latter's level of control is often low and the un-certainty is high. This contributes to high-intensity stress reactions. Paradoxi-cally, central exposure may sometimes allow a high level of control and low level of uncertainty. Such aspects of the exposure go a long way towards explaining why the traditional scaling of exposure according to the degree of danger cannot precisely predict posttraumatic psychopathology.

4.3.6
Time Phase and Geographical Zone Models

In more extensive potentially traumatizing events, it is important to be familiar with the geographical zone model and the time phase model.

Table 4.1 gives a schematic description of the time phases that may be identified in the course of a disaster. There are other, more detailed phase patterns than this. The value of such a time phase model is that it makes it possible to make certain predictions about human response patterns in later phases if the circumstances during an earlier phase are known. A common experience is that if the steady-state phase, the calm common everyday, has been characterized by denial of risk, the delayed awareness of actually finding oneself in a crisis situation may provoke only partial or even no stress reactions. The appearance of a calm and undisturbed leader should cause awareness. Alternatively a psychic shock reaction due to lack of mental preparedness may cause exaggerated stress reactions. Both these response patterns have negative effects on the capacity for crisis management. From a stress response perspective, the reaction might be seen as various degrees of central ner-vous system (CNS) activation, where the opposite extremes consist of underactiva-tion and hyperactivation respectively.

Research has shown that competent persons often react with adaptive prepara-tory responses earlier than the untrained in the course of events, and are more calm, cool and collected when the critical moment is imminent. Central concepts in mental preparedness and coping with stress are "positive response expectancy"

Tab. 4.1. Time phases of disaster.

Types	Threat	Counter
Steady state	Far away	Preparedness
Crisis	Approaching	Crisis management
Disaster impact	Present	Survival, rescue, salvage
Aftermath	Passed	Preventing psychiatric aftereffects
• shock phase		
• reaction phase		
• repair/reorientation		
• new orientation		

and "positive result expectancy." This implies an expectation of being able to control at least to some extent a threatening event. It seems that expected control allows a person to concern himself on beforehand on worst case scenarios than the unprepared whose negative response expectancy is more likely to foster denial of future dangers.

The postdisaster phases should not be seen as a precise sequence of reactions, rather as a fluctuation and back-and-forth movement of posttraumatic stress reactions. The shock phase, with its denial and sense of unreality, yields to intense reexperiences of the impact signifying the start of the reaction phase. The transition from the reaction phase to the repair/reorientation phase is characterized by an active willingness to confront the passed event rather than the passive involuntary reexperiences of the former.

The geographical zone model divides the disaster area into geographical zones within which people, both victims and rescue personnel, often show characteristic response patterns. The filter zone is the membrane through which people, material, and information will be filtered in and out. One common problem, not least in the developed part of the world, is the so-called convergence phenomenon that causes the pores in the filter zone to be blocked. The convergence makes rescue work and disaster medical work more difficult. Various groups contribute to convergences: people searching for their close ones, persons who need to be convinced that family members have not been affected, others motivated just by curiosity, representatives for the mass media, volunteer helpers, emergency medical and rescue personnel and other professionals who have a role to play. The problem in the filter zone is often magnified by an uncontrolled flight or evacuation from the disaster area.

4.3.7
Individual Versus Collective Trauma

As seen from Table 4.2 there are certain important differences with regard to stressors and coping possibilities both during and after exposure, between a severely stressful event that hits the single individual and one which is experienced by a person who is part of a collective. What type of collective one belongs to is naturally of importance. The loyalty is stronger within a family or other types of primary group, than if one finds oneself in a mass of strangers. In a pressured situation, however, loyalty and willingness to make altruistic sacrifices may develop as a part of a survival strategy, even between people who otherwise are strangers to each other.

The possibility of being forewarned about a danger also increases when one is together with others: Many eyes see more than two. The size of the group and who are its members are of importance for discovery and identification of a threat, but only to a certain point. If the group becomes too big, much internal activity may distract so that an imminent threat may go unnoticed. The single individual's reaction to a warning is to a high degree influenced by the reactions of others. Responsibility for the safety of others, for example children or patients, or some form

Tab. 4.2. Collective vs. individual trauma.

	Collective trauma	Individual trauma
Impact phase/isolation phase	**Death threat** Intensity, duration	**Danger to life** Intensity, duration
	Physical injury/exhaustion Severity, localization	**Physical injury/exhaustion** Severity, localization
	Witness experience Threat to next-of-kin, degree of helplessness – own and others	**Witness experience**
	Responsibility stress Responsibility of care, impossible choices	**Responsibility stress**
Rescue phase	Need > resources	Need ~ resources
Posttraumatic phases	Symptom contagion Synchronization of stress reactions Working through in group The altruistic society/loss of/ or conflicts in the group	Isolated fate
Involvement of media	++	+
Politicians	++	0
Royalty	++	0
Clergy	++	+
Medical personnel	++	++
Police/rescue personnel	++	++

of leader role, all have positive effects. Flight behavior is very much influenced by how other people react by others. Such reactions were illustrated by the 2004 tsunami. Preliminary findings from our studies show the following: for some competent people the earthquake was a warning about an oncoming tsunami; for others, the sudden lowering of the water level functioned as a warning. For those unfamiliar with these natural hazards the latter phenomenon rather created curiosity and exploration of the appearing seabeds as a fascinating phenomenon. Behavioral responses were influenced by caretaker responsibility; the response of key people in the local environment to whom one ascribed authority and competence was important for how the situation was perceived, and their immediate response once in proximity tended to have a dominating effect. To initiate evacuation all by oneself, when nobody else shows sign of such behavior, demands considerable psychological strength.

Contagion is also considerable: During the crisis at the Three Mile Island nuclear power plant in Pennsylvania the government advised all pregnant women and all who lived within an area of 5 miles from the nuclear power plant to evacuate. The result was that half of the population within a radius of 20 miles, 300 000 people, chose to evacuate immediately. A crisis situation thus developed into a sociological catastrophe.

As seen from Table 4.2 there is an important difference related to the exposure, i.e., the impact/isolation phase in collective stress situations as compared to individual trauma. The witness experiences often imply a considerable stress experience. Witnessing mass death creates a strong feeling of powerlessness and hopelessness. Several studies show that to be present when close ones are injured or killed is an extremely traumatizing part of the stress exposure. We have coined the term "double helplessness" for the helpless victim who is witnessing the helplessness of a close one in an extremely threatening situation. This experience is certainly one of the most stressful events a person can encounter. Such an aspect of the collective event also contributes to the fourth psychological dimension which constitutes a risk factor, namely the burden of responsibility. In two of our disaster studies we found that approximately 25% had been confronted with impossible choices, i.e., incompatible and conflicting needs to act, for example to have to choose between saving oneself and trying to rescue others.

The situation in the rescue phase is, as mentioned, a basic criterion for labeling the situation as a mass accident or disaster, and for deciding about mobilization of medical resources. Injured persons in accidents are treated on-site according to the principles of emergency medicine. They are not exposed to the triage of disaster medicine, which labels the lightly injured as patients who may wait. The ultimate prioritization in disaster medicine is that the most heavily injured should not be treated at all. The limited resources are to be spent on those whose lives can be saved with limited, rapid and simple interventions. For the next-of-kin and even for professionals, this paradoxical prioritization often is extremely painful. It is tempting to continue to practice emergency medicine at the high level instead of practicing disaster medicine: do only that which is strictly necessary for as many as possible, as rapidly as possible, as simply as possible.

In the posttraumatic phase, observations have been made that indicate that a collective handling of survivors and bereaved family members may cause a certain synchronization of the posttraumatic stress reactions as a consequence of mutual interactions. There is also a risk of symptom contagion.

There is sometimes a dramatic difference between the responses of society to disasters and to accidents in everyday life. This is among other things expressed in the enormous interest from mass media, politicians, representatives of royalty and the collective memorials arranged by religious institutions. For victims of individual traumas perceptions of equality and justice may often be provoked by such differences. Ideally the health services, the police and rescue services should provide as good a service to people exposed to everyday trauma as collective events.

Lazarus and Folkman were less interested in studying the most severe stressors when they formulated their cognitive stress theory. Accordingly their theory emphasizes that the individual's perception and interpretation of the threat, his primary and secondary appraisal, have great importance for which stress reactions will develop. During massive collective exposure, the variance of how people appraise the threat situation is less.

Partly this is because these situations are so unambiguous and overwhelming that the individual variations are small, and partly because the individuals in the collective situation are influenced by each other reciprocally in their understanding of the situation.

Stressors that create traumatic effects challenge/threaten/attack/crush the individual's assumption of a safe, predictable and just world. Those stricken have naturally strong needs for safety, predictability and justice. This is expressed in their wish for physical protection and safety, care, acknowledgment, attention, sympathy, understanding and acceptance. Their need for justice is expressed in positive expectations about being seen as innocent, and not responsible for what happened, and about investigation, legal processes that lead to sentence and punishment, about not losing social acceptance or suffering economic losses. They also expect public restoration and when appropriate, financial compensation for tort and losses. The possibility that these expectations will be fulfilled is greater after collective trauma. It has, for example, been found in Sweden that the economic compensation to affected persons has been higher after accidents of great magnitude than comparable accidents that affected few. Such a legal practice involves a threat to the Nordic ideals about equality and justice.

The support groups for survivors and bereaved families have during recent years become prominent players in the public arena after catastrophic events. They often get wide coverage in the mass media, where they forcefully express their opinions about lack of preparedness, legal aspects, the role of the legal system, the health services, etc. In the wake of the tsunami in Asia 2004, several governments have come to realize that such an organization provides the government with a channel to reach all affected and that the support organization may also function as an effective and representative spokesman for the victims. The third function for such organizations is to provide mutual support between its members.

4.3.8
Four Types of Danger

The risk for psychological traumatization increases with the degree of human involvement in the causation of danger (Table 4.3). In otherwise comparable circumstances measured after mortality rate, etc., violent traumas have been found to cause a higher prevalence and more severe posttraumatic stress sequels. Nature is dangerous, but not evil, at least not to those who have a scientific view of the physical world. In the third world, certain natural disasters may still be interpreted as wrath of the gods, as a punishment.

Natural disasters are therefore not experienced as being as insulting as interpersonal violence.

Tab. 4.3. Four types of dangers – common reactions among victims.

Natural disasters	Accepted as accidental, fatalistic acceptance. Nature is dangerous, not evil. Poses no threat to self esteem (own worth).
Human failure	Blame for loss of control and lack of preventive measures. Questions self esteem.
Human negligence	Strong blame, loss of trust Challenges self esteem.
Human malice	Fight (aggression). Flight (fear), surrender (shame), humiliation, narcissistic injuries, hatred, eventually revenge, cycles of violence. Attack on self esteem.

However, as illustrated by the angry responses of western victims of the tsunami, victims may feel strongly humiliated if their governments are unable to establish adequate information support and evacuation services. This anger arose in spite of the fact that western governments carried no responsibility for the disaster as such or the rescue services. Accidents place themselves somewhere in between, dependent on what failures in safety precautions that become evident.

Disasters caused by safety failures often lead to a loss of trust in the product or the service and may seriously affect customer behavior. Accident victims may develop phobias that reflect the harmful event. In contrast, victims of violence run the risk that their relationships with other people are changed so that distrust, fear and subparanoid attitudes lead to withdrawal, social isolation and agoraphobia. For example, refugees from war have a highly increased prevalence of psychosis, most frequently paranoid conditions.

The degree of irritability and aggression and even the search for financial compensation and desire to have punishments executed, increases with the degree of interpersonal involvement in the causation of the trauma. This may indicate a cycle of violence in which the victim legitimizes his violent retribution that may follow. These mechanisms may occur at the national level as well.

Summing up, an important, perhaps decisive dimension in the psychic trauma is to what degree it threatens the individual's sense of worth. This aspect of humiliation and insult may represent an attack on the individual's integrity. The combination of exposure to life-threatening danger and/or loss of a loved one and a blow to ones self-esteem seems to represent a massive risk for psychic traumatization.

4.3.9
Shock Trauma

Concrete danger is manifest, accompanied often by strong perceptual stimuli for both vision, hearing, smell, tactile perception, etc. These stimuli often have an

Tab. 4.4. Natural disasters.

Natural disasters
• Flood
• Tidal wave
• Storm/hurricane
• Cyclone
• Tornado
• Forest fire
• Tsunami
• Earthquake
• Volcano outbreak
• Land slide
• Snow avalanche
• Drought

Tab. 4.5. Man-made disasters.

Man-made disasters
• Fire in large buildings and places
• Collapse of constructions (bridges, mines, dams, buildings, roads)
• Transport systems (ships, railway, airplanes, motor vehicles)
• Technological (oil rig, toxic chemical, nuclear explosions)

invasive quality. If the danger appears suddenly, without forewarning and with high intensity, the result is usually a relatively acute development of posttraumatic stress reactions. When there are no escape possibilities, so-called inescapable shock, the risk for development of a posttraumatic stress disorder (PTSD) is particularly high. During brief acute danger exposures, there is usually no time for either mobilization of psychological defense mechanisms or problem- or emotion-focused coping strategies. The stress reaction then appears immediately or after a brief delay caused by a shock reaction.

The pure form of PTSD usually develops after severe stress danger exposures in individuals who have not previously been exposed to trauma or suffered from other psychiatric conditions.

4.3.10
Longlasting Danger and Threat

If the danger is expected and/or of a more long-lasting nature, mobilization of psychological defense mechanisms is often necessary if the person is to endure.

Strong fear, anger or depressive reactions may be incompatible for survival. Dissociative mechanisms help to split off emotions. When the danger is over, the reaction is often characterized by a sense of relief and even euphoria. Such long-lasting and extreme exposure may be followed by a latency period, i.e., symptom-free intervals that may last several years, sometimes decades, before the so-called late psychic sequelae appear. This course of reactions has been studied in survivors of concentration camps (CCs).

Exposure to highly dangerous situations may in many persons result in psychological traumatization, particularly when the risk is long-lasting, and accompanied by a high degree of uncertainty and a low degree of control. A group illustrating this type of stress exposure are the sailors in the Allied Merchant convoys during the Second World War. A combination of high risk, high degree of uncertainty, lack of defense and long duration turned out to be a particularly virulent combination of risk factors. A majority of the sailors developed psychological problems after this type of war service, and these became apparent only after many years of latency, up to 30–40 years after the exposure. One mechanism that probably was harmful was the constant, high level of CNS activation necessary in order to be prepared for a possible attack while the sailor at the same time had to suppress his anxiety in order to cope with the situation. Very few of the sailors could in the aftermath remember that they had experienced fear. They probably applied effective displacement techniques, for example total concentration about something else and other dissociation strategies. This way of manipulating one's awareness and avoiding thinking about the danger by focusing on the activities of the moment, certainly was useful and necessary in a short term, but likely to be harmful in the long perspective. The psychological late effects in persons who are exposed to this type of threat are characterized by delayed PTSD. The threat was precise enough to create a relatively specific symptom picture.

It is interesting that researchers who first studied the CC syndrome were doctors who had themselves survived the CCs. Likewise the war sailor syndrome was first described by a doctor who had himself survived torpedo attack in convoy service in the North Atlantic.

When the threat has a less precise character, more general fear and anxiety symptoms usually dominate the eventual psychic illness.

4.3.11
Silent Trauma

Environmental dangers such as ionizing radiation cannot be perceived either by means of vision, smell or other sense organs. The stress develops only when the individual is made aware of his exposure. In such situations the individual is exposed to two stressors: the knowledge of the risk and the actual exposure. In contrast to manifest and threat of danger, silent traumas do not cause a posttraumatic stress syndrome. The reactions consist often of increased awareness of one's own physical health condition, reduced threshold for symptom identification and a tendency to enter into patient roles. Attribution is a common phenomenon. After exposure to ionizing radiation the stressors are persistent, future oriented, somatically based and not limited to an isolated perceptible event that may be processed. The resulting syndrome with somatization, depression, depression, anxiety symptoms and compulsive preoccupation with safety aspects has been given the name "the informed about radioactive contamination syndrome." Legitimization in the form of such a new diagnosis may reinforce psychic contagion.

4.3.12
Disaster Behavior

A person's behavioral responses during a life-threatening situation are important. Immediate responses to impact frequently determine chances of survival, ability to rescue other victims, and whether he is to contribute to rational collective behavior or to group panic. His responses during the traumatic impact phase may also deeply affect the type and intensity of his posttraumatic stress reaction.

Maladaptive or psychiatric reactions to a severe danger, such as immobilizing fright, uncontrolled flight behavior or breakdown of reality testing may be incompatible with survival in situations where immediate rational action is mandatory. However, the exact proportion of deaths caused by maladaptive responses to a danger trauma never been established. Psychiatrically disturbed behavior may also tax rescue resources and severely affect the behavior of others.

As described in Table 4.2 there are four aspects of disaster trauma which the exposed person has to cope with: (a) danger to life, (b) physical injury/exhaustion, (c) witness experiences, and (d) responsibility stress. In a study of a massive industrial accident with explosion and fire it came out that certain factors protected the individual and were related with optimal functional level during the disaster exposure. These factors are: previous disaster training and/or experience, strong group cohesion, and trust in leadership. Previous experience with leadership roles also predicted on the coping capacity. No particular personality dimension appeared to be of particular value, but a nondeviating personality and good intellectual capacity correlated with optimal disaster behavior. A high degree of disaster competence predicted an optimal or adaptive immediate disaster response (disaster behavior) with a sensitivity of 81% and a specificity of 85%. The vulnerability factors during the disaster exposure were low level of training/preparedness and the personality dimensions of denial and passivity. The psychotraumatization already appeared during the stress exposure in the form of acute disturbances or total loss of cognitive functions, emotional storm or emotional paralysis, foremost anxiety. These disturbances were associated with a reduction in controlled behavior with resulting maladaptive disaster behavior in the sense that the behavior increased risk to one's own or others' lives. Some of these persons were rescued thanks the to effort of others.

Those who coped well during the disaster impact had a low risk for development of PTSD, in the short and in the long term. That coping capacity during dangerous situation presented a protective factor indicates that perceived control prevented the death threat from overwhelming the person during the exposure. Real control over the situation was not possible, but a high level of training appeared to help the person to do whatever was possible. Concentrating on this helped them to avoid the helplessness and powerlessness that had traumatic effects in those who were unable to cope. Thus, some real control and considerable perceived control was possible. Posttraumatic stress disturbances appeared therefore, at least partly, to be a result of a failure to cope with a stress during the exposure, not so much as a failure recovering from "normal reactions to an abnormal event" in the aftermath. The results are important for what preventive strategies to recommend: The most important primary prophylaxis in high risk professions is a high level of preparedness. Several studies of disaster workers have also documented that competence built on education, training, exercise and real experiences is protective both when it comes to coping with the disaster stressors during the rescue operation and towards post traumatic stress reactions.

4.3.13
Collective Stress: Causal Mechanisms of Psychopathology

Severe and collective stressful events such as war and major disasters affect the individual in various ways:

- Collective stress reactions, i.e., mass phenomena such as panic and psychological epidemics. Individual stress reactions contribute to mass phenomenon and are in turn reinforced by the individual's participation in the collective.
- Large numbers of posttraumatic-stress-related conditions may develop, of which PTSD is the most common.
- Social disintegration of societies and local communities may result. War and disaster are not the only risk factors for such developments. They both imply a threat to the conditions for maintenance of a society, namely control of the forces of nature and external threat, health, economy and a certain stability in norms and value systems. In actuality it is often an interaction between factors that have a negative effect on each other in a destructive social process. Social disintegration is a process in the local community in which both formal and informal social structures are more or less dissolved. Such societies are characterized by a high prevalence of broken homes, few and weak organizations, few and weak leaders, small possibilities for recreation, small and fragmented social networks, high degrees of distrust and hostility between people and high prevalence of crime. These societies have a very high level of mental illnesses/problems with breakdown of the active and reciprocal fellowship and spirit of community. One of the end results is a degree of social disorganization.

The threat that social disintegration represents for the mental health of the individual is presumed to be dependent on disturbing effects upon the primary group, for example the family, and in reduction of the level of social support so leaving the individual more vulnerable to stress.

4.3.14
Psychological Epidemics

The ideas that le Bon presented upon his studies on mass behavior during the Paris commune in 1870 has repeatedly led to discussions of the so-called psychological battle field. It is a well-known fact that increased suggestibility followed by development of infectious hysteria may lead to psychological epidemics. War and disasters may also result in disturbed mass behavior.

Medical doctors may come to contribute to this phenomenon. It has repeatedly been observed that wrong diagnosis of somatization disorders as real somatic disorders has a legitimizing effect and provides considerable primary and secondary gain.

One example of this is the cardiological symptoms in the combat stress reaction, first described by Da Costa (1871) during the American civil war. Doctors with a great interest in cardiological symptoms and without great insight into symptoms of anxiety, later contributed to iatrogenic epidemics. During World War I, a particular syndrome was labeled as "soldiers heart", "neurocirculatory asthenia", "disordered action of the heart" or "effort syndrome." More than 20 years later, in 1939, 44 000 British soldiers still collected invalidity pension for this syndrome. It had already been established that this "mystical cardiological disorder that soldiers developed" was a manifestation of fear and anxiety.

During World War I twice as many soldiers broke in down in gas hysteria than of gas poisoning. The concept of shell shock is also assumed partly to be an evacuation syndrome, saving both the soldier's life and, temporarily at least, his self esteem.

Group panic is a feared phenomenon. There are many examples of mass panic in war. Panic is an uncontrolled flight behavior characterized by egocentric thinking, overwhelming fear, and loss of control over behavior. Panic development is also associated with a series of biological, psychological and social risk factors. Among others, these are sleep deprivation, fatigue, reduced group cohesion and loss of trust in leadership. The triggering factor for panic behavior is often that possibility of escape is disappearing. Group panic may be prevented, but is difficult to control once it has erupted.

4.3.15
Toxic Disasters

The sarin attack in the Tokyo underground killed 12 people and poisoned an additional 50. However, 10 000 persons had an immediate need to be medically examined. Thus, fear of having been exposed and failure in differentiating between somatic anxiety symptoms and early signs of poisoning created a vast number of worried-well persons that overwhelmed the health services. In the USA during the anthrax terror in 2001, more than 50 000 people were treated with antibiotics, while only 5 died of the infection.

Environmental disasters can involve chemical substances or ionizing radiation. The latter is not a time-limited event. Ionizing accidents elicit a chain of events that may continue for many years and thus create a chronic stress situation for many people. That type of accident does not have a clearly defined low point from which the situation will gradually improve, which is the case with most other disasters. The insecurity following exposure to ionizing radiation has given rise to a series of psychological traumas, observed among survivors in Hiroshima and Nagasaki. The survivors felt trapped in an endless sequence of potential death threats. Bystanders considered them as sentenced to death, and stigmatization increased the stress and contributed to social isolation.

Man's contamination of the biosphere is a relatively new type of danger. It implies not only an ecological emergency, but also creates a social and political crisis. It often creates a culture of uncertainty, especially when the pollution is "silent." To be poisoned or to believe oneself to be poisoned is a very different psychological experience from being wounded or injured by concrete external forces.

Social isolation may also accompany epidemics that transmit from person to person. This necessary countermeasure to prevent spreading of epidemics undermines the group cohesion which is so important in coping with stress. It has been described how many people construct their perception of reality in concert with others. People experience contamination of soil, water and air – under ordinary circumstances vital elements of life – in a strongly loaded atmosphere of uncertainty. When the toxic threat cannot be perceived by our senses, the individual becomes completely dependent on others for information. When the authorities do not react and behave as if they are attempting to conceal the facts, certain groups may become convinced that there exists a hidden, but serious, threat.

In toxic exposure in contaminated communities the self, the basis of our sense of worth and self-respect, becomes the first victim of the contamination. Contaminated persons risk being treated as contagious and may feel rejected and marginalized by their fellows. This is a direct contrast to the altruistic society that develops after natural disasters, when "everybody helps everybody." The result is loss of trust in institutions and a feeling of being an outcast. Those exposed feel that they are being influenced by forces outside their control and understanding, and experience the authorities as being able to act, but unwilling. When the authorities at last yield to the demands for an investigation, activist groups are convinced that they have already for some time been exposed to poisoning. The authorities on the other hand see a crowd of hyperactive citizens and sensation-hungry journalists and demand the population to react in more rational and responsible way in a crisis situation which very well may prove to be no danger at all. This "engineering" thinking does not acknowledge the subjective perspective and the importance of emotions, but rather sees emotions as the opposite of reason.

When the group dynamics are developed as far as described above it is too late for the authorities to achieve a balanced perception among those involved. The perception then has become selective, so that members in the group are most receptive to information that confirms their own conviction and avoid information which does not fit this.

There is an increasing need for risk communication in many types of risk situations in society. The target group should often be reassured and calmed down, because the risk is small at the individual level. Too often the message from societal leaders and authorities in effect is denial of danger, in contrast to the exaggerations of the alarmist tabloid media. Successful risk communication is characterized by the following criteria: (a) the communicator is seen as a competent expert concerning the risk at hand, (b) he has earned a reputation for being honest, open and available, and (c) he is capable of emphatic communication.

References

DYNES RR. *Organized Behavior in Disaster.* Disaster Research Center, Ohio State University, Ohio, 1974.

FULLERTON C, URSANO RJ, WANG L. Acute stress disorder, posttraumatic stress disorder and depression in disaster and rescue workers. Am J Psychiatry 161:8, August 2004.

Institute of Medicine. Preparing for the psychological consequences of terrorism. A public health strategy. National Academic, Washington DC, 2001.

LEIGHTON A. Social disintegration and mental disorder. In: ARIETI S. (ed.) *American Handbook of Psychiatry, vol 2, 2nd edn.* Basic Books, New York, pp 411–423, 1974.

National Institute of Mental Health. Mental Health and Mass Violence: Evidence-Based Early Psychological Intervention for Victims/Survivors of Mass Violence. A Workshop to Reach Consensus on Best Practices. NIH Publication No. 02-5138, US Government Printing Office, Washington, DC, 2002.

NORRIS FH, FRIEDMAN MJ, WATSON PJ, BYRNE CM, DIAZ E, KANIASTY K. 60 000 disaster victims speak: part I. An empirical review of the empirical literature, 1981–2000. Psychiatry 65(3):207–239, 2002.

NORRIS FH, FRIEDMAN MJ, WATSON PJ. 60 000 disaster victims speak: part II. Summary and implications of the disaster mental health research. Psychiatry 65(3):240–260, 2002.

PYNOOS RS, FREDERIC C, NADER K, ARROYO

W, STEINBERG A, ETHS S, NUNEZ F, FAIRBANKS I. Life threat and post-traumatic stress in school-age children. Arch Gen Psychiatry 44:1056–1063, 1987.

RAPHAEL B. *When Disaster Strikes. How Individuals and Communities Cope with Catastrophe.* Basic Books, New York, 1986.

TØNNESSEN A, WEISÆTH L. Terrorist events using radioactive materials: lessons for bioterrorism. In: URSANO RJ, NORWOOD AE, FULLERTON CS (eds.) Bioterrorism: Psychological and Public Health Interventions. Cambridge University Press, Cambridge, pp 165–199, 2004.

URSANO R, FULLERTON C, NORWOOD AE, URSANO, RJ, FULLERTON, CS. *Psychiatric Dimensions of Disaster: Patient Care, Community Consultation, and Preventive Medicine.* Harv Rev Psychiatry 3:196–209, 1995.

WEISS MG, SAXENA S, OMMEREN M. Mental health in the aftermath of disasters: consensus and controversy. J Nervous Mental Dis 191(9):611–615, 2003.

WEISÆTH L. Preventing after-effects of disaster trauma: The information and support centre. Prehosp Disaster Med 19(1):86–89, 2003.

WEISÆTH L. A study of behavioural responses to an industrial disaster. Acta Psychiatr Scand [suppl] 335:13–24, 1989.

WEISÆTH L. Disasters: psychological and psychiatric aspects. GOLDENBERGER I, BRENITZ L, S (eds.) *Handbook of Stress.* The Free Press, New York, 1993.

WEISÆTH L. Psychological and Psychiatric

Aspects of Technological Disasters. In: URSANO RJ, MCCAUGHEY BG, FULLERTON CS (eds.) *Individual and Community Responses to Trauma and Disaster.* Cambridge University Press, Cambridge 1994.

Worlds Health Organisation. *Resolution on The International Decade for Natural Disaster Reduction.* Geneve: WHO A/44/832/Addl., 1998.

5
Stress – Why Managers Should Care

Bengt B. Arnetz

5.1
Introduction

The focus of this chapter is stress at an aggregate organizational level, and it is written from an organizational and management perspective. The simple question is: why should line managers, production managers as well as chief executive officers (CEOs) care about stress? After all, stress is primarily a concern for human resources.

The short answer is: it affects the bottom line. Stress impacts not only the individuals' health and well-being, it is an important determinant of organizational performance, change capacity, flexibility, product and service innovation, competitiveness and profitability.

Contrary to the common management belief that stress is conducive to productivity, unhealthy stress is unproductive stress with a low return-on-energy-invested by management and employees. It is simply an inefficient use of human resources. Organizations with optimal stress perform at a sustainable level, from both business and employee health perspectives. Under- or overstressed organizations fail to deliver their full potential. The challenge for managers is to find the optimal level of organizational stress where human resources are engaged at their full potential without threatening their own, or the organization's long-term well-being.

5.2
Stress – An Organizational Perspective

Stress is often viewed from an individual or group perspective, mostly focusing on psychosocial, behavioral and physiological/medical issues. Those aspects of stress, in addition to the societal aspects, e.g., socioeconomic disparities and stress, are indeed important. Organizational or workplace stress, however, also has implications for the health and well-being of the organization, its productivity and its competitiveness. Regardless of their industry, size or geographic location, organizations and companies today face some major challenges that might easily turn into severe

Stress in Health and Disease. Edited by Bengt B. Arnetz and Rolf Ekman
Copyright © 2006 WILEY-VCH Verlag GmbH & Co. KGaA, Weinheim
ISBN: 3-527-31221-8

threats or stressors. If these challenges are handled in a proactive way, the organization will flourish; if not, the future of the organization and its employees might be bleak.

5.3
Organization – A Biological Entity

Organizations are no different from individuals in the way they react to stressors and challenges in their environment. When a company or organization faces a major stressor, e.g., a situation that could disrupt and fundamentally change the business basics, the way managers perceive the situation influences how they interpret the stressor and describe it to others in the organization. The management perception of the stressor also impacts their decisions about how to manage and adapt to the situation, as well as how they choose to allocate scarce resources. If they see the stressor or the disruption in their markets as a threat, they tend to overreact. Managers may commit too many resources too quickly. If they perceive the situation as an opportunity, they are likely to commit insufficient resources. Managers' perceptions and interpretations of the challenges are critical to the strategy applied to cope with the situation. There are numerous examples of how managements' initial perceptions and reactions to a potentially disruptive change in their markets impacts on the long-term prospects of the company. For example, when digital photography started to reach consumers in the mid 1990s, Kodak's senior management realized that eventually the new technology might disrupt their core business. Kodak responded accordingly but its initial innovations in digital photography failed in the traditional market and did not create a new market. Hewlett-Packard, Canon, and Sony entered the market for digital photography as new players. They launched products based on home storage and home printing of pictures. Framing digital technology as a threat, i.e., an organizational stressor, helped Kodak free up resources for the new technology, but were the allocations of resources optimal? Most likely not.

AT&T, another once mighty business leader, was recently bought by a rapidly growing competitor. The rapid development in the areas of information technologies, e.g., mobile phones, SMS messaging and Internet, has resulted in dramatic changes in the basic business conditions. Could AT&T have been in a more envious position today, had management perceived potential stressors earlier in the market disruption process and managed the challenge differently?

Rosabeth Moss Kanter has been inside a number of companies in turnaround situations and observed how new leaders brought distressed organizations back from the brink of failure and setting them on a healthier course. Cutting expenses is a characteristic turnaround move. "But how this is done has a big impact on whether the turnaround is a temporary fix or a path to sustainability" [1]. To a large degree this is a matter of management skills and ability to handle unhealthy organizational stress reactions.

5.4
Drivers of Constant Needs of Organizational Changes

There are some basic factors driving the need to constantly change organization and business structures and processes. The way managers perceive and manage these drivers of change determines to a large degree whether the employees will view them as stressors or challenges. Collectively, these challenges or stressors require organizations to develop new capabilities.

Some of the major challenges facing organizations today are globalization, profitable growth, technological innovations, management of knowledge and intellectual capital, employee motivation, commitment and health. Management and employees also need to handle change and still more change. Change creates new opportunities but also new stressors. One of the most difficult things for management is to create a culture conducive to continuous change and adaptation. Customers have become more demanding and value-conscious. There is an emergence of a global capital market and the rate of deregulation is fierce. Most organizations have to deliver more services and products for the same or lower cost. In the service and knowledge-based economy, healthy adaptation to constantly new circumstances requires "organizational capabilities such as speed, responsiveness, agility, learning capacity, and employee competence" [2].

5.5
Organizational Stressors' Impact on the Bottom Line

Concerns over the effects of organizational stress on productivity, absenteeism, and health-related problems and consumption have increased substantially during the past two decades. The overall cost of stress to industry in the United States alone has been estimated to be between $150 billion to $180 billion a year.

It is obvious from the reasoning above that employee health and well-being are important assets to organizations and businesses, often grouped under the larger and more general heading "intangibles." Intangible assets of corporations are a skilled, healthy and motivated workforce, patents and know-how, software, strong customer relations, brands, unique organizational designs and processes, and other related areas. Intangible assets generate most of the corporate growth and shareholder value. "They account for well over half the market capitalization of public companies. They absorb a trillion dollars of corporate investments fund every year. In fact, these 'soft' assets are what give companies their hard competitive edge" [3].

Studies from Swedbank, one of Scandinavia's largest bank corporations, estimate the bank's total cost for stress-related disorders to be in the vicinity of $40 million per year. The bank's annual revenue in 2004 was approximately $3.5 billion with a net profit of $160 million. Based on this information, the CEO and the senior management of the bank have launched a comprehensive project aimed at decreasing stress-related costs and improving well-being. Management considers this initiative a business-critical effort to secure the future commercial success of the bank as it steps up initiatives to secure their success in new business areas. Swedbank received a prestigious work environment award in 2004 for their efforts to improve health and well-being simultaneously with improving business processes. The bank was also awarded the prize for being Sweden's best commercial bank of the year.

In summary, "In an era when physical assets have essentially become commodities, the benefits intangibles investment yields – increased productivity and processes – are the only means companies can use to escape intensifying competitive pressures" [3].

In the following issues concerning management, workplace stress, employee health and well-being and productivity will be discussed. The focus of the chapter is on the most important intangible of any organization: the human beings, in their roles as managers, employees, investors or customers.

5.6
Optimal Organizational Stress and Slack

From a management perspective, it is important to make optimal use of available resources, including human resources. The challenge is to define the optimal level of stress in an organization, i.e., the level at which performance is optimal as a factor of stress and employee well-being. A variation of the Yerkes–Dodson Law from 1908 is the oldest model of stress and performance. The model suggests an inverted U-shaped relationship between stress and performance. At low to moderate levels of stress, the relationship between stress and performance is positive. Increased stress results in improved performance. At moderate to high levels of stress, the relationship is negative. If management increases the aggregate level of employee stress, i.e., organizational stress, performance will decrease. The inverse association between stress and performance at moderate to high levels of stress is typically explained by the "activation theory." With increasing stress, there is a narrowing of the employees' attention, which causes them to neglect, or be blind to relevant as well as irrelevant information and tasks. The end result is decreased quantitative and qualitative performance.

Organizational theorists have presented the term "slack" which is related to organizational stress. Slack has been defined as "the pool of resources in an organization that is in excess of the minimum necessary to produce a given level of organizational output" [4]. A study by Nohira and Gulati, concerning the relationship between slack and innovation, found that too little slack inhibits innovation because any kind of experimentation with uncertain results is discouraged. An abundance of slack also inhibits innovation by fostering complacency and lax controls. Thus, the authors concluded that the real challenge is to find the optimal level of organizational slack. The notion of organizational slack and the inverse U-shaped association between slack and innovations are very much in line with the ideas presented in the revised version of the Yerkes–Dodson law, which relate to performance in general, not only innovation.

Recognizing the inverse U-shaped relationship between organizational slack/stress and innovation/performance is of more than just theoretical interest. Organizations and businesses are "increasingly forced to juggle simultaneous demands to be innovative and efficient" [4]. Companies that participated in the cost-cutting programs of the 1980s, such as lean production, downsizing, and business process reengineering are today feeling the negative consequences of too much organizational stress and too little innovation and investment in future products and services. It has been reported that organizational stress not only impacts the future health of businesses but also the health of its employees. There are studies reporting a significant association between major downsizing and absenteeism as well as musculoskeletal disorders and occupational accidents.

5.7
Organizational Stress Models – Concepts and Definitions

There is no generally agreed upon definition of stress. The same is true for such concepts as organizational stress, workplace stress or occupational stress. Rather than focusing on better definitions of these terms, definitions of occupational stress and the operationalization of stress measures have continued to proliferate. Rarely is it possible to do crosscomparison studies, due to different definitions of stress and stressors as well as the way different researchers define and conceptualize stress *per se*.

In this chapter, the term "organizational stressors" will be used for situations determined to be a potential threat to the *status quo* of organizational operations and processes. For example, digitalized photography was an organizational stressor to Kodak, which management had to perceive, evaluate, interpret and develop an efficient strategy to cope with and adapt to. A mismatch between production demands and available human resources or lack of necessary skills and technology might also be organizational stressors.

Organizational stress is the collective or aggregate consequence within an organization stemming from organizational stressors. That is, organizational stressors are situations of potential threat to which management and employees have to react in order to prevent unwarranted organizational reactions, e.g., decreased productivity, or increased turnover and quality problems. The way management and employees cope with and adapt to these stressors will determine the collective organizational stress level. Organizational stress can be measured as the aggregate level of employee mental and physical stress, for example self-rated stress, energy, ability to concentrate as well as stress-sensitive hormones, such as blood levels of cortisol from the cortex of the adrenal glands, prolactin from the pituitary or blood levels of testosterone and estradiol, two important anabolic and restorative sex hormones.

The United States' National Institute of Occupational Safety and Health (NIOSH), has been concerned with workplace stress issues since at least the 1980s. The moderate stress response is described by NIOSH as "challenge." NIOSH defines stress as the harmful physical and emotional responses that occur when there is a mismatch between job requirements and employees' capabilities, resources and needs. This is in line with the definition used here. Furthermore, NIOSH suggests that the concept of stress is often confused with challenge. These concepts are different, however. "Challenge energizes us psychologically and physically, and it motivates us to learn new skills and master our jobs. When a challenge is met we feel relaxed and satisfied. Thus, challenge is an important ingredient for health and productive work" [5].

The collective level of organizational stress, is the aggregate sum of stress stemming from the workplace as well as from the employees' private sphere, e.g., from spare-time activities and the family arena. The aggregate level of organizational stress, regardless of its source, affects the long-term health and performance of the organization. Therefore, stress is a management issue, as are workplace-based intervention programs aimed at mitigating unwarranted stressors and stress in the organization. Organizational stress relates to important organizational issues, such as productivity, performance, quality, and absenteeism, as well as customer satisfaction. Later on in this chapter, an integrated model describing the interrelationships between management, organizational stress and its relationship to organizational performance and employee health will be presented.

A number of occupational stress theories and models have been presented over the years. In this section there is a brief description of some of these stress theories. Many of these theories also provide suggestions as to how to attenuate unhealthy stress and create healthy and productive workplaces.

There are basically three schools of thoughts concerning workplace stress. One group of researchers has focused on the person/employee and her or his individual characteristics, such as coping ability, skills, stress resiliency, genetic make-up and prior experiences, as well as the specific job tasks to be carried out.

Another school focuses more on the workplace environment and organizational characteristics as the major source of workplace stress.

The third group of researchers uses a transactional theory of stress. This school recognizes that the environment might be the source of stress but an individual's interpretation or appraisal of the situation, properties of the organization as well as the person determine the mental and physiological stress response as well as long-term health consequences.

The most influential and widely accepted theory of workplace stress is probably the Person–Environment Fit theory. This theory posits that strain and stress in the workplace result from the interaction of an individual with her or his work environment. Job demands perceived by the employee as a personal threat contribute to an incompatible person–environment fit. This incompatibility between the employee and the environment elicits psychological strain that may cause stress-related psychological and somatic disorders.

The Person–Environment Fit theory has stimulated a rich array of research aimed at characterizing and measuring the work environment, various jobs, employee skills, individual differences in coping, and personality traits, as well as attitudes, including job satisfaction and relation of these areas to health and well-being. Concepts such as role ambiguity and role conflicts stem from the Person–Environment Fit theory and have been the subject of a large amount of research.

The Job Diagnostic Survey (JDS), developed by Hackman and coresearchers, is closely related to the Person–Environment Fit model, even though it also has bearings on the Demand–Control and Effort–Reward Imbalance models as well, described in the following. The revised form of the JDS contains 15 items rated by the employee, encompassing 5 core factors: skill variety, task significance, task identity, autonomy, and feedback.

The Person–Environment Fit model allows for interventions at the organizational and job design level, the individual level, including skills development, as well as improving employees' ability to cope with a demanding environment. However, it might be difficult for managers to draw any firm conclusions as to worthwhile interventions at the organizational level since much of the stress, according to the model, is a product of the interaction between the person and the environment. One exception might be where there is strong evidence that environmental conditions are behind much of the psychological strain in a large proportion of the employees at a specific workplace. In those cases, managers might be able to introduce efficient mitigation programs. For individual interventions, the model offers a rich array of opportunities. However, managers need to have a predominantly organizational perspective, rather than individual, in order to achieve across the border improvements in terms of organizational stress.

Another model of occupational stress is one originally described by Karasek. Karasek's model consists of two major factors. In the model, Karasek proposed that there are two critical factors of relevance to workplace stress: demand (e.g., worker production and flexibility demands) and control or lack of control over workplace processes. Karasek labeled the term lack of control "lack of decision latitude." An interesting aspect of Karasek's Demand–Control theory is that the possibilities to utilize and develop new skills are related to authority over decisions. This is in line with earlier research by Gardell who suggested that jobs that entailed relatively little worker autonomy or skills utilization tended to be associated with lower mental health.

Karasek's Demand–Control model has been further developed in collaboration with other researchers, foremost Theorell, in which links between jobs with high demands and low decision latitudes, so called high-strain jobs, and major public health issues, including cardiovascular diseases and musculoskeletal disorders, as well as job satisfaction and absenteeism have been demonstrated. The original Demand–Control model has been expanded to also include workplace social support. Thus, there are three important dimensions of the model: workplace demands made upon employees, the individual's ability to control and influence workplace processes, and social support at work. The Demand–Control model has been validated in a number of studies, using either self-rated data about employees' work conditions or data inferred from job titles, e.g., employees are assigned demand–control scores based on what is typical for that specific job category. Most studies lend support to the Demand–Control model and its predictive value for the risk of future cardiovascular diseases, even though there has been some challenges to the notion that (occupational) stress is a cardiovascular risk factor.

The Demand–Control model offers managers concrete avenues to manage workplace stress issues by improving the ratio between workplace demands and decision latitude. There have been studies showing the beneficial effects of applying the Demand–Control concept as well as enhancing managers understanding of employees psychosocial needs with regard to mental and physiological stress responses.

The third theory of relevance to managers is the Effort–Reward Imbalance model by Siegrist. This model suggests that stress occurs when there is a lack of reciprocity between efforts that an employee puts into a job and the potential rewards she or he receives. Work stress from this perspective is the consequence of high work pressure and effort, from the external work environment as well as from within the person, and low potential for rewards, such as promotions, pay raises and recognition. The model posits that Effort–Reward Imbalance contributes to work stress and health-related problems.

The Effort–Reward Imbalance model also offers some rather concrete means for managers to create a healthier balance between employee efforts and rewards. For example, improving skills or decreasing external pressure to produce will contribute to a healthier balance, as will increased recognition, enhancement in the pay scheme or clear rules for career advancements.

5.8
Organizational Inefficiency and Organizational Stress

Lately, Arnetz and coworkers have introduced the Quality–Work–Competence (QWC) method of assessing organizational working conditions, management structure, occupational stress, quality and employee competence. The QWC model was developed in close cooperation with management and employee representatives from a range of organizations and businesses representing areas such as healthcare, federal and local agencies, telecommunications, pharmaceutical research and development, biotechnology, banks and other financial institutions, insurance businesses, automobile producers and educational institutions.

The QWC consists of 44 items that are aggregated into 11 scales. It is a questionnaire-based method but only aggregate data for groups or entire workplaces are used in the feedback of results and enhancement processes. These scales cover areas such as employee health and well-being, work tempo, performance feedback from management, and participatory management. In addition, organizational goals, efficacy and leadership are assessed. The QWC model takes employee health and motivation, work climate, management and organizational aspects into consideration. That is, occupational stress is theorized to be the result of both individual, job task-specific and organizational issues. For example, the same production demand might result in quite different occupational stress levels in different departments of an organization due to different organizational efficacy and goal clarity.

QWC is a management tool and individual managers are supposed to use the data and the targeted recommendations in their efforts to improve workplace health and productivity in collaboration with the employees. The QWC method includes statistical analysis identifying the most important areas for improvement with regard to impacting on areas such as employee health and energy, efficacy and performance.

There are two reasons for providing managers and the work group with this statistically based analysis. First: managers, as well as groups, tend to shy away from the most pressing areas; for example, let us assume that the QWC analysis has identified leadership or employee commitment as the most crucial areas to work on in order to improve organizational performance and health. If the group works with other, less important areas, they are less likely to achieve the necessary results. Apart from suboptimal use of human resources, this might lead to frustration and less interest in improving work processes in the future.

The second reason is that managers need to direct their energy, a scarce resource, to the most important areas. With highly reliable instruments for organizational assessments, managers are basically offered a diagnosis of the workplace with concrete suggestions for "treatment." For example, high work tempo is often found to be improved by enhancing performance feedback and organizational efficacy.

QWC also includes a weighted summary or aggregate measure of organizational health and performance, the Dynamic Focus Score. The score offers managers an easy and reliable means to view the entire organization on one graph, pinpointing units or divisions with outstanding Dynamic Focus Scores as well those with immediate need of corrective actions (Fig. 5.1).

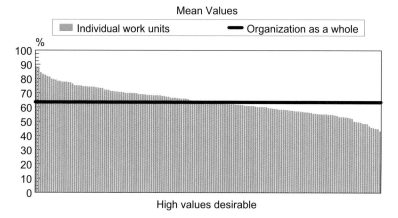

Fig. 5.1. Dynamic Focus Scores across different units in a major knowledge organization with more than 7000 employees.

The QWC method has been validated using both subjective and objective measures, including stress and anti-stress hormones, independent management ratings of groups' production demands, stress, and performance, and productivity, as well as customer perceptions [6–8].

5.9
Ingredients for Healthy and Productive Work Environments

Jackson and coworkers have pointed out the need for complementary measures to assess job characteristics salient to stress, employee well-being and behavior. These complementary areas might be of special relevance to employees engaged in more complex work, such as advanced manufacturing technology, service and knowledge-based work. The proposed measures include timing and method control, monitoring and problem-solving demand, and production responsibility.

Various models of work stress clearly point to a causal association between work stress and employee health and well-being. The following discussion will focus on the relationship between work, stress, employee health and well-being and organizational and business performance in terms of productivity and quality of products and services.

5.10
Work, Stress and Productivity

Productivity enhancement has been seen as an important means to improve quality of life and the economy, as well as a competitive position in the world marketplace. It has been argued that in order to compete against low-wage countries, and to cope with rapidly changing business environments, organizations need highly skilled employees who are both able and motivated to expand their role in the organization. Bill Gates, the chairman of Microsoft, also points out the importance of productivity enhancement measures: "The productivity area is probably the most important franchise we have" [9].

Productivity enhancement is vital for the welfare of individuals, organizations, and countries as a whole, but it is important to achieve it without causing increased unhealthy stress, "soft" costs that are not readily apparent and increased socioeconomic discrepancies. This is no easy task. As productivity of organizations and companies increases, so do stress-related symptoms and health disorders. An increasing proportion of employees also complain about the negative impact of stress on their quality of life. The Washington Business Group on Health has found that 46% of all employees are severely stressed to the point of burnout. Occupational and societal stress at these levels is of concern to individuals, families and organizations, as well as to society at large.

There is little doubt that with restructuring and the adoption of new technology as well as reductions in staff, productivity has increased in most sectors of society. Based on existing findings, however, productivity can be enhanced without causing unhealthy stress. As discussed in the introduction of this chapter, an important issue concerning productivity enhancement in the face of organizational stress, is the current level of organizational stress, the reasons behind the stress and reasonable means for managers and employees to ameliorate stress. The issue of stress and productivity should be expanded and viewed from the standpoint of healthy and productive workplaces. Traditionally, there has been a debate as to whether financially sound and productive workplaces that also promote healthy individuals are an oxymoron. An abundance of findings suggests quite the contrary; organizational stress needs to be controlled and managed in order to achieve productive and financially healthy workplaces.

"Healthy" work organizations have both financial success and a healthy workforce [10]. Research on healthy work organizations suggests that some of the same factors that affect employee outcome, e.g., quality of work life, also affect organizational outcomes, such as performance and profits. There is still only a very limited amount of actual research that has actually looked at both employee and organizational well-being. There is even less research that proactively and over time evaluates the interrelationship between stress, health and productivity. However, there has been some interesting research of relevance to managers who wish to foster both organizational and employee health.

5.11
Organizational Effectiveness and Perceived Stress

A NIOSH study in a large manufacturing company in the United States focused on organizational effectiveness and perceived stress. Management practices that predicted both organizational effectiveness and low levels of employee stress were continuous process improvement, career development, strategic planning, human resources planning, and fair pay and rewards.

Factors related to the organizational climate predictive of both employee stress and organizational effectiveness were innovation, cooperation, diversity, conflict resolution, and sense of belonging. The NIOSH study also looked at organizational attributes that predicted organizational effectiveness and employee stress. These were commitment to technology, employee growth and development, and valuing the individual employee. The study thus suggests that technology, properly designed and implemented, might mitigate stress at the same time as the financial health and productivity of organizations are enhanced.

There is a void in intervention research focusing on the possible beneficial health effects of modern information technologies and its applications in working life. Studies assessing the impact of modern information technologies on productivity rarely expand their horizons to include health, employee skills development, and quality of life issues.

A study by Hendric and coworkers looking simultaneously at organizational and employee outcomes reported that task significance predicted performance and that poor supervision and quantitative workload predicted emotional exhaustion. Emotional exhaustion mediated the relationship between job stress and job performance. The study by Hendric and coworkers was an exploratory study and did not look at factors that were predictive of both employee and organizational outcomes. The study did find, however, that job stress was inversely related to organizational performance.

In a similar line of research, Arnetz and coworkers found that stressed employees had a higher degree of musculoskeletal symptoms in the arm, wrist and hand region. Furthermore, employees scoring lower organizational efficiency, reported higher levels of mental stress. This suggests that issues related to productivity, such as employees skill levels and organizational efficiency also relate to employee stress levels. Job satisfaction was inversely related to symptoms of mental stress and cognitive fatigue, i.e., symptoms such as mental fatigue, irritation and difficulty in concentrating [11]. Job satisfaction, an overall indicator of an employee's perception of work, has also been reported by others to be related to perception of health, which in its turn is a strong predictor of healthcare utilization, an important organizational and business cost issue.

A study by Forsberg and coworkers looked at the effects of performance-based reimbursement in healthcare versus an annual fixed-budget kind of model. Their study showed that the performance-based system increased productivity and efficiency to a larger degree but at the cost of decreased professional autonomy and organizational influence for physicians. The system seemed to have caused the physicians to have to "run faster but not smarter." The long-term health consequences of new forms of reimbursement, based more on "actual performance," are not known.

There is a need to improve healthcare efficiency but the challenge is to achieve this without negative effects on organizational stress and other important work conditions, including professional autonomy and power. The study by Forsberg et al. shows that over the short-term, improvement in efficiency and productivity might be achieved, even though organizational stress indicators move in an adverse direction. As reported later in this chapter, this is not a necessity. Productivity and occupational stress might be improved simultaneously.

It has been suggested that quality improvement (QI) methods, used successfully within manufacturing and service organizations to improve quality and financial outcomes, might also be applicable to improve employee health outcomes. Typically, when traditional QI methods are implemented, the focus has been on organizational processes and product and service quality. Employee health and other outcome facts, such as quality of working life (QWL) have rarely been considered. Studies to date have not demonstrated any significant and consistent effects on employee well-being and work-related attitudes from total quality management (TQM) and QI efforts, but much work remains to be done in these areas as they relate to enhancing employee well-being and other relevant outcome factors. Sainfort and coauthors state in their review of QI efforts and their impact on organizational and employee outcomes that "research has shown that TQM/QI can have positive, negative, and/or no effects on different aspects of work design, and, consequently, on QWL" [10].

A critical issue appears to be the implementation process of TQM/QI, as well as other methods to enhance organizational performance. Reasons for failures in the areas of TQM/QI have been reported to be unrealistic targets and expectations by senior management, inappropriate structural support, and insufficient training. Lack of commitment and sustained support from top management also contributes to implementation failures [11].

5.12
Stress Intervention and Implications for Organizational Health and Productivity

There have been only a few prospective studies to date focusing on organizational productivity and effectiveness while looking at working conditions, such as health, employee attitudes and stress.

Jackson carried out an oft-cited study with three overall questions: (1) does increased employee participation in decision-making processes within their organization reduce psychological strain/stress? (2) If so, how does participation in decision-making counteract stress? (3) Does reduced psychological strain benefit the organization financially, e.g., by reducing turnover and absenteeism [12]?

The Jackson study is interesting since it considers occupational stress and financial benefits simultaneously. But, in addition, it is prospective and includes control conditions, in which employees were offered no systematic intervention. In order to be able to draw any firm and generalizable conclusions from this type of organizational intervention experiment, the use of control or comparison groups, offering no or alternative interventions, is critical. Jackson also attempted to identify why participatory management, offering employees an increased opportunity to partake in decision makings, might reduce organizational stress and mental strain. The condition, offered to members of the intervention groups only, was increased frequencies of staff meetings. They increased from once- to twice-monthly. Managers of these staff meetings participated in a 2-day training workshop prior to the initiation of the intervention. The aim with these workshops was to provide ideas on how employee participation can be improved, as well as concrete topics to discuss at the staff meetings. Managers in the control condition did not receive any group process training. Participants were followed up at 3 and 6 months following the initiation of the program.

At three months, 9 of the 10 control units had held one or fewer meetings per month, while in the intervention units, 11 out of 12 had held 2 or more meetings per month.

Results at the 6-month follow-up revealed that the intervention had been successful in increasing employees' feelings of being able to influence specific workplace and corporate topics as compared to the control group.

Statistical modeling demonstrated that employees who participated in enhanced decision making felt increased influence, which was predictive of higher overall job satisfaction and decreased turnover intention. Job satisfaction was inversely related to turnover intention and absence frequency. Prior research in nurses has demonstrated that the intention to leave a job is a predictor of actually leaving the organization in the future.

The study gives support to the notion that objective changes to enhance decision making and participatory management result in psychological changes in employees, which in turn influence behaviors, job satisfaction and turnover, important to organizational effectiveness.

During a 4-year period, Parker and coworkers studied employee stress within a context of strategic downsizing. The authors suggest that strategic downsizing is different from reactive downsizing [13]. Thus, "reactive downsizing refers to reduction in the workforce undertaken mainly in response to external events and short-term need, typically for reasons of cost-containment" [13]. Reactive downsizing is suggested to be instituted "without concern for process and outcome consistency with business strategy, mission and goals" [14].

In contrast, strategic downsizing is described as a process that is well-articulated and designed to support the long-term organizational strategy. The process is suggested by Parker et al. "to promote organizational benefits while minimizing negative individual impact. Although the strategy involves the shredding of labor, as a result of the fact that this can be planned ahead of time and often without recourse to compulsory redundancies, downsizing can be achieved gradually. Moreover, it often involves changes to the responsibilities of the employees who remain" [13].

Parker and coworkers studied the effect of strategic downsizing on work characteristics such as demand (monitoring as well as problem-solving demands), control, clarity, participation in change, job satisfaction, and employee well-being. The study was carried out within a site of a multinational company producing specialty chemicals, involving pre- and poststrategic downsizing assessments. The company needed to downsize to remain cost-effective but without negative effects on product quality and development. The strategy adopted to achieve these aims was to introduce new technologies while introducing new work practices, in particular worker empowerment. The management program basically involved continued emphasis on employee multiskilling, the removal of management layers, and a restructuring of the organization into business and support teams. There was a closer integration of engineering with production. Managers were trained in the principles of empowerment and greater attention was given to individual development.

During the study period, organizational performance improved, measured as tonnage per operator, absenteeism decreased along with recorded accidents (from seven accidents per year across the site to one). Reports of near-misses increased, however. Work characteristics, demand, control, and participation all increased significantly over the study period. Clarity did not change. Employee well-being was measured by an integrated "job-related strain" scale. Despite an increase in demand, job-related strain did not change over time. Job satisfaction, however, increased significantly over time, specifically for operators in the plant, but not for the supervisor and support staff. Results showed that an increase in demand did not predict a decrease in well-being, i.e., did not relate to an increase in job-related strain. However, increased control, clarity and participation related to decreased strain or improved well-being. There was no significant interaction between the two work characteristics, demand and control, in the final model predicting changes in job-related strain or well-being. Moreover, a limited increase in demand over time interacted with increased control in its positive association to job satisfaction. The most important predictors of changes in job-related strain were changes in organizational clarity and participation. Employees that improved awareness of their role, results expected of them, understanding of department and business aims, and performance criteria increased their well-being, i.e., decreased their job-related strain.

The results suggest that by improving role and business clarity among employees, as well as by improving participatory management, the negative effects of increased demand following downsizing might be offset. The study points to means by which management can implement proactive policies to mitigate some of the negative effects of the current drive to create ever more effective and productive organizations.

Pritchard and colleagues carried out a prospective and controlled study concerning the effects of group feedback, goal-setting, and incentives on organizational productivity. Measuring group performance is more difficult than assessing individual performance, and less research has been done in the area of group effectiveness than on measures to improve the individuals' performance. There is, however, overwhelming support for the beneficial effects of feedback, goal-setting, and incentives to alter motivation, behavior and performance. Pritchard's study is of interest for the management of occupational stress and productivity. Given that productivity and effectiveness must increase, how might this be achieved without causing negative health effects among employees? The basic design included the introduction of monthly feedback, showing each of the five participating units their achievements in specific areas. After 5 months, each of the five units began setting productivity goals in addition to receiving feedback. After 5 months of feedback and goal-setting, incentives were added as the final component of the intervention. Time off from work was chosen as the incentive. Results on productivity, measured as effectiveness, were that the average increase over baseline productivity was 50% during the feedback period, 75% for goal-setting, and 76% for incentives. Looking in more detail at the temporal changes in productivity revealed that feedback had the largest effects, followed by goal-setting. Incentives added very little further improvement in productivity. Employee ratings of job satisfaction, morale, and evaluation clarity improved significantly as well as differed between treatments. The productivity gains were achieved with the same or somewhat reduced number of employees.

Pritchard et al. discuss the reasons for these findings in detail, and the interested reader is encouraged to read the original article, which considers important methodological and other issues relevant for the design and interpretation of the study.

Herzberg reported similar improvement in employee performance (a shareholder service index was used) among stockholder correspondents from a job enrichment program focusing on enhancing employee responsibility and achievement, recognition, growth and learning, as compared to a control group. The basic theory behind the job enrichment program was Hertzberg's theory of intrinsic motivators as the major cause behind individuals' motivation and drive, not hygiene factors, such as salary, work conditions, and supervision.

In summary, various intervention studies focusing on productivity-enhancing measures indicate that the same factors that drive performance enhancement also contribute to a healthy workplace with a positive job attitude. Furthermore, psychosocial work characteristics including high job demands, emotional demands, and conflicts with supervisor and/or colleagues are risk factors for being injured in on-the-job accidents.

In order to demonstrate how managers might use psychobiological stress models to improve not only the bottom line but also organizational energy, stress and employee well-being, the following section discusses the Quality–Work–Competence (QWC) method in more detail. At first the theoretical background and model guiding the development process of QWC will be presented. Subsequently, the effects on occupational stress, employee health and productivity from using QWC in organizations will be presented.

5.13
QWC – Theory, Model and Applicability

5.13.1
Introduction to QWC

The QWC, Quality–Work–Competence, method assesses organizational leadership, stress and efficacy. The QWC method provides senior managers with valid data in areas traditionally considered nontangible or soft, i.e., assessment of organizational leadership, stress and its relationship to productivity and efficacy. Leadership is of fundamental importance in creating efficient work conditions, which in turn fosters job satisfaction. Job satisfaction is an important determinant for quality and bottom line results.

The overall goal of QWC is to optimize organizational stress in order to maximize sustainable productivity and efficiency, while allowing for a healthy, creative and innovative work climate. Organizational stress is rarely explained merely by the basic workload. Typically, poor leadership, organizational inefficiencies and unclear goals in times of a rapidly changing business environment are more important determinants.

5.13.2
Theoretical Model

QWC is based on modern transactional stress theory. Stress is a complex biological response aimed at ensuring that our mental and physical capacities are ready to handle an anticipated challenge. Short-term stress reactions are critical for our survival. The biological responses include increased blood pressure and blood glucose, as well as higher circulating levels of stress hormones such as adrenaline (epinephrine), noradrenaline (norepinephrine) and cortisol. We become more focused and capable of handling the challenge. Once the challenge or threat has passed, we are programmed to relax and recover.

In the modern world, it is all too common that the activation of the stress response is not adequately shut off. Rather than recovering from one challenge, we continue to be in a mode of mental and biological hyperactivation. In this situation, the stress response actually increases the wear and tear of the organism and our long-term health as well as the ability to successfully manage future challenges is decreased. Long-term stress, with insufficient time to recover and wind down, results in increased catabolism, that is, break down of bodily resources, such as energy supply and muscle fibers. The restorative process, anabolism, which is driven by hormones such as testosterone, dehydroepiandrosterone (DHEA) and estradiol is attenuated. Long-term stress is characterized by an imbalance between anabolic and catabolic processes. The body trades long-term well-being for short-term survival. The end result of this unhealthy and unproductive stress is fatigue, stress intolerance and, finally, poor health and even death.

The stress system is constructed to protect us from threats to our well-being. Our brain constantly surveys the surroundings by means of our senses, e.g., hearing and vision. Once the basic structures of the brain, the so-called limbic system or the central stress coordination center, register a potential challenge or signal of unknown importance, the stress system is activated.

Long-term stress creates individuals that are worse performers, mentally and physically fatigued and less open to change and innovation. On an organizational level, stress results in lower productivity and quality and an increased rate of errors. Poor leadership is a major cause of organizational stress. Stress is also an important indicator of organizational inefficiencies. Employees working in less efficient organizations are forced to spend more energy to achieve the same end results as employees in more efficiently run operations.

Organizational stress is thus an indicator of a poorly functioning organization. The most common reason for organizational stress is directly or indirectly related to leadership issues, often open to different enhancement initiatives.

5.13.3
QWC Development

The aim in developing the QWC method was to identify the most important and causally relevant areas in understanding the relationship between leadership, stress and organizational efficiency.

The QWC development process included four steps.

- Literature review. A review of the international literature on leadership, stress and efficacy. In addition, detailed interviews with managers and employees representing service and knowledge-based organizations were carried out.

- Piloting and scaling down of questionnaire. Based on the above work, an extensive questionnaire including some 350 questions was assembled. A large number of mostly service and knowledge workers responded to the questionnaire. Questions measuring similar areas, for example, leadership, work climate or stress, were grouped together and formed specific scales. The groups' ratings on the questionnaire were related to the groups' biological stress profiles. Groups with high stress levels, according to the questionnaire assessments, were also expected to exhibit higher levels of stress hormones and lower levels of the anti-stress hormones, i.e., restorative hormones including testosterone, estradiol, and dehydroepiandrosterone. After extensive work, the 350-plus questions were reduced to the 44 most important ones. The 44 questions created a total of 11 scales or QWC enhancement areas. These were: mental energy, work climate, work tempo, work-related exhaustion, performance management, participatory management, skills development, goal clarity, efficacy, leadership, and employeeship.
- In addition, based on follow-up studies, an overall, aggregated, weighted measure of organizational health – the Dynamic Focus Score – was developed. It is a weighted summary of most of the individual QWC scales. This measure offers senior managers a singular score, identifying strong and weak units/departments in their organizations.
- Validation and refinement. The QWC scales have been validated using biological measures, independent assessments of workload, productivity, employee as well as customer ratings of quality (patient ratings of quality of care). In the health-care sector, departments with the highest employee QWC ratings also rated highest among the patients [15].

The QWC system offers managers a valid tool for internal and external benchmarking. Extensive research has been able to identify target levels for the various scales. The target level indicates the desired level for each respective scale. Organizations surpassing these targets are most likely also efficient, productive and healthy, able to handle stress and change, and to have sufficient energy to cope with today's rapidly changing business environment. Organizations and units that show suboptimal results need to institute corrective measures in order to counteract future problems. In occupational stress effectiveness studies, these recommended target levels might be of interest for comparing the cost-effectiveness of various kinds of occupational stress intervention programs. Overall, these target levels define the optimal organizational stress level. Hyperstressed and overchallenged organizations are one type of challenge, but underchallenged and understressed organizations are another important issue.

As reported earlier in this chapter, job satisfaction has been linked to important employee attitude issues, such as motivation, commitment and health, as well as to productivity and bottom line results.

Figure 5.2 depicts the relationships between QWC enhancement areas as well as individual characteristics and job satisfaction. Individual characteristics including self-esteem, coping style, and self-rated health explained less than 10% in the vari-

Pathways to Job Satisfaction

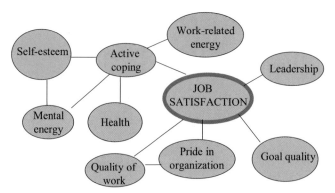

Fig. 5.2. Relationships between individual and organizational characteristics and job satisfaction. Modification of Fig. 5.1 in [16]. Reproduced with kind permission from the Royal College of Psychiatrists.

ance in job satisfaction, compared to some 40% for organizational characteristics, such as leadership, efficiency and goal clarity.

The QWC analysis provides the equivalent of a diagnosis of organizational and employee health. The analysis suggests concrete means (treatment) by which to improve the values. That is, QWC offers managers a picture of the current shape of their organization as well as a predictive risk assessment of the future. It also identifies the most efficient intervention areas to enhance the various QWC areas measured.

5.13.4
Application of QWC in Organizational Stress and Productivity Studies

QWC has been used to assess and manage organizational stress, health and productivity issues in a range of different settings. Some of these are described below.

5.13.4.1 Organizational and Employee Health Intervention in a Bank
QWC was applied to some units of one of Europe's most efficient and profitable banks, related to the number of employees. The 6-month intervention to improve organizational and individual stress consisted of two arms. One focused on improving organizational stress and productivity. It consisted of repeated QWC analyses that identified areas for improvement, such as performance feedback, organizational focus as well as efficacy. Managers met with their team and developed specific measures to improve in areas identified in the QWC analysis. In addition, there were five general meetings over a 5-month period that touched on more general organizational and individual issues. The second arm was an individually tar-

geted stress management program. Participants met seven times for 4 h each in groups of ten. The study only included pre- and postintervention assessments using both biological and subjective ratings. In addition, administrative efficacy data was used. Efficacy was measured as the number of projects handled times each project's degree of complexity. In total, the program consumed 28 h per each participant. Follow-up was carried out 3 and 6 months after the termination of the formal intervention program. Results revealed a statistically significant decrease in personnel-rated workload and increased ratings of organizational efficacy. Biological measures of stress [serum levels of the stress-sensitive hormones prolactin and thyroid stimulating hormone (TSH)] decreased significantly. The administrative and objective measure of efficacy increased by approximately 15%. The total cost of the program, including personnel time for group meetings, was $100 000. The net benefit, after considering the cost of the intervention program, was $50 000 over an 11-month period. Follow-up with management at the bank's units 3 years later revealed that they still perceived positive results from the program: 32 employees could handle the same amount of work that had required 40 before the intervention. None of the surplus employees were let go. They were offered other positions in the bank, where their skills and energy were better needed.

5.13.4.2 Organizational and Employee Health During Organizational Changes

A university hospital, that has been followed for over 10 years with regular QWC analyses, offers an interesting case study on the importance of senior and middle management in handling financial cut-backs, structural changes relating to organizational stress, employee well-being and productivity. The senior management of this university hospital decided in the early 1990s to measure employee perception of organizational and employee well-being. There were various reasons behind the decision to initiate regular surveys. Professional groups, foremost physicians, indicated that their professional role and work conditions were changing. Organizational stress indicators were on the rise. Finally, senior management predicted that the future financial conditions would be more dire, requiring improved efficacy, structural changes as well as a leaner organization. In addition, management initiated regular surveys directed to the hospital's healthcare consumers. An interesting aspect of these employee surveys was that they also included questions on how staff perceived the quality of the care environment. The patient surveys included questions of how patients perceived the work environment of employees in the units they had visited. In that way, it was possible to demonstrate similarities and differences between employee and patient perspectives, as well as pointing out the interdependency between the two [15].

External researchers were used for data analyses and interpretation. Aggregate results at the hospital and department-specific level, as well as by age, gender and professional group were fed back to the board of directors, senior and middle managers, as well as to all employees and their supervisors. Managers, as well as team leaders, at each organizational level were supposed to analyze and discuss their own aggregate results with their team, for example, coworkers on a specific ward. They were encouraged to choose no more than 3 areas out of a total of 11 for fur-

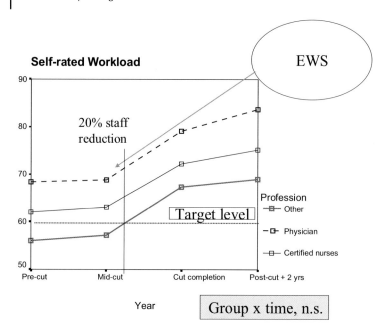

Fig. 5.3. Workload before and following a 20% reduction in staff by professional group. There was a significant increase over time in workload ratings ($p < 0.01$). *EWS* Early warning signs. *Other* paramedical professionals, administrative staff, and other categories. n.s. = non-significant.

ther enhancement. The kinds of enhancement initiatives chosen for individual QWC enhancement areas were guided by the results from statistical analysis. The analysis might show that in order to improve the QWC enhancement area organizational efficacy, the group should focus on goal clarity, decision-making processes and participatory management.

Following the first assessment, a 20% reduction in staffing was announced as part of a general cut-back package. Prior to the announcement of cut-backs and at the time of the first survey, there had been no official discussions about cut-backs. Figure 5.3 depicts the development of staff-rated workload before and following the announcement of cut-backs. Time between the precut and mid-cut measurements was 1 year. For the subsequent measurements, the time intervals have been 2 years. As shown, the announcement *per se* did not impact on self-rated workload. At this time there had not been any actual cut-backs. However, once cut-backs had been implemented and completed ("cut-completion"), workload had increased significantly and reached levels well above the recommended optimal stress levels of 50–60%, on a 0–100% scale. However, the relative differences in workload between staff categories did not change. The group "other" consists of paramedical profes-

Tab. 5.1. Mitigation factors related to improved employee well-being during organizational changes and staff cut-backs.

Healthy change by balancing organizational stress

- Increase
  - Participatory management
  - Work climate
  - Employee commitment
  - Goal clarity
- Optimize
  - Workload

➡ Improved organizational mental energy and health

---

sionals, administrative staff, and other categories excluding physicians or certified nurses, by far the largest professional group.

Hospital departments that optimized their workload, and improved their participatory management and goal clarity increased employees mental energy and productivity over the same period that there was 20% cutback in staffing (Table 5.1).

Department managers that did not consider work characteristics and organizational issues, such as efficacy and goal clarity, exhibited a continuous worsening both in their organizational performance, customer ratings, and employee health data. A key factor for successful adaptation to the new circumstances, with structural changes and a leaner organization, was participatory management, facilitating employee skills development, and clarifying goals. Successful units also strived to define what they should and should not do, and aimed at optimizing, not maximizing, workload.

5.13.4.3 Organizational Health, Biological Markers and Productivity

In another study, under the project leadership of Dr. Ingrid Anderzén, in our laboratory, we carried out an organizational performance and employee health assessment and intervention study within 22 local offices of the Swedish Internal Revenue Services (IRS). The project was initiated by the senior management in collaboration with the researchers. The overall aim of the intervention study was to create "a health-promoting and efficient organization with healthy employees." The Swedish IRS is undergoing major changes, including the introduction of new information technology software, work routines, and a continuous demand for improved effectiveness.

Briefly, the study involved 22 offices in different geographical areas of the IRS, both in the larger Stockholm region, as well as in cities to the north and west of Stockholm. The units chosen represented both the tax administrative and collection arm, as well as units involved in securing payment in cases where a person or organization had failed to pay taxes or other claims.

The study was undertaken during the period 2002 and 2003 with final reporting in 2004. Baseline data included QWC surveys, productivity, health, sickness and disability absentee data, and biological measures. Follow-up data was collected 1 year after the baseline assessment and included similar measures to the initial assessment [17].

A total of 383 employees received the baseline QWC questionnaire. Of these, 306 choose to respond to the survey (response rate 80%). The equivalent numbers for the second survey were 381 and 291, respectively (76%).

Following the analyses, the researchers identified the following QWC key enhancement areas: leadership, participatory management, employeeship (motivation and commitment among employees to drive change, actively search out relevant information, and stimulate one another to develop skills and work habits), management performance feedback, and work-related exhaustion. Each of the 22 units received specific recommendations. The recommendations included areas to focus on as well as a manual outlining the process of analyzing key improvement areas, focusing the process of identifying concrete improvement measures, and ensuring the implementation of the group's ideas into everyday work processes.

At the 1-year follow-up, 80% of the respondents stated that the QWC results were in agreement with their own view of their workplace, while 70% stated that they had utilized the results to improve the work environment and 64% felt that the data had been helpful to do so. Nine out of ten respondents stated that they had not used an external consultant in the change process and of these, 60% stated that they did not desire external support. The group and its leader had sufficient capacity and facts to enact efficient changes.

Improvements were noticed in a range of important organizational and employee health indicators. Participatory management increased from 69% at the first assessment to 74% at the second. The target level for participatory management for healthy organizations has been calculated at 80%. Employeeship improved from 76% to 79%. This is just below the target level of 80%. Skills development improved from 69% to 73%. The latter value even exceeded the target level of 70%. Management feedback to employees also improved from 58% to 64%, which is close to the target level of 65%. Organizational efficacy increased from a pre-intervention value of 63% to 68% after the 1-year intervention. The target level for efficacy is 65%. In addition to organizational performance improvement, employee health and well-being improved from 68% to 72%. The target level for employee health/mental energy is 70%. Work-related exhaustion decreased from 42% to 38%; the target level for work-related exhaustion is 30% or less. Leadership ratings improved from 65% to 69%, which is close to the target level of 70%.

The Dynamic Focus Score, the overall, aggregated, summary measure of organizational and employee well-being increased from 65% to 68%. The target level for the Dynamic Focus Score is 70%, a level at which organizations have capacity to handle change and other potential organizational challenges.

With regard to biological markers, serum levels of total cholesterol, a risk factor for cardiovascular disease, decreased from a mean of 5.5 mmol/L to 5.3 mmol/L. Serum cortisol, an important stress hormone, increased from a mean of 376 nmol/L to 432 nmol/L. Serum cortisol has been shown to be decreased in burnout and severely mentally fatigued patients. In the current study, we noticed an increase in employee well-being/mental energy at the same time as work-related fatigue decreased. These changes are in agreement with the change in serum cortisol levels. Serum testosterone increased as well, from a mean of 3.7 nmol/L to 4.6 nmol/L. Overall, these changes in the biological profile of the employees suggest a normalization of the stress response capacity. This is indicated by the increase in serum cortisol level at the same time as testosterone levels increased. One of the earliest signs of unhealthy organizational and individual stress is decreased levels of serum testosterone. Interestingly, in line with these changes, was the observation that an important risk factor for cardiovascular disease, serum levels of total cholesterol decreased. This study is the first to our knowledge that links improved employee biological and self-rated health and well-being to organizational performance.

Looking at the relationships between changes over time in the various outcome measures of interest, significant associations were found between increased ratings of self-rated health and decreased work-related exhaustion (an inverse correlation r of -0.49, $p < 0.05$). Changes in self-rated health was also positively related to changes in self-rated sleep quality ($r = 0.70$, $p < 0.01$). Improvement in self-rated health was related to decreased sickness absenteeism ($r = -0.60$, $p < 0.01$).

Changes in the anti-stress, restorative hormone testosterone in serum was related to a number of positive changes in QWC organizational and employee health measures. Thus, increased serum testosterone related to improvements in the following organizational health indicators: participatory management ($r = 0.67$, $p < 0.01$), workload/tempo (inverse association, $r = -0.37$, $p < 0.05$), skills development ($r = 0.47$, $p < 0.05$), internal communications quality ($r = 0.45$, $p < 0.05$), and Dynamic Focus Score ($r = 0.51$, $p < 0.05$).

Figure 5.4 depicts the association between changes in the Dynamic Focus Scores from before to after the intervention and changes in serum levels of testosterone during the same time period.

Overall productivity was measured only at the unit collecting nonpaid taxes and other fees. Productivity, measured as document cases handled, increased from a site mean of 69 cases in 2002 to 164 cases in 2003. Productivity increased measurably in two out of three sites. The last site was exposed to a major organizational change, possibly contributing to the fact that work-related exhaustion increased while social climate and self-rated health decreased during the study period at that site.

The Swedish IRS study is based on data from 22 sites and 1-year follow-up. It needs to be replicated and further studies are needed to understand the mechanisms linking organizational and employee health data to productivity and biological outcomes. However, it suggests how management and organizational theorists and consultants could collaborate with psychologists and medical/

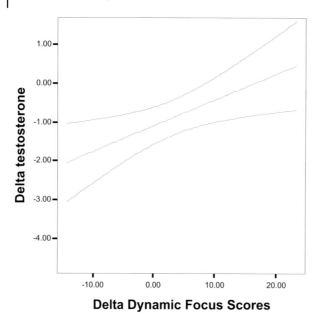

Delta Dynamic Focus Scores

Fig. 5.4. Associations between changes in Dynamic Focus Scores and changes in serum levels of testosterone (delta testosterone). Delta was calculated by subtracting values at start from values following 1 year of intervention. Mean results for individual work sites. The regression line and 95% confidence intervals are depicted.

physiological professionals in studies of organizational performance and employee health and well-being.

5.14
Multiorganizational Assessments of Organizational and Employee Well-Being

Much of the intervention research in the area of organizational and employee well-being has been done in single organizations and then mostly at a single site or a limited numbers of different sites within the organization. This poses a challenge as to the generalizability of results. Similar problems have been pointed out for research concerning effective management tools and practices to achieve superior business results [18].

Dr. Vanja Blomkvist in our research group led a study analyzing QWC data collected at least twice during an extended period from four different large organizations, representing three different regions. A total of approximately 10 000 employees responded to the QWC questionnaire twice during the period 1998–2002. The response rates ranged between 60% and 77%. Data was analyzed at the organization, department and professional group levels. The study focused on changes in organizational and employee health. The three outcomes of interest were leadership, efficacy, and employee health/well-being. These three areas were chosen as good indicators of organizational performance and employee health.

There were large differences between, and especially, within each organization in organizational health and employee well-being. Organizations developed differently over time in organizational efficacy and leadership. Important determinants of improved efficacy were improvements over time in participatory management and goal clarity. Improvement in management feedback to employees was an important predictor of increased leadership ratings. In general, focusing on enhancing employee skills developments and performance feedback during periods of change enhanced organizational performance and employee well-being.

Looking specifically at changes in the respective organizations, units within each organization, and within each profession, important differences in organizational and employee health promoters appeared. Thus, within an organization different professional groups reported significant differences over time in how they rated changes in important outcome measures. Similar findings held true when studying different units within and between organizations.

The results from the study suggest that there are, indeed, some common factors promoting organizational and employee well-being. However, there are some organizational and site-specific factors that appear to be of importance as well as, that requires further research.

5.15
Leadership and Employee Job Satisfaction and Organizational Performance

Based on research to date, there is support for linking leadership, specific organizational characteristics, and job satisfaction to employee health and organizational performance. However, less is known of the causal relationship between the various input factors to outcome measures of interest. Substantially more multidisciplinary research is needed in order to better define which factors are of the greatest importance to create healthy and productive organizations, and under what circumstances.

Figure 5.5 summarizes the current QWC model linking leadership to job satisfaction, performance quality and bottom line results.

From Figure 5.5 it is apparent that the number one factor in creating healthy and productive organizations is leadership. Leadership refers to the immediate leadership at each level of the organization. Given high-quality leadership, issues such as efficiency, participation and goal clarity clearly become important mediators to achieve high work satisfaction. Employee work satisfaction has a direct impact on enterprise quality and customer satisfaction. Employee work satisfaction affects the employees' pride in working for the organization, which in turn relates to the bottom line.

Figure 5.6 is a theoretical description of the leadership–bottom line performance axis. Leadership, in the model, is seen as the fundament for organizational health

Organizational efficacy and customer satisfaction

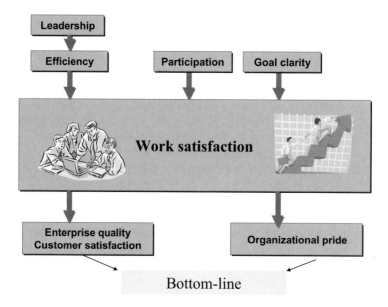

Fig. 5.5. Theoretical model linking leadership, job satisfaction, to organizational performance (the bottom line).

and employee well-being. Resources, including employee skills, motivation and overall energy, technology, know-how and other nontangibles are important mediating variables. Process quality and the ability to run efficient processes with clear and well-defined goals and routines with optimal use of available resources deter-

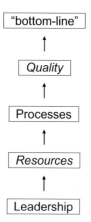

Fig. 5.6. The leadership–bottom line performance model.

mines, together with leadership, the overall quality of services and products rendered. The net effects of all these factors are organizational well-being in the form of profitability or other measures of an organization's bottom line.

5.16
Implementation of Productive and Healthy Work Practices

Based on a range of studies carried out within the areas of organizational and employee health, there appear to be some major challenges to achieving the desired end results. The implementation process, for example, of various proposed management tools and practices is one key factor. Even within one organization, the ability to implement and really make use of tools to improve organizational and employee health varies substantially. There is sufficient knowledge about effective tools and practices warranting the start of a process of creating healthier work organizations. The practices and tools are just not put into practice. We have therefore initiated a study aimed at evaluating how different management strategies used in the implementation process might influence the actual utilization rate of these tools in the organizations, as well as its relationship to actual organizational changes.

Nohria and coworkers [18] also point to the importance of not only looking at specific management tools and practices in understanding organizational health and performance. They carried out a large and very ambitious study in which they examined more than 200 well-established management practices as they were employed over a 10-year period in 160 companies, representing a variety of branches. They reported "Most of the management tools and techniques we studied had no direct causal relationship to superior business performance. What does matter, it turns out, is having a strong grasp of the business basics. Without exception, companies that outperformed their industry peers excelled at what we call the four primary management practices – strategy, execution, culture, and structure" [18].

Thus, it appears that issues relevant to achieving superior financial performance in organizations also relate to successful health promotion and anti-stress interventions, such as a clear strategy, a goal-oriented culture focusing on performance, and a flawless operational execution.

Senior management plays an important role in initiating and reinforcing practices conducive to organizational health and productivity. If senior managers follow both traditional as well as softer indicators of organizational performance when assessing managers and units, the motivation for middle managers and team leaders to adapt healthy and productive work practices increases.

Senior managers must be personally convinced about the benefits of this new approach, but by measuring and holding managers accountable for the development of soft indicators of organizational and employee well-being, the likelihood of fostering the right environment and work practices increases.

Motivation to adopt revised work practices is needed at all levels of the organization. Short-term financial or other benefits might well be counterproductive to long-term gains in organizational and employee health. Motivation is a psychological process that stimulates and sustains behavior. As suggested by Herzberg, the most important factors contributing to positive job attitudes might be intrinsic motivators, such as achievement, recognition, work itself, responsibility, advancement, and growth. It is therefore logical to further consider how such intrinsic motivators could be strengthened in future intervention studies to achieve healthy work organizations.

Our indicators of healthy work organizations need further refinement. Health and work productivity assessment is a research area that is developing rapidly, but there are still a number of issues that need to be resolved in order to estimate the true costs and benefits of healthy and productive work organizations as well as means to measure productivity in the service- and knowledge-based economy.

These caveats aside, there is substantial empirical and scientific evidence that it is possible to create both productive and healthy workplaces; organizations where employee health, participation in decision-making processes and skills development go hand-in-hand with a healthy bottom line.

References

1 Moss KANTER R. Leadership and the psychology of turnarounds. Harv Bus Rev 2003; 81(6):59–67.
2 ULRICH D. A new mandate for human resources. Harv Bus Rev. 1998; 76(1):125–134.
3 LEV B. Sharpening the intangibles edge. Harv Bus Rev. 2004; 82(6):109–116.
4 NOHRIA N, GULATI R. What is the optimum amount of organizational slack? A study of the relationship between slack and innovations in multinational firms. Eur Manag J. 1997; 15(6):603–611.
5 KALIA M. Assessing the economic impact of stress – the modern day hidden epidemic. Metabolism. 2002; 51(6), Suppl 1:49–53.
6 ARNETZ BB. Physicians' view of their work environment and organization. Psychother Psychosom. 1997; 66:155–162.
7 ARNETZ BB. Staff perception of the impact of health care transformation on quality of care. Int J Qual Health Care. 1999; 11(4):345–351.
8 ARNETZ BB. Techno–stress: a prospective psychophysiological study of the impact of a controlled stress-reduction program in advanced telecommunication systems design work. J Occup Environ Med. 1996; 38(1):53–65.
9 LOHR S. Pursuing growth, Microsoft steps up patent chase. N Y Times. 2004; 153(52,926):C3.
10 SAINFORT F, KARSH B-T, BOOSKE BC, SMITH MJ. Applying quality improvement principles to achieve healthy work organizations. J Qual Improv. 2001; 27(9):469–483.
11 ARNETZ BB, WIHOLM C. Technological stress: Psychophysiological symptoms in modern offices. J Psychosom Res. 1997; 43(1):35–42.
12 JACKSON SE. Participation in decision making as a strategy for reducing job-related strain. J Appl Psychol. 1983; 68(1):3–19.
13 PARKER SK, CHMIEL N, WALL TD. Work characteristics and employee well-being within context of strategic downsizing. J Occup Psychol. 1997; 2(4):289–303.
14 KOZLOWSKI SWJ, CHAO GT, SMITH EM, HEDLUND J. Organizational downsizing: Strategies, interventions,

and research implications. In: Cooper CL, Robertson IT (eds.), International Review of Industrial and Organizational Psychology. Wiley, London, 1993, pp 264–332.

15 ARNETZ JE, ARNETZ BB. The development and application of a patient satisfaction measurement system for hospital-wide quality improvement. Int J Qual Health Care. 1996; 8(6):555–566.

16 THOMSEN S, DALLENDER J, SOARES J, NOLAN P, ARNETZ B. Predictors of a healthy workplace in Swedish and English psychiatrists. Br J Psychiatry. 1998; 13:80–84.

17 ANDERZÉN I, ARNETZ BB. The impact of a prospective survey-based workplace intervention program on employee health, biological stress markers, and organizational productivity. J. Occup Environmed. 2005; 47(7): 671–682.

18 NOHRIA N, JOYCE WW, ROBERSON B. What really works? Harv Bus Rev. 2003; 81(7):43–52.

6
The Empowered Organization and Personnel Health

Töres Theorell

6.1
Introduction

The individual's ability to exert control over his/her situation is of fundamental importance to health. When individuals lack control they can be exposed to a multitude of humiliations which could provoke psychophysiological reactions. If these are repeated for long periods, illnesses may arise. This is a general theory which underlies the main messages in many systems of thinking. The main proponents of existential philosophy, for instance Sartre, have formulated the theory that the surroundings should not be allowed to take command over the individual's existence.

Freud's psychoanalytic theory deals in a similar way with the ego's fight to exert control over primitive parts of itself (the id) as well as over the the sometimes too-demanding superego. One conclusion from this is that a good society should build an environment which helps citizens to exert control over their own lives. Of course, this a complex task because every individual has to take into account that *other* individuals must be allowed to exert control over their lives.

A common statement is that it is anxiety-provoking for many individuals to make decisions and that many simply do not want to make decisions and want to be told what to do. Such "decision anxiety," however, may have arisen due to previous experiences. If an individual has never had any possibility to influence his/her life situation he/she may internalize the thought that others have to decide. Figure 6.1 shows some of the key concepts and how they are related to one another.

6.2
A Historical Perspective

Empowerment is the process that leads to increased power for the organization and/or the individuals. To "own power" is the desired result of empowerment. The "locus of control" is the "place" for the exertion of control. Internal locus of

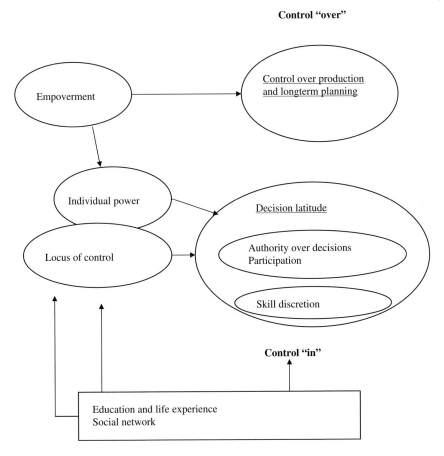

Fig. 6.1. Concepts related to decision latitude.

control refers to the individual's own feeling that he/she can control the situation himself/herself. External locus of control, on the other hand, refers to the feeling that "others" have to exert control. Locus of control is greatly influenced by experiences in adult life [1] and can change as a consequence of external conditions [2].

Control "in" refers to the concept "decision latitude" (see [3]) which has two components: authority over decisions, and skill discretion. Both of these can be influenced by means of organizational change (see also below). During the 1970s and 1980s, Swedish working men and women reported that they experienced more and more opportunity to influence their work (working tempo, planning of work). During the same period, they also reported that their work became more and more intellectually challenging (increasing the possibility to learn new things at work). That work entails increased opportunities to learn new things means that the employees develop better possibilities of exerting control.

According to the survey of living conditions (ULF) Swedish working men and women reported improved skill discretion and authority over decisions during the 1970s and 1980s.

The work environment surveys have shown that authority over decisions has deteriorated for employees in counties (regions with responsibility for public transportation and health care) and communities (with responsibility for public schools and care of the elderly) during the 1990s.

Psychological demands increased during the whole of the 1990s. This was reflected in the percentage of working men and women who reported "too-high demands". For both men and women, there was a continuous increase over the whole decade of approximately 10% in the proportion of subjects who reported too-high demands.

Accordingly, during the late 1990s there was a combination of continued increase in demand and a decrease in decision authority for most working men and women in Sweden. The worst development was seen for women employed in counties and communities.

Since there was an unfavorable development with regard to demands and decision authority, particularly during the latter half of the 1990s, it is interesting to study possible changes in illness patterns during this period. Figure 6.2 shows the development of total sick-leave from 1955 to 2001 in Sweden according to official statistics. The Swedish state insurance system covers everybody.

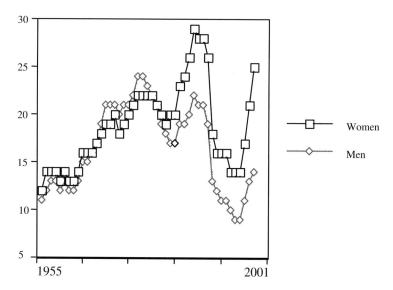

Fig. 6.2. Average number of sick-leave days per working person and year in Sweden for each year 1955–2001. Separate data for men and women respectively.

During the late 1990s, long-term sick-leave increased mainly in the groups who reported the most pronounced loss of control at work, namely women employed in counties and communities, i.e., women employed in health care, care of elderly and education. This could be interpreted as a confirmation of the hypothesis that a low decision latitude increases the risk of long-term sick-leave. There are many caveats to such a conclusion, however.

It should be pointed out, however, that reduced benefits (which were effected during the first half of the 1990s, and which were followed by reduced sick-leave) may result in increased long-term sickness. The mechanism behind this is that workers who go to work when they are sick may expose their physiology to wear and tear causing regulatory disorders resulting in long-term illness (see below). "Sickness presenteeism" has been studied in Sweden [4], and the results of this research show that sickness presenteeism and a high sick-leave rate often exist in the same occupations.

Mortality (including successful suicides) and incidence of myocardial infarction have not been dramatically affected yet.

The prevalence of mental symptoms (worry, stressy or bullying) due to work, which is followed every year in the official statistics (Arbetskraftsundersökning, AKU, labor force survey) is shown in Fig. 6.3. The prevalence of mental symptoms due to work is stable in the early 1990s but rises steeply during the second half, both for men and women. This coincides with the development of "lack of control", the prevalence of which started to rise during this period. In addition, the mental symptoms rose more sharply in those branches which had the most unfavorable development of decision authority (health care and education).

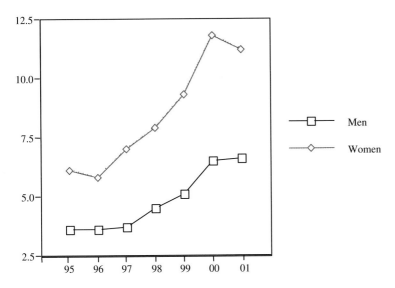

Fig. 6.3. Work-related mental ill health symptoms. Prevalence in working Swedish men and women.

Finally it should be pointed out that women have reacted with more long-term sick-leave than men. One of the reasons for this may be that women often have more obligations at home than men. The combination of an adverse home situation and an increasingly uncontrollable situation at work with increasing demands may become unbearable. This may explain why women have had a more adverse development of health and sick-leave than men: unpaid work is still more extensive for women than for men.

6.3
Concepts Related to Work Control

Many concepts are used in this field; it would be impossible to cover them all. The reader is referred to a review by Ganster [5]. According to the terminology proposed by Karasek [3], the overriding concept related to possibilities that the work environment gives the employees to make decisions regarding their own situation is decision latitude. This has two components:

- The first component corresponds directly to everyday democracy at work, *authority over decisions*. This is firstly related to the opportunity given the employee to influence work tempo, timing of pauses and meals and other conditions directly related to the work day, and secondly to everyday decisions regarding work, such as who is appointed as supervisor or workmate. An important part of authority over decisions is regular department meetings which aim at the provision of information about ongoing changes and which give the employees openings to discuss important aspects of their work.
- The second component is *skill discretion* or *intellectual discretion*. The employee who has got the opportunity to develop relevant competence may exert control over unexpected situations at work.

The two components in decision latitude were both reduced for the workers in the development of the principles of scientific management according to Taylor [6].

Decision latitude is closely related to power distribution at work. If the boss has all the power, he/she will be troubled by the number of decisions that he/she has to take, and their subordinates will be frustrated by the many situations in which activity is hindered by the fact that the boss does not have time to make a decision.

There is a substantial difference between micro- and macroperspectives in decision latitude. The microperspective could be referred to as "control in" the work situation whereas the macroperspective corresponds to "control over". It is more difficult to measure control over, and few studies have dealt with the macroperspective. It has been pointed out recently that the framework for creating justice and resolving conflicts may be one crucial aspect of this, and one study has shown a relationship between organizational justice and employee health. Other concepts that are useful in the discussion are described below.

Locus of control refers to the individual's perception of ability to exert control over a situation [7]. According to this terminology, internal locus of control refers to the individual's feeling that he/she can control most situations himself/herself while external locus of control means that the individual expects persons in the environment to take care of the problem. Locus of control accordingly corresponds to an attitude to problem solving. Both extremes may be harmful since an extremely internal locus of control may create a destructive feeling of self-blame in situations that the individual – for external reasons – cannot possibly deal with. An extremely external locus of control may correspond to passivity and fatalism. A large epidemiological twin study has shown that locus of control is determined to a great extent by experiences in adult life and only to a lesser extent by genetic factors and childhood experiences [1]. Locus of control has a counterpart in work psychology, work locus of control, which has been shown to differ in managers across various countries. In the western hemisphere, work locus of control was shown to be more internal in managers than it was in managers in Asia and Africa. This finding indicates that locus of control is influenced by tradition and culture. One interpretation is that countries with strong democratic work traditions may give its citizens the feeling that they can influence their own work situation. Locus of control is only one aspect of coping. There are also other aspects of coping that may be influenced by working conditions. The degree of openness in coping with situations that implied unfair treatment at work was studied in an epidemiological study of working men and women in Stockholm. Questions were made about what the participants would typically do if they were treated in an unfair way at work. Subjects with a *covert coping* pattern would not show the person who treated them in this way what they thought, whereas those with the *open pattern* would do so. Participants who reported that they had a poor decision latitude at work typically reported covert coping patterns [8]. These examples amplify the potential importance of the work environment in the development of coping patterns. An environment with a high decision latitude stimulates more open coping patterns and possibly also a more internal work locus of control.

The so-called demand–control–support model was introduced by Karasek [3, 9] who developed the theory behind the model with Theorell and Johnson. The model has three dimensions, psychological demands (including quantitative as well as qualitative demands), decision latitude, and social support from workmates and superiors. All these dimensions are conceptualized as environmental factors and all of them could be improved by means of organizational changes. The level of psychological demands should be reasonable. This means that the number of employees and the competence in the employees should be appropriate for the tasks. If the load is too demanding staff resources should increase or demands decrease. Decision latitude can be improved in several ways (see below).

Figure 6.4 illustrates the time effects of working in the different areas of the demand–control model. Working with job strain means an accumulation of psychological strain that could in itself inhibit learning. This could mean that employees who have been living for a long time with high demands and poor decision latitude (low degree of democracy) may have difficulty in obtaining benefits from

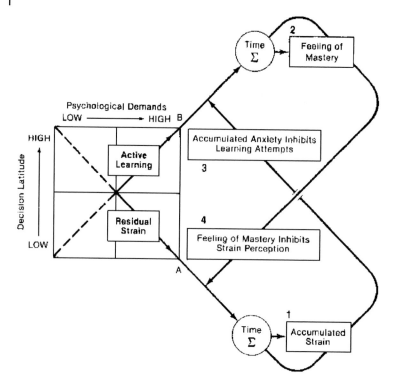

Fig. 6.4. Accumulated effects of long-term exposure to strain work and active work. Source: Karasek and Theorell [3].

an improved work organization. Such a workplace needs a long time for adaptation to an improved situation. Conversely the active work place (high demands and high decision latitude) may make it possible for the employees to improve their coping strategies. This means that the employees in such a workplace may develop improved coping strategies, and thus may be able to manage in a better way than employees in other workplaces to cope with a temporary deterioration in working conditions.

Social support is often associated with good friendships at work and good relations among workmates and between superiors and subordinates. It is emphasized that the employees should have good opportunities to solve conflicts. Education in solution of conflicts is often arranged in order to improve social support at work. Social support is not a matter only of group psychology, however. For instance, it is important that the employees have a joint image of the goals of the production/ activity in the workplace. If they have such an image it will be more possible for them to give support. The goals could be discussed with the employees at regular intervals. Protocols for raising salaries should be based upon principles that are accepted by the majority and understood by all employees. Otherwise a bad social climate and lack of support may arise.

As indicated by Johnson [10] the concepts of decision latitude and support are close to one another, especially when they are regarded in a collective perspective. If the employees support one another, they may also collectively obtain more influence over decisions at work – mainly because mutual understanding may lead to a unified workforce.

Accordingly, the ideal workplace makes reasonable demands on its workers, and has good social support and good decision latitude for the employees. There are many studies that show that employees in workplaces with these characteristics have better health. The most pronounced health problems mostly exist in workplaces with job strain, a combination of high psychological demands and poor decision latitude. If the social support is also bad (isostrain) the health problems tend to increase even more.

The active workplace (high psychological demands and good decision latitude) may also imply health risks. In recent years, several studies have shown that younger white collar workers who report an active work situation may have a high prevalence of health problems. Extremely high levels of psychological demands alone may decrease the possibility to exert control and to use the opportunity that the environment provides. Some groups in the modern labor market may believe that they have good decision latitude despite small real possibilities to influence decisions. One such group may be information technology workers, who typically report that they have a very high level of decision latitude.

6.4
How to Evaluate Decision Latitude?

Conceptualization and assessment are two different things. Although a concept may be theoretically clear, it may be very difficult to assess it in practice. In particular it is very difficult to separate the individual component from the organizational. The most commonly used methodology is to ask the employees themselves about different aspects of democracy in their workplaces. Standardized questionnaires are mostly used in these assessments. This makes it impossible to eliminate the individual's interpretation of the situation and this interpretation could be flavored by experiences that may have nothing to do with the work situation. An alternative way is to ask experts to do ratings. They could be external experts who make judgments on the basis of general knowledge about working conditions. They could also be occupational health staff with experience in psychosocial assessment who are asked to rate different aspects of authority over decisions and intellectual discretion. A third way is to use imputed assessments from national surveys. The latter method has been used in several publications. It means that decision latitude is assessed on the basis of means from all individuals in a given occupation who have participated in a national survey. The imputed measures are specified not only on the basis of occupation but also on the basis of age (older and younger workers), number of years in the occupation and gender. Such assessments are, of course, crude. The underlying assumption behind "imputation" (the average from the national survey is used as measure of decision latitude for this particular group) is for instance that all male carpenters above age 45 years who have been working in this occupation for less than 5 years have the same decision latitude.

A direct comparison between expert ratings performed by members of occupational health care teams and self-ratings has been performed with regard to decision latitude in 3804 men and women employed in different kinds of workplaces in Stockholm. The results showed that there was in general a good correlation between expert and self-ratings. Greiner et al. (2004) have shown that objective measures of stressful working conditions are associated with blood pressure and blood pressure variations in bus drivers, whereas no such associations were found when subjective stress measures were used.

6.5
Questionnaires

Authority over decisions has been assessed by means of two types of questions. The first type of question deals with the influence that the employees have over what they should do at work and how it should be done; these are very general questions. The other type of question deals with special conditions such as the appointment of workmates, working hours, vacations etc. General questions of the first type are included in the most widely used questionnaire, the Job Content Questionnaire (JCQ), but also in the shorter Swedish version. The more specific questions have been included in some national surveys such as the Swedish ones referred to above (National Board of Work Environment and Statistics, Sweden [11]) and also in American surveys [5].

Intellectual discretion is usually illuminated by means of questions about monotony and repetitions, about possibilities to learn new things and whether work requires creativeness, etc. JCQ includes such questions, as does the NIOSH questionnaire.

It should be pointed out that the higher level decision latitude which relates to long-term planning and decisions of profound importance, control over work [4], has not been assessed extensively in research. JCQ includes such questions but they have not been used in many studies. The framework relating to possibilities to ensure justice has been assessed in a newly constructed Finnish questionnaire.

Accordingly it is possible to describe several aspects of skill discretion and decision authority in different workplaces. These different kinds of assessments are useful for different purposes. The more objective observations (systematic observations, expert ratings, imputations) have the advantage that they are not influenced by irrelevant individual experiences. Self-ratings, on the other hand, are of course more valid from the individual's point of view but may be less relevant from a job organizational point of view.

6.6
Relationship Between Decision Latitude and Health

There are many situations in which we react physiologically because we fear that we are losing control. This may be an important reason for the consistent and strong relationship between loss of control and illness onset. Such situations arise, for instance, in the case of job loss. There are several studies indicating that illness risk increases when there is threat of unemployment and when employees lose their jobs [12, 13] although there is also a discussion regarding the direction of this relationship. There is agreement that both forward and backward associations exist together. Thus, there is both an increased risk among employees with illness of becoming unemployed and an increased risk of becoming ill after the onset of unemployment [14, 15].

Even when subjects have a job, they may of course lose opportunities to exert control at work. This could also be of significance to the risk of illness. This has recently been explored in two different epidemiological studies of the risk of coronary heart disease. One was a prospective examination of state employees in England [16]. Health was measured by means of registers and self-reported data. Biological data such as serum lipids and blood pressure were also measured. All these measurements were performed approximately at 2-year intervals. Among other things the participants were asked how much decision latitude they had at work. It could be shown that subjects who had lost a significant amount of decision latitude at work between two examinations had a significantly greater risk of developing new coronary heart disease (without having had symptoms previously) during follow-up. The risk was approximately doubled even after adjustment for accepted biological risk factors such as smoking habits, serum lipids and blood pressure. The other study was a case control study of first myocardial infarctions in Stockholm, the Stockholm Heart Epidemiology Program (SHEEP). All men and women aged 45–65 years who had suffered a first myocardial infarction [17] in the greater Stockholm region were invited. A matched group of men and women without coronary heart disease were invited as referents. The myocardial infarction patients were examined within 3 months of their infarction. The same medical and psychosocial examinations were performed on all subjects. Occupation was recorded for every year during their whole working career. This made it possible to impute a measure of decision latitude for each year and subject (specified with regard to occupation, gender, age and duration of employment in the occupation) from the Swedish classification system [18]. The hypothesis was tested that subjects who had lost decision latitude during the 10 years preceding the examination would have a greater likelihood of belonging to the myocardial infarction group than others. There was support for this hypothesis in men and particularly so in the age group 45–54 years. Significantly lowered decision latitude was operationally de-fined to have occurred among the 25% who had had the least favorable (lowered) decision latitude during the period. After adjustment for accepted biological risk factors the odds ratio of belonging to the myocardial infarction in this group was 1.8. Thus there was almost a doubled risk of having a first myocardial infarction in this group. Among men between 55 and 65 years there was no such excess risk associated with lost decision latitude at work. This difference between the middle-aged and the older men could be due to expectations: after the age of 55 years men in the modern world of working may expect decreasing rather than increasing de-cision latitude. Accordingly a decreased level of decision latitude may be perceived as normal and not such a negative event as it could be in men below age 55. An-other explanation could be that a large proportion of men between the age of 55 and 65 years have stopped working, and thus those remaining in the working pop-ulation may be a selected group.

That loss of decision latitude may also have importance for the risk of developing acute neck/shoulder pain has been illustrated in a recent case control study of low back pain and neck/shoulder pain. In this study physical as well as psychosocial conditions were examined at work and outside work. During an interview the par-ticipants described their situation at the time of the examination. Afterwards they were asked to assess whether the situation had changed with regard to for instance decision latitude at work during the past 5 years. Those who reported that they had experienced decreased decision latitude had an increased likelihood of belonging to the neck/shoulder pain group even after adjustment for a number of possible con-founders, such as previous neck/shoulder pain episodes, socioeconomic status and age. In this particular study the associations between loss of decision latitude and illness risk were stronger than the one between a low level of decision latitude and illness risk.

That loss of decision latitude may induce increased illness risk is something to consider when jobs are reorganized. If many persons go through work changes that mean less decision latitude, lower status and less possibility for development of competence, there is obviously an increased risk that the prevalence of certain illnesses will arise. Accordingly there is reason to contact those who are in these risk situations and try to help them find new, meaningful and dignified tasks.

Another possibility is to explore whether a low level of decision latitude *per se* is associated with increased risk of developing illness, without any loss of decision latitude. In the longitudinal study of state employees in England it was tried in a systematic way to shed light on this question [16]. Several questions about the work environment were posed, on several occasions (approximately every second year). On these occasions a medical examination was performed and blood sam-ples were drawn for the assessment of serum lipids and other relevant biological parameters. The part of decision latitude that was studied in this examination was authority over decisions. In men as well as in women, a significant relationship was found between a small degree of authority over decisions and increased risk of developing new coronary heart disease during the follow-up period. In this study it was possible not only to adjust for accepted biological risk factors, but also for socioeconomic factors (education and social class) and a number of individual psychological characteristics as well. The most important psychological trait was "negative affectivity", which is the tendency to complain about conditions in general.

In a study of the long-term effects of exposure to low decision latitude [19] the working career of a large number of Swedes was related to risk of dying a cardiovascular death during follow-up. The subjects had participated in a survey study that is performed by the governmental Statistics Sweden [Survey of Living Conditions (ULF)]. They responded to a question regarding what occupation they had had during each year of their working career. By means of the classification system, decision latitude was imputed for each individual for each year. The results indicated that there may have been a cumulated beneficial effect of high decision latitude which was evident up to a period of 15–20 years. After 20 years there was no additional cumulative effect.

Thus, in the British study of the state employees, as well as in the Swedish study of cardiovascular deaths in the general working population, there was evidence of a protective effect of a high decision latitude on the risk of developing cardiovascular disease.

Most studies of the association between low decision latitude have been focussed upon the combination of a small decision latitude and a high level of psychological demands (job strain). The demand–control model [3] stipulates that this combination is particularly dangerous in relation to illness risk. The results of these studies have been summarized recently by Belkic and others. A more recent review has analyzed the quality of published studies. The conclusion was that job strain should be regarded as an established risk factor for coronary heart disease. Several of these studies show no association between psychological demands and the risk of cardiovascular disease, but in most of the studies the precision of the predictions increase when psychological demands and decision latitude are combined compared to when decision latitude is studied separately. The excess risk associated with job strain is between 40 and 150% in most of the studies that are based upon self-ratings. In studies based upon imputed scores when the only information available has been occupation the excess risk has been lower – between 20 and 100%. The strongest explanatory factor has been decision latitude.

Three different studies in the Nordic countries have shown similar results with regard to etiologic fraction [17]. According to the most recent one, the SHEEP study, the proportion of myocardial infarctions occurring in the working population that could be prevented if the work environment among those 25% with the most pronounced job strain could be improved to the level of the remaining 75% is in the order of 7% for men and 13% for women. This was shown after adjustment for accepted biological risk factors and social class. In men below age 55 years, the etiological fraction was 11%.

Job strain has been more consistently associated with heart disease risk in studies of blue collar workers than among white collar workers. There are more studies of men than of women, and the associations are less clear for women than for men. The relationship between low decision latitude and the risk of developing musculoskeletal disorders has not been as strong and consistent as the one between decision latitude and cardiovascular disease risk. The relationship seems to vary between different study populations and may also between men and women, as well as between social groups and occupational groups [Scientific Committee for Musculoskeletal Disorders of the International Commission on Occupational Health (ICOH) 1996]. There may also be differences in the relationship between different types of musculoskeletal disorders (neck/shoulder pain or low back pain are the largest groups). In some studies psychological demands are more important and in others one of the two basic aspects of decision latitude. In a recent study [20], lack of decision latitude (in particular the intellectual discretion component according to a systematic interview) was associated with low back pain in men and also with elevated interleukin-6 concentration in serum. Interleukin-6 is related to inflammatory activity in tissues and also to stress reactions. In women, on the other hand, the patterns of associations were different. There were also different patterns of associations for neck/shoulder pain than for low back pain in this large case-control study. An interesting observation in this examination was that particularly in women, the most powerful predictions were made when there were both physical and psychosocial adverse working conditions. The likelihood of having low back pain, for instance, was threefold among women who reported both job strain and physical load compared to women without this combination. Women with the combination of low decision latitude and physical load had a doubled risk compared to those without these joint loads. Lack of decision latitude may thus be significant in combination with other factors in the etiology of low back pain.

Functional gastrointestinal disorders such as dyspepsia or irritable bowel syndrome have also been related to low decision latitude at work.

Sick-leave, in particular very long spells of sick-leave (exceeding 60 days), is strongly associated with lack of decision authority. This has been shown in Swedish, British [21], and Finnish studies [22]. In a recent Swedish study, the combination of lack of decision authority and lack of workmate support (both self-reported) was associated with between 60 and 90% excess risk of at least 60 days of sick-leave during a 1-year follow up [23], in both men and women.

In summary, lack of decision latitude has been related to the risk of developing cardiovascular disease and functional gastrointestinal disorders. It may be of importance in the development of musculoskeletal disorders. Conversely, a high level of decision latitude may be protective. But how do these relationships arise? The relative risks associated with a low decision latitude may not be very great, but since low decision latitude is a widespread phenomenon at work the association does have considerable impact on public health.

6.7
Decision Latitude and Physiological Reactions

In principle there are two ways in which decision latitude could influence illness risk. The first is related to lifestyle factors, such as smoking and dietary habits as well as use of alcohol and drugs. Such life style factors could be influenced by psychosocial factors at work as well as by factors outside work. The second path is related to direct effects of psychosocial factors on endocrine systems and metabolism. Opinion is divided regarding the relative importance of these paths among researchers. Israeli studies of a large cohort of industrial workers have indicated that there are significant effects of decision latitude on smoking habits, and there are similar findings in a study in Sweden. Other studies have shown that there are such relationships between lack of physical exercise and low decision latitude. Despite these results there are many studies which have shown that the relationship between low decision latitude and cardiovascular illness risk remains after adjustment for lifestyle factors [16, 17], and there are even studies which indicate a strengthened relationship after adjustment for such factors. This indicates that the second pathway may be of importance.

Fighting for control should be reflected in physiological reactions. There is considerable support for this notion [24]. Lack of decision latitude makes it necessary to mobilize energy in order to restore control in many situations. In such situations those systems are activated that supply us with fuel in the threatening situation. At the same time those systems that facilitate our adaptation to a physically demanding situation are activated. Sensitivity to pain is diminished, coagulation of blood is facilitated and water and salt are retained in order to maintain the blood volume intake during the fighting stage. In this situation, mobilization of energy and adaptation to physical effort are given the highest priority at the expense of anabolism – the body's processes aimed at restoring and repairing of worn out cell functions. There is a continuous breakdown of bodily tissues. The muscles and the skeleton are being constantly rebuilt in order to be adapted to the needs created by our pattern of bodily movements. Muscle cells are worn out and have to be replaced. There are corresponding processes going on in the white blood cells, for instance. If the anabolism is neglected the condition of these organ systems will deteriorate and accordingly the risk of injury will increase. Anabolism is stimulated by deep sleep (stage IV) in particular. Therefore deep sleep is essential to anabolism. In the long run this is very important to our protection against damage in periods of crisis. Furthermore there is a relationship between anabolism and reproduction. Some of the same hormones are responsible for these functions. The most obvious examples are the sex hormones in men and women. It has been shown that the serum concentration of testosterone decreases in white collar workers when their level of job strain (demands in relation to decision latitude) increases. Police superintendents who lost their jobs had a lowered serum testosterone concentration when this happened. Their concentration was normalized 3 years later, when most of them had new, similar jobs. Correspondingly, female caring personnel had lowered estradiol 1 year after they had been subjected to downsizing and reorganization in a large regional hospital in Sweden [25] – a situation in which they lost control over part of the caring process.

The mobilization of energy is mirrored in many ways in the body [8]. The acute mobilization could be assessed as elevated heart rate and blood pressure but also as increased electromyographic activity in the muscles. There is also elevated excretion of adrenaline and noradrenaline in blood and urine. As soon as the activation has been going on for some minutes the hypothalamo–pituitary–adrenocortical

(HPA) axis is activated. This can be measured as an elevation of the concentration of cortisol in blood and saliva. If the mobilization of energy is pronounced and repeated frequently during a long period of at least several months, other changes may arise, so-called disturbances of regulation. This can be summarized under the umbrella term allostasis. Some examples with particular relevance to the exertion of control:

- One such disturbance is common in subjects who suffer from a classical psychiatric depression: the concentration of cortisol is high in saliva and blood both in the morning and the evening, as if the inhibition mechanism is not functioning. The opposite pattern – low concentration both in the morning and the evening with small variations in relation to stressful situations – is frequently observed in chronic fatigue syndrome. In the latter case the accelerator function seems to be disturbed. Studies of British civil servants have shown that low decision latitude is associated with elevated saliva cortisol levels [26].
- Effects on coagulation. Several different epidemiological studies have shown that the concentration of fibrinogen in blood plasma is elevated in subjects with a low level of decision latitude at work. An increase of fibrinogen is an accepted risk factor for coronary atherosclerosis development and, in the longer perspective, also a risk factor for early myocardial infarction development. This seems to be particularly true when indirect assessment (imputation of scores from national surveys or expert assessments) is used.

The most extensive studies on a physiological function in relation to decision latitude have been the studies of blood pressure. Blood pressure elevation during daily activities – recorded by means of fully automated equipment – has been shown to be related to a combination of high demands and low decision latitude in several studies both of men and women. In these studies the combination of high demands and low decision latitude has turned out to be crucial.

6.8
What Can Be Done for the Improvement of Decision Latitude?

The feeling of being in control is fundamental. Several attempts have been made to increase authority over decision-making at work, and evaluations of such attempts have been made. These studies investigated whether there is any relationship between change in the experience of control at work and improved health of the employees. For example, in one study [27] hospital outpatient facilities were randomly allocated to an experimental and a control population. In order to increase decision latitude for the employees, the frequency of staff meetings was substantially increased to two per month. In order to improve social support, the staff were trained in participatory group problem techniques. Follow-up data in the two populations after 6 months showed that there was a significant drop in role ambiguity and role conflict in the experimental population, but not in the control population. As a result the staff in the experimental population experienced significantly reduced emotional strain, job dissatisfaction, absenteeism and intention to leave the job. In another study which represents a less conclusive but useful kind of evaluation [28], mail deliverers were offered the opportunity to move to a new postal office in the same region, an adaptation to a marked increase in the size of the population in the area. The employees in both stations were subjected to a follow-up study. When the new station started a number of psychosocial work environment changes were instituted, aimed at increased decision latitude and improved social climate for the employees, for instance more responsibility for a particular area for the working group with the aim of increased cohesiveness. The results indicated that the development of physical ergonomic conditions did not differ between the groups during the year of follow-up but that social climate improved more in the new station. Possibly as a consequence, the prevalence of symptoms from the neck/shoulder region decreased in the new station but not in the old. In a third study, the occupational health care team offered a 2-day course in psychosocial stress for employees in offices, and also explored the psychosocial work environment as well as individual conditions by means of standardized questionnaires. On the basis of the findings a number of changes involving the employees were started, all aimed at improving decision latitude and social support. The findings after 8 months indicated significantly improved autonomy and intellectual discretion, as well as almost significantly improved social climate in the experimental group and no changes in the control group. No significant changes in personal habits (such as smoking and diet) were found. Despite this, a significantly improved serum lipid pattern, indicative of reduced coronary heart disease risk, was found in the experimental group but not in the control group. In a practical experiment with two different work organizations in car industry, the more flexible organization was associated with better unwinding of catecholamines after work shifts than the less flexible organization [29]. There are several other experiences in the field that indicate psychosocial improvements of this kind take time, usually several months, and that collective feedback and support belong to the necessary conditions for successful organizational changes.

A new British study was designed specifically to test the effect of increased employee participation in decisions [30]. After a screening phase, work sites with poor scores indicating a problematic psychosocial work situation were identified. Two of those work sites were randomly selected to belong to the experimental group and two were allocated to the control group. The program, Participation Activation Research (PAR) was instituted over several months, and the employees in the two groups were examined before and after the year of intervention with regard to sick-leave and (by means of questionnaires) mental symptoms as well as self-reported effectiveness. There were [30, Fig. 7a and c] significant two-way interactions for all three outcomes, with improved mental health and effectiveness as well as decreased sick-leave in the intervention but not the control work sites.

In addition, statistical analyses showed that the difference in outcomes between the two groups was accounted for by the difference in the development of decision authority.

Usually, simple organizational solutions constitute the framework of the changes. One example would be an attempt to change the role of a foreman to become more of a coordinator rather than a supervisor, or (as in the first example described above) introducing regular, structured meetings for organized information exchange.

There have been attempts to increase cohesiveness in a work team by allowing the group to take responsibility over a large number of diverse tasks in the working process – accordingly less specialization results – as in the second example. A common result with such an approach is an improvement in perceived authority over decisions as well as improved social support.

Thus, whereas several studies have evaluated the health effects of psychosocial interventions involving the whole staff and also interventions focusing on foremen, no studies have evaluated the employee health effects of interventions specifically focused on higher level managers.

In a study of an insurance company there was an anxiety-provoking social situation at the company during the spring of 1998. The whole company was affected by a thorough discussion about the basic conditions. A program for the improvement of the managers' psychosocial competence was started. It lasted from the August 1998 until May 1999. Participation in the program was mandatory for the managers who had to attend 30-min lectures every second week. The lectures were followed by group discussions lasting for 90 min based upon the themes discussed by the seminar leaders. The 2-week intervals were intended to be periods of practical application of the knowledge in the organization. Psychosocial processes always take time to develop. The program was evaluated by means of a follow-up of managers and their employees in the experimental division as well as in a comparison sample in the same company (where no similar program was ongoing). There were 300 participants in the evaluation. The results indicated that compared to the levels preceding the experimental period, authority over decisions had improved after 1 year in the experimental group (in managers as well as in other employees). During the same period the serum cortisol concentration had decreased in the experimental group – not among the managers themselves, but among the other employees. No similar changes had taken place in the comparison group. Since the work demands and the tempo in this organization were high the interpretation was that the lowered cortisol level in the experimental group reflected a lowered physiological arousal level.

The examples that I have described illustrate that it is possible to improve decision latitude. Social climate and support may change at the same time and it is often very difficult to disentangle these effects from one another. In addition it may be very difficult to know whether it is the organizational effects that are important, or whether effects on individual coping patterns are responsible for the beneficial effects.

When such improvement efforts are planned it is important to be systematic. If there are problems at a work site, one has to discuss how to do the initial exploration and all parties have to be sympathetic to it. After this the use of the results of the exploration should be actively planned. There must be resources and time for follow-up (not only week and months but actually years) and possible redesign efforts. The results of the exploration should be fed back to the work sites to both the managers and to the employees. After this, those responsible should be aware that there will always be discussions and conflicts regarding the solution of practical problems. One has to work with the redesign in a structured way – groups have to be selected for formulating solutions. The planning includes deadlines and feedback to managers. The feedback should be thoroughly planned.

Attention both to individual and organizational aspects of the psychosocial working conditions seems to be important in improvement efforts. This always makes it more difficult to evaluate which are the beneficial components. On the other hand, practical experiences have indicated that the likelihood of success increases when individual and organizational attention is combined [3].

References

1 Pedersen NL, Gatz M, Plomin R, Nesselroade JR, McClearn GE. Individual differences in locus of control coping during the second half of the life span for identical and fraternal twins reared apart and reared together. J Gerontol. 1989, 44(4):100–105.

2 Lökk J, Arnetz B. Psychophysiological concomitants of organizational change in health care personnel: effects of a controlled intervention study. Psychother Psychosom. 1997, 66:74–77.

3 Karasek RA, Theorell T. *Healthy Work*. Basic, New York, 1990.

4 Aronsson G. *Work Contents – Decision Latitude – Stress Reactions. Theories and Field Studies, Part I*. Doctoral thesis. Department of Psychology, University of Stockholm, 1985.

5 Ganster DC. Worker control and well-being: a review of research in the workplace. In: Sauter SL, Hurrell JJ Jr, Cooper CL (eds.) *Job control and worker health*. Wiley, Chichester, UK, 1989, pp. 3–23.

6 Taylor F. *The Principles Of Scientific Management*. Norton, New York, 1967.

7 Rotter JB. Generalized expectations for internal vs. external control of reinforcement. Psychol Monogr Gen Appl. 1966, 80(1):1–28.

8 Theorell T, Alfredsson L, Westerholm P, Falck B. Coping with unfair treatment at work – what is the relationship between coping and hypertension in middle-aged men and women? Psychother Psychosom. 2000, 69:86–94.

9 Karasek RA. Job demands, job decision latitude, and mental strain: implications for job redesign. Admin Sci Q. 1979, 24:285–307.

10 Johnson JV. Collective control: strategies for survival in the workplace. Int J Health Services. 1989, 19:469–480.

11 National Board of Work Environment and Statistics. *Negative stress and ill health. Information on education and labour market, 2*. National Board of Work Environment and Statistics, Sweden, 2001.

12 Janlert U. Unemployment as a disease and diseases of the unemployed. Scand J Work Environ Health. 1997, 3:79–83.

13 Hammarström A, Olofsson B-L. Health and drug use – relations to unemployment and labour market position. In: Julkunen I, Carle J (eds.) *Young and Unemployed in Scandinavia – a Nordic Comparative Study*. Nordic Council of Ministers, Copenhagen, 1998, pp 93–114.

14 Isaksson K, Hellgren J, Pettersson P. Repeated downsizing: attitudes and well-being for surviving personnel in a Swedish retail company. In: Hogstedt

C, Eriksson C, Theorell T (eds.) *Health Effects of the New Labor Market.* Kluwer/Plenum, New York, **2000**, pp 85–101.

15 Hallsten L. Mental health and unemployment. Mental health selection to the labour market. Arbete Hälsa. **1998**, 7:1–224.

16 Bosma H, Marmot M, Hemingway H, Nicholson A, Brunner E, Stansfeld S. Low job control and risk of coronary heart disease in Whitehall II study. Br Med J. **1997**, 314:558–565.

17 Theorell T, Tsutsumi A, Hallquist J, Reuterwall C, Hogstedt C, Fredlund P, Emlund N, Johnson VJ, SHEEP Study Group. Decision latitude, job strain, and myocardial infarction: a study of working men in Stockholm. Am J Public Health. **1998**, 88(3):382–388.

18 Fredlund P, Hallqvist J, Diderichsen F. Psychosocial job exposure matrix. An updated version of a classification system for work-related psychosocial exposure. Arbete och hälsa, vetenskaplig skriftserie (Scientific series), 11, Arbetslivs-institutet, **2002**. (In Swedish).

19 Johnson J, Stewart W, Hall E, Fredlund P, Theorell T. Long-term psychosocial work environment and cardiovascular mortality among Swedish men. Am J Public Health. **1996**, 86:324–331.

20 Vingård E, Alfredsson L, Hagberg M, Kilbom Å, Theorell T, Waldenström M, Wigaeus Hjelm E, Wiktorin C, Hogstedt C, MUSIC-Norrtälje Study Group. To what extent do current and past physical and psychosocial occupational factors explain care-seeking for low back pain in a working population? Results from the Musculoskeletal Intervention Center-Norrtälje Study. Spine. **2000**, 25(4):493–500.

21 North F, Symes SL, Feeney A, Shipley M, Marmot M. Psychosocial work environment and sickness absence among British civil servants. The Whitehall II study. Am J Public Health. **1996**, 86:332–340.

22 Vahtera J, Kivimäki M, Pentti J,

Theorell T. Effects of change in the psychosocial work environment on sickness absence: a seven year follow up on initially healthy employees. J Epidemol Community Health. **2000**, 54:484–493.

23 Oxenstierna G, Ferrie J, Hyde M, Westerlund H, Theorell T. Dual support and control at work in relation to poor health. Scand J Publ Health. 33; 455–463, **2005**.

24 Theorell T. Fighting for and losing or gaining control in life. Acta Physiol Scand. **1997**, 640:107–111.

25 Hertting A, Theorell T. Physiological changes associated with downsizing of personnel and reorganization in the health care sector. Psychother Psychosom. **2002**, 71:117–122.

26 Steptoe A, Willemsen G. The influence of low job control on ambulatory blood pressure and perceived stress over the working day in men and women from the Whitehall II cohort. J Hypertens. **2004**, 22(5):915–920.

27 Jackson S. Participation in decision making as a strategy for reducing job related strain. J Appl Psychol. **1983**, 68:3–19.

28 Theorell T, Wahlstedt K. Sweden. Mail processing. In: Kompier M, Cooper C (eds.) *Preventing Stress, Improving Productivity. European Case Studies in the Workplace.* Routledge, London, **1999**, pp 195–221.

29 Melin B, Lundberg U, Söderlund J, Granqvist M. Psychophysiological stress reactions of male and female assembly workers: a comparison between two different forms of work organizations. J Organ Behav. **1999**, 20:47–61.

30 Bond FW, Bunce D. Job control mediates change in work organization intervention for stress reduction. J Occup Health Psychol. **2001**, 6:290–302.

31 Theorell T, Emdad R, Arnetz B, Weingarten A-M. Employee effects of an educational program for managers at an insurance company. Psychosom Med. **2001**, 63:724–733.

7

Can Health be Subject to Management Control? Suggestions and Experiences

Ulf Johanson and Andreas Backlund

7.1
Introduction

The idea of visualizing the financial consequences of health/sickness and health promotion at an organizational level is not new. Such an idea has been about in different forms for a long time. As early as the beginning of the 20th century, industrial safety engineers tried to prove the profitability of investments in the working environment. For instance, 100 years ago US Steel claimed that the return of every dollar spent on health investments was 2.3 times as high [1]. There has been a number of different ways of calculating profitability with the purpose of motivating investment in the working environment. The simple notion has been that if the profitability could be proved then change might occur. More recent studies on management and management control change have demonstrated that this idea is a bit naïve [2]. A representation of a phenomenon is hardly enough to establish change in the organization. The interplay amongst humans in an organization is very complex and takes place in cooperation with external factors (e.g., the surrounding community and customers) and internal factors (e.g., organizational structure and history). Organizations are sluggish and are characterized by habits and routines. The focus has now been directed away from representation to influence and a more relevant research question today might be: how should a management control system be built in order to influence people's behavior in the organization in a desired direction?

In recent decades, important steps have been taken to develop management and management control models that can be used relative to intangible resources such as health and competence. An important early step was the development of human resource accounting (HRA) e.g., [3–6]. HRA highlighted the question of the role of accounting as a means for change, even if the problematization was weak. During the 1970s, the term behavioral accounting emerged. This concept addressed the purpose of accounting and the conflicting ideas of precise measurement versus behavioral influence were discussed. What are the implications for accounting if the relevance of accounting is based on the second proposal? During the 1980s

Stress in Health and Disease. Edited by Bengt B. Arnetz and Rolf Ekman
Copyright © 2006 WILEY-VCH Verlag GmbH & Co. KGaA, Weinheim
ISBN: 3-527-31221-8

and 1990s, new management and management control models of intangibles were developed. Some of these were the balanced scorecard, intellectual capital, and in the early years of the new millennia, health statements. The latter were proposed in the Nordic countries.

In this chapter we will account for the ideas of, experiences with and possible futures for some of these models. We will draw upon experiences from Sweden. One of the reasons for doing so is that Sweden has been the subject of numerous initiatives and efforts regarding management and management control of different intangible resources. We have selected models that address health or human resources in a working environment context. The pedagogical idea underlying our selection is to illuminate problems and possibilities regarding management control and organizational change targeting health as an intangible resource. After a brief summation of the research on the correlation between health and profitability, we pass on to discuss experiences with and possibilities of the different models. The models discussed are health in the balance sheet, health in the profit and loss account, human resource costing, recent management control methods and health statements. After presenting a case, we conclude with a summary of different dilemmas.

In the present chapter we will frequently use the concept of management control. This often refers to activities related to controlling and governing an organization (the control process) and to the information sources/areas that the control activities are mainly based on (the control system). The management control process comprises formal as well as informal elements and is a process of (1) understanding, (2) communicating, and (3) encouraging action in accordance with the organization's vision and objectives. A precondition for a management control process that encourages action in accordance with organizational goals is a widespread learning that includes not only the top management team but also all employees. To facilitate learning and adaptive action, continuous follow-up is essential. Indicators of intangibles could be used to support understanding, communication, action and follow-up.

7.2
Health and Profitability

For the past 15 years there has been increasing interest in investigating the correlation between health and health promotion on the one hand, and profitability on the other, partly because of the increasing costs of absenteeism. Pelletier [7] holds that there are a number of problems with the published studies in this area. Often an evaluation of a health promotion activity is performed only *after* an intervention, which makes comparisons with data from before the intervention impossible. A second problem is the difficulty of collecting data from several and noncoordinated information systems, such as accounting, production, sales and personnel systems. A third problem is the difficulty of getting objective results because the causal link between investment and effect can be tricky to prove. Ozminkowski et al. [8] adds that most evaluations focus on effects only 1 or 2 years following the implementation of the project, which is too early. In long-term evaluations it has been shown that the main effects of the program arise 4–5 years after the intervention.

A number of published studies have been subject to a critical review in six literature surveys [9–14]. The surveys can be summarized as follows: there are strong indications of a correlation between health hazards and financial performance, although the direction of the correlation is unknown. Aldana [11] stresses that most *health hazards* are not connected to higher costs for health and medical services, with the exception of stress, excess weight and a number of cooperating risk factors. In many studies health *promotion* has had a positive effect on medical costs for the firm. Studies addressing return on investments show a positive yield. For example, in 13 studies surveyed by Aldana the average return was four times the investment in health programs because of improved health and decreased medical costs.

One example of a study is an evaluation of the Johnson & Johnson "Live for Life" program. This program was realized between 1979 and 1983 and consisted of health inventory, changes in the physical working environment and different life altering programs such as antismoking treatment, handling of stress and exercise programs. The experimental group consisted of more than 8000 employees and the control group of 3000 persons. The results indicate that the group participating in the intervention program had a lower increase of medical costs and fewer sick days than the control group. These differences were equivalent to a US$980 000 saving during the 4-year period. Another evaluation of the Johnson & Johnson health program is a pre-postlongitudinal study revealing that most of the profits occurred 3–4 years after the initiation of the program [8].

It is worth observing that the most significant costs with respect to changes in employee health, i.e., productivity and quality losses, have not been subject to high-quality studies with an experimental and control group design and with pre- and postmeasurements. In a Swedish study [15], we showed that the effects on productivity were the most significant perceived effects of health promotion programs. The effect on productivity in monetary terms was assumed to be five times as high as the effect on changes in costs for absenteeism. The respondents were more assured in their estimation of productivity effects than on other effects (e.g., absenteeism).

However, knowledge about the correlation between health and profitability is not enough to reach a sufficient investment level (whatever the level might be) with respect to health promotion. There is also a need to look at and try to change the habitual behavior in the firm regarding management and management control addressing health issues.

7.3
Health in the Balance Sheet

7.3.1
Idea

An idea that has been around for quite some time concerns the visualization of the value of human resources (HR) and its corresponding HR investments in the accounting documents. In the 1960s and 1970s the balance sheet was given a salient role within HRA. Many models were developed, some of which were based on the expected future use of the personnel, while others concerned accounting for personnel investment costs, (e.g., in recruitment, training or health promotion). The pedagogical idea underlying the HR balance sheet was that the managerial attention and behavior would be different if the content of what is accounted for was changed.

For about 5 years, the Swedish telecommunication company Telia published extra balance sheets in which recruitment and training costs were treated as assets in the 1990s. The assets were written off over a 3-year period in the profit and loss account.

Current assets Billions SEK (Swedish Kronor)	13 164
Recruitment capital	666
Training capital	653
Fixed assets	44 210
TOTAL	**58 693**
Liabilities and nontaxed reserves	36 205
Owners Equity	
Restricted equity	17 403
Recruitment capital	666
Training capital	653
Unrestricted equity	3766
TOTAL	**58 693**

A similar example can be taken from a Swedish management consulting firm with about 100 employees. In this firm, a balance sheet valuation of competence investments is used to emphasize that continuous competence development is as important as earning money in the short-term perspective [2]. This firm included investments, for example, in training programs and recruitment in its balance sheet for more than a decade. The preciseness of this balance sheet valuation is not the important issue; rather, the message is that the owner appreciates intangible investments for the future as much as he appreciates tangible investments. This message filters down to the employees through the balance sheet valuation.

7.3.2
Experiences

HRA textbooks normally comprise different suggestions on balance sheet models. However, with minor exceptions, practical applications are hard to find. The main reason for this could be the conflict with accounting regulations concerning what can be treated as an asset in the balance sheet. Assets that cannot be owned do not fulfil asset criteria, but there is nothing that prevents organizations from providing HR balance sheets. Nevertheless, the latter has not been accomplished other than by a few exceptions from the sports industry.

7.3.3
Possible Development

Theoretically, there is a possibility of having a post in the balance sheet labeled health capital. The value of the post could be based on health-promotion costs. However, this avenue is presently closed because of different accounting regulations provided by, e.g., FASB (Financial Accounting Standards Board) and IASC (International Accounting Standards Committee). These regulations are restrictive for different reasons e.g., fear of inflated balance sheets, especially if the organization is financially weak, lack of good methods for valuation of intangible assets apart from historical costs, and the difficulty of separating an intangible asset from other assets.

7.4
Health in the Profit and Loss Account

7.4.1
Idea

At the end of the 1980s, the idea was introduced in Sweden that expenses for recruitment, absenteeism, competence development, and other personnel related costs could be shown in the profit and loss account together with the more traditional posts. The proposed model for this was as follows [6]:

Income
– supplier costs
– depreciation
= added value

– costs for recruitment
– costs for absenteeism
– costs for competence development
– employee benefits

– costs for rehabilitation/improvements in the working environment
– production salary
= operating profit

Production salary refers to salary costs required in order to achieve production. It is calculated as salary less what is included in other personnel cost components. It should be observed that the operating profit is identical to similar results in a traditional profit and loss account.

This approach has been extensively practised in Sweden and Finland over the past 15 years. One of many organizations that established HR profit and loss accounts on a yearly basis was the Stockholm County Council Public Dental Care Service [16]. Using a detailed profit and loss account (this was possible because of a well-functioning time-reporting system), the costs for different personnel activities are calculated in monetary terms as well as in percentages of total personnel costs. This is accomplished for different departments, and used in the management control process. The figures are used for comparisons between units as well as between years.

Billion SEK (Swedish Kronor)	Year 1	Year 2
Replacing employees	3.0	2.3
Employee redundancies	1.0	3.3
Training	6.0	4.5
Absence	2.0	1.1
Rehabilitation		0.1
Physical work environment		1.0
Trade union relations	1.0	0.6
Employee benefits	1.0	1.0
Annual leave	9.0	8.5
Miscellaneous	2.0	1.2
Wages for production	75.0	77.4

7.4.2
Experiences

Since the early 1990s, many Swedish organizations have practised HR profit and loss accounts. The pedagogical idea underlying HR profit and loss accounts is the same as for HR balance sheets, i.e., if the cost of, say, absenteeism is made visible to the management, then the incentive for action would be obvious. An organization's profit and loss account is always debated at the board meetings and with partially new content, the problem with absenteeism should be noticed. Generally, if an old established routine (accounting), which directs most of the firm's daily activities, is given a new content, change might occur.

The experiences have shown, though, that the routines for accounting are difficult to change [17]. It has not been easy to enter new information and numerous problems have appeared. One of the problems concern definitions, e.g., what is rehabilitation? What should be included in the calculation of costs that are due to absenteeism? The lack of time reports has been another factor hindering the establishment of profit and loss accounts because the loss of working hours is often the biggest cost in HR calculations, regardless of whether the focus is absenteeism, development of competences or rehabilitation.

Most of the organizations that started using HR profit and loss accounts have abandoned them; apparently it is too difficult to integrate them into the existing management control system. In most cases, the HR profit and loss account has ended up as an appendix to the annual report.

7.4.3
Possible Development

The idea of HRA accounting is a good one. In most organizations, accounting language dominates or even controls discussions and actions taken. This means that the notion of bringing personnel-related issues into the accounting routines is compelling. Financial consequences of employee behavior and efforts are required, which has been the case for decades and is even more so today. Yet the experiences of HRA have shown that changing accounting routines is not a "quick fix" because it involves changing people's and organizations' habitual behavior [17]. We don't think that the concept of performing HR profit and loss accounts should be abandoned, but the question is: how to get on with it?

7.5
HR Costings

7.5.1
Idea

Closely linked to HRA is HR costings, which has the same aim as HRA, i.e., to focus attention on the financial aspects of human resources and to motivate HR investments. Sometimes the approach has been labeled utility analysis (e.g., [18, 19]) and sometimes human resource costing. Gröjer and Johanson [6] proposed the concept human resource costing and accounting (HRCA) in order to embrace both HRA and costing HR. HR costings have often been applied to absenteeism, rehabilitation, employee turnover, recruitment, competence, and other working environmental issues.

A common model for calculation of the costs of sick-leave is shown below [16]. The model takes into account direct and indirect costs, together with costs for loss of productivity and deteriorations of quality.

1. Direct costs	Sick-leave payment
	Holiday compensation
	Payroll tax
2. Indirect costs, visible in the accounting books	Overtime
	Substitutes
	Employee surplus
	Administrative costs
3. Indirect costs, invisible in the accounting books	Effects on production
	Effects on quality
	Effects on sales
	Effects on new recruitment

In situations in which absenteeism can be handled on a short-term basis by giving less priority to certain assignments, or by working overtime or even delaying the production, the cost of sick-leave and possible costs because of overtime might be the larger part. In other cases the cost of disturbances in production because of sickness might be considerable, which would reduce the sick-leave payment to a smaller amount. The two extremes might level out in the long run. In order to avoid the risk of losses in productivity and/or quality, new personnel may be recruited. Then the cost of absenteeism is equal to the sum of sick-leave payments and recruitment of substitutes. The latter may prove to be rather high. New recruitment, and above all teaching new employees, takes time. Smaller organizations are more likely to face higher costs than larger organizations. Smaller organizations cannot parry by moving about personnel or changing their priorities.

The pedagogical idea underlying HR costing differs from that of HRA in the sense that in HR calculations are not based on any fixed formula that has to be followed. Calculations can be performed separately from accounting. There is, in fact, no real limitation at all and this is the strength as well as the weakness of costings. The weakness is in terms of not having a formula to fall back on and to give it weight; the strength is that it is free and not hindered by any norms. Costings, or cost estimates, can be used anytime, anywhere and in any way.

7.5.2
Experiences

There are varied experiences with HR costings. Experiments on decision-making indicate that decisions are changed in accordance with the HR information and studies of individual learning propose that individual managers are positive to and learn a great deal from HR costings [17]. The managers in the studies hold that their way of thinking and their attitude towards HR-related issues have been influenced. Further, Macan and Highhouse [20] hold that even if the costings do not always provide the management with the information they want, sometimes it is the information they need. Those managers who demonstrated the highest interest in the organization's profitability also considered the costings to be of more use than other kinds of information.

However, HR costing also has problems. The assumed demand from people that costings should be performed in a certain standardized way has deterred many from carrying them out. A general assumption exists that there is a right or a wrong way of doing a cost estimate. There is also the problem that some financial consequences could not be achieved from the accounting books. Losses in productivity or sales are such examples. The question then is: should items that are accounted for as well as those that are not be included in the costing? A cost estimate on future efficiency comprising, e.g., productivity is meaningless if the principles for management control are solely based on costs that are accounted for in the books.

Another problem is that the trust for cost estimates is often lost when productivity effects are included because of the immense financial consequences that very often occur, despite the proposition that productivity is the most common and the most influential HR cost item. In a study based on 108 HR costings on health promotion [15] the connection between investments and effects on productivity was the one that the respondents were sure it was the most important item to consider in the costing. The impact on the costing from productivity was, in financial terms, twice as high as the impact from reduction of absenteeism.

An anecdote from a conversation with Stig (fictitious name) concerning HR costings reveals a lot. Stig first came in contact with HRCA 20 years ago as a rehabilitation and health promotion officer in a company with 1000 employees. During all these years, Stig has employed financial arguments in order to motivate rehabilitation and health promotion.

"Well you know, we don't use costings in a formal sense and we don't do systematic follow-ups. I try to get the people in charge to understand that it is crazy not to invest in rehabilitation and preventive actions. Imagine what the cost is of having an employee not performing 100% or worse – just having them loitering around. It's easier to spend $18 000 on a new gadget then to invest $3000 in rehabilitation or new equipment to increase performance. A coworker that is loafing with a salary of $2000 would cost around $50 000 per year, including all expenses. If a person has an injured hand and a certain tool costs $3000, then in order for it to be profitable he just has to work 4% of his normal performance. Since I convinced the management about this way of reasoning, we have profited a lot and many have avoided to be put on the sick list. But it takes time. You have to changes attitudes and that isn't easy. Some people think that it is a quick process but it took me 10 years."

The routines and the talk about financial aspects are mainly influenced by the accounting language, a language that is also very technical. This means that the mentality of an organization often hinders new ideas about economy, finance, and action. Stig demonstrates a movement forward by helping others to see a new reality they have never seen before. Stig learned from the financial language and has since then used it on his own terms in a powerful manner.

7.5.3
Possible Development

Despite all their pros and cons, costings will always be performed. HR costings have and will continue to be done on an *ad hoc* basis. However, if we believe that organizations are managed by routines then *ad hoc* costings are not enough to obtain change. To achieve change the routines have to be altered, which is a complex process. An alternative is to be satisfied with the way that Stig shows us. He employs HR thinking on a daily basis in order to prevent financial folly, and that is what is most important.

7.6
Recent Management Control Methods

7.6.1
Idea

Although HRA might provide valuable background information, it is of little or no use as a tool for prognostics. The same is true of historically based HR costings. The aim with HR costings as preestimates is, however, to show a possible movement forward before taking action. That is fine but there is a big drawback regarding the connections between effort and effect, i.e., investment and outcome. The latter could be improved if longitudinal data in vast quantities were collected. Examples of this can be found in various organizations. One example is the Swedbank, which has practised a management control system addressing such intangible resources as competence for the past 15 years [2]. More recently they have also addressed health as an intangible resource. Because it serves as a good illustration of contemporary efforts to develop management control systems that address intangible resources, we will devote considerable space to this example. Some may call this an example of intellectual capital, whereas others would probably refer to it as a balanced score card. However, as with Swedbank, we will not use either of these concepts.

The idea of the Swedbank's management control system is that good management and empowered workers influence the entire human capital value, which in turn generates high market capital and high profitability in the end. The Bank continuously measures human capital (HC), market capital (MC), productivity and profitability. HC measures the notion of empowerment, i.e., what employees want to do, what they can do, and what they actually do; HC does not measure how well employees get on in the organization. How well people enjoy their work is, according to the bank, no guarantee of success in business. Four core HR areas are addressed: meeting with customers, competence, organization, and leadership. MC is a concept comprising the way customers gauge a company's appreciation of them, how satisfied customers are with the company, and how loyal the customers feel toward the company.

The results of the comprehensive and systematic measurements are coordinated into a single large database. Of particular significance in the database are the interrelationships between HC, MC, and profitability. Among other things, the analysis has demonstrated that leadership affects all other parts; i.e., if leadership fails, so does everything else. A qualified leadership leads to increased HC, MC, and profitability. On the other hand, banks that are without solid leadership will find it difficult to show a profit margin. Offices that obtain lower scores on business-minded personnel have lower profitability. A large gap often exists between how customers perceive competence and how employees perceive their own competence.

The measurements result in three types of report: the senior executive report focusing on common strategic issues, the local bank report, and a report with the results for all 800 bank offices. When the report is ready to be passed on to the director of the bank, the lower and regional bank directors each receive a "box" that is referred to as "tools for the future." A three-person group comprising the bank director, a controller, and a regional market analyst evaluates the results. The local bank directors obtain figures for their region, as well as the results from the open questions in the measures taken of the customers and employees. The results are then discussed within the "developmental contract." The highest-ranking director, together with his or her subordinates, exchanges ideas and opinions about the results and compare them with earlier measurements, and steps for improvement are planned and discussed. Initially, only supportive steps are taken but if development is not moving in a positive direction, discussions about a voluntary job transfer can be initiated.

It is primarily the local leaders who own the material and thus it is these individuals who are supposed to be the driving force when it comes to determining any changes that need to be made. The three components, MC, HC, and profitability are used in contracts with the leaders: salaries are directly linked to the development of MC, HC, and earning capacity.

The management control process itself is also subject to continuous adjustment to improve the understanding of the specific value-creation chain of the bank. It is also subject to a follow-up routine: first, response rates on attitude surveys are followed and analyzed; second, statistical analysis is done on the consequences of using the measurement results; and third, statistical analysis regarding the effects of providing feedback on measurement results is provided.

The second item is strongly correlated to improvements on the HC index, MC index and financial performance at the local bank level. The third item reveals that work satisfaction and performance are significantly higher in organizational units where employees have had feedback on earlier measurements. The follow-up routine is a significant support routine to the measurement routine in order to ensure learning, action, and change.

Economic evolutionary theory proposes that firms are characterized by relatively constant patterns of behaviors or rules. These rules are subject to an evolutionary process in the sense that they are evaluated, reproduced, eliminated, varied, and selected. The Swedbank can serve as an example in which old management control routines have been changed to include even HR or IC (Intellectual Capital) routines. In the present case and a number of other cases, Johanson et al. [2] identify the following routines that ensure the survival of the HR management control system and process:

1. recognition and measurement routines
   - human capital surveys
   - market capital surveys
   - accounting
2. reporting routines
   - continuous internal reports
   - informal information to financial analysts
3. evaluation routines
   - evaluation of single indicators by each manager
   - statistical analysis
4. attention routines
   - meetings
5. motivation routines
   - benchmarking
   - dialogues
   - salary bonus
6. commitment routines
   - ownership, contract
7. follow up routines
   - analyses of response rates
   - consequences of using results
   - effects of providing feedback.

The subroutines listed above could be related to the action model of Weick and Swieringa [21] in that meetings and dialogues direct the attention of managers and employees to the results from the measurements. These results, in combination with statistical analysis, affect knowledge. Motivation is further addressed by a clear top-management demand, benchmarking, and salary bonuses. Finally, commitment to change is made possible by means of a contract between managers at different levels. The empirical data reveal that organizational learning processes have been affected in such a way that dominating cognitive schemes and coordinated action have been obtained.

7.6.2
Experiences

Experiences drawn from the Swedbank and other Swedish firms (e.g., NCC, Xerox, and Telia) that have used regular HC and MC surveys were the object for a study conducted over several years [2]. Conclusions based on this study indicate that the new model of management control has brought about considerable changes in the organizations. The dominating concepts have been influenced and there have been collective and coordinated actions because of the new management control model.

The Swedbank has used its model for nearly 15 years, and has recently laid the foundations for the bank's health management system. A representative for the managerial body claims that they know more about what is important for customers and coworkers (e.g., what managerial qualities lead to sales). "The tool gives plain information about an individuals driving force. At the foremost the tool's usefulness is in local altering processes." This representative also notes that if you only measure HC, ignoring MC and financial aspects, you easily end up in a cosy corner. "If no connections are made to financial results, the measurements become rather trite. It is at the local operational level that the tool is of highest importance."

7.6.3
Possible Development

A development of databases such as the Swedbank's is important. A well-developed longitudinal database might provide opportunities to study correlations between notions of health and profitability as well as the profitability of different health promotion activities. But it is not sufficient just to create databases; the data must also be used. The Swedbank demonstrates that such a database can prove useful not only on an *ad hoc*, but on a regular basis. In Section 7.7, we further examine this area on how to integrate measurements in management control. Later, we will return to the Swedbank for a case study of their work on health and management control.

7.7
Health Statements

7.7.1
Idea

In Sweden a proposal has been made by the government to develop the health statement (HS) in order to focus attention on and motivate action in decreasing the costly (both at the firm level and at the societal level) sick-leaves among the work force. By directing attention to healthy or unhealthy situations in an organization, preferably with a connection to profitability, it should be possible to get health issues onto the management's agenda and thus decrease sick-leave. One of many activities that have been performed is a 3-year research and development project addressing HS and involving seven Swedish municipalities. The general idea of the project is to let these organizations, all of which claim to have serious problems with absenteeism, develop their own HS model. The focus is not only on substance but also on usefulness. What will the municipalities do with the HS concept? How will they manage it so that it can come to use in improving the health situation amongst their coworkers? We will give an account of our experiences from this project.

7.7.2
Experiences

The experiences are very different among the seven local authorities and even between different departments. Many state that the HS project has meant that issues on health, well-being or HR policies have had more attention and successful processes of change have started. There is a general opinion that HS is important – in some cases crucial – for the municipality's future. The upcoming need for recruitment of new personnel is one of the main challenges to which the HS project can contribute. If the need for more manpower can't be solved through decreased sick-leave and increased status as an attractive employer, the organizations will face some serious problems in a couple of years time.

However, in many ways the project has also been characterized by ambivalence. Many believe in the strengths of sequential planning and that they can realize the change project in that way. The flip-side of this common sense methodology is that reality doesn't always arrange itself in an orderly fashion. Actually, it's an understatement to say "not always." How many projects follow this roadmap? But to abandon the idea of sequential planning of a project is unthinkable in projects as extensive as these. The duty of planning is mainly to create a feeling of control and thus manageability. Without this feeling, anxiety will spread through the organization like wildfire. Therefore, it is not difficult or strange to state that there is a strong feeling of ambivalence in the alteration processes. The ambivalence doesn't exist only within the local authority's own process to develop a HS or achieve health improvements but also applies to the contents of the report, attitudes towards measurability, and especially the basic use of concepts.

There is no generally accepted definition of the HS concept. It is the local authorities' task to give the concept substance and evaluate its usefulness. The term "health statement" has provoked numerous reactions. The term as such is short, smart, promising, and innovative. At the beginning of the project it was easy to attract the attention of different municipalities using this concept; latterly, though, it has started to feel a bit more problematic, possibly because it's difficult to interpret, and leaves room for many different associations. Some of the organizations have chosen not to use the HS concept and instead selected more easily communicable concepts such as "the good workplace" or "attractive workplace." For others, HS has become a part of the general work for managing health. In short, the HS concept has different functions in the different local authorities. Sometimes it is used as a representation of a certain method or technique of reporting while other times it is used as a way to signify the ambition of creating better places of work or as a means of announcing the ambition to integrate the different initiatives that are being made as a whole in the personnel domain.

Furthermore, the concept of HS could be understood as implying a final report of something that has been, rather than an ambition of improving something. The most positive aspect of the concept is that it signals gravity. The concept as such is interpreted as being able to put health issues on the agenda and give health as a resource a place in the regular management control system. However, even with this argument, there are many that are doubtful whether the HS will secure an understanding of health improvements being an investment for the future.

What should a HS contain? What should a HS report contain? One of the organizations has concluded that HS should:

- complement traditional accounting
- be based on HR statistics and HR costing
- contain measurable facts as well as experienced states
- visualize the attitudes and values in an organization
- show the coworkers' health in a broad perspective
- visualize the strengths and weaknesses of the work environment and organization.

Another organization is of the opinion that HS is an elaboration of HRCA. The organization stresses the following:

"The basis for HS is the HRCA that provides an understanding to the HR structure. An example of key ratios is number of employees, distribution according to gender, age distribution, level of education, and so on. In the HS we develop the accounting with ratios concerning the employee's work effort from a health and economic perspective ... the statistics is then completed with some sort of measurement on perceived working situation."

By visualizing the connection between heath issues and financial control, a foundation for action is made. The HS should therefore be a plan for action. Even though the project isn't finished as of the writing of this chapter, the model produced by the participants will probably have following structure:

1. vision
2. strategies
3. health components (e.g., elements of success)
4. goals for each health component
5. activities for each health component
6. follow-up and measuring methods for each health component
7. indicators (could be ratios and statements/testimonies but it could also be illustrative HR calculations) for each health component.

The proposition of the model will be accompanied by reflections on the means of implementation.

The magic of numbers has clearly made the work difficult. Indicators and key ratios based on executed surveys are seen as a necessity: "The numbers and the key ratios have become a holy grail." The term "key ratio" is one of the most frequently used expressions in the project. There have been debates and questions about which key ratios to produce, what they are, and what they represent. Why is this causing such alarm? It should not be such a problem to define key ratios if a sequential manner is executed where each of the seven steps shown above is formulated and defined. One problem is that the sequential manner of work, as proposed by all the participants, hasn't been implemented. Therefore, it is hardly surprising that problems have arisen in selecting which key ratios to develop and how they should be defined.

Some of the organizations became stuck on the question about what can be measured. These organizations sought scientific truth on how to measure health. The project groups have debated the question of what health is and the components that can describe and measure it. They haven't reached a decisive answer though. Because of a lack of answers, one local authority has abandoned this path and chosen to measure activities with the aim of improving health, i.e., the assumption is made that health-promoting activities result in good health. The vague answers from the scientific community on the practical questions regarding what needs to be managed to achieve better health should lead to a perceived freedom of experimentation. In some cases the effect has been the opposite. The absence of scientific solutions on how health and its prerequisites should be measured and managed has created frustration and a complete inability to act instead of the joy of exploring new territories. One might speculate whether it is that the norm concerning measurements and exactness being associated with science is so strong that it hinders the development of a HS based on practical experiences. None of the project groups will relinquish the chance of making measurements, but the real question is whether it is important to perform surveys if you don't know what to measure or even dare to experiment?

7.7.3
Possible Development

To develop models as a basis for the HS is of little or no use if the report itself will not lead to any improvements. As our seven municipalities have done, it is highly important that an effort is made to integrate the HS into the daily management and the regular planning, managing, and follow-up. This is to say that a future HS model has to address the HS report as well as what kind of change with respect to organizational routines needs to be altered. This is a complex and an ambitious task, which, to a great extent resembles the approach taken by the Swedbank.

7.8
Health and Management Control in the Swedbank: A Case Study

Today, the Swedbank has around 10 000 employees, 450 bank offices, and about 4.5 million customers. The Swedbank has a long tradition of performing customer and personnel surveys, which have been described and analyzed above. From the beginning, the purpose of the surveys was to increase customer satisfaction and thereby increase the company's profitability; today however, they are also used for analyzing health and absenteeism.

Traditionally, absenteeism in the company has been 2–3%, but during the early years of the 21st century the situation had altered. At the beginning of 2003, absence because of sickness had increased to 4.9% and was costing the company about US$50 million. In the cost estimation that was made the following directly measurable costs and calculated costs were considered:

- direct costs for sick-leave
- costs for recruitment and other expenditures for substitutes
- costs for reduction of productivity and teaching
- costs that remain even though a person is on sick-leave.

Although it is difficult to draw any firm conclusions as to why sick-leave increased, contributing factors might be general changes that took place in society, that the company had halved its working staff in less then 10 years, and that it had made significant alterations in the composition of assignments. As a result of the increasing absences among employees, management initiated a project with the initial aim of decreasing sick-leave below the 4% level.

The Swedbank has defined two quantitative measurements originating from personnel statistics. These are percentage of long-term health and sick-leave. The definition of a long-term healthy person is an employee with 5 days or fewer of sick-leave per year. The goal is that 80% of the work force should be long-term healthy. For sick-leave, the goal is, as mentioned above, less then 4%.

Further to these two measurements, are two measures from a personnel survey: well-being and risk. The term well-being is based on the statement, "Generally I feel fine," a summarizing term in Swedbank's survey. The definition of risk relates to personnel in a working situation that will endanger their health if no counter-

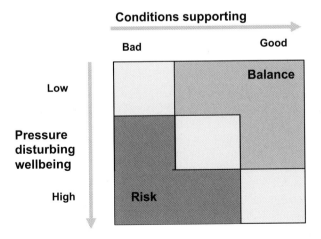

Fig. 7.1. Matrix of how the Swedbank defines employees of being in risk.

measures are carried out. No more then 20% of the coworkers in a unit are allowed to be in a risk zone. Those individuals inside the risk zone have either poor conditions for managing their job or have a workload that is too heavy.

Pressure refers to the individual's experience of pressure, and conditions to the individual's experience of work conditions.

Since the beginning of 2003, the Swedbank has conducted regular personnel surveys through web-based questionnaires in an effort to deal with the sick-leave problem. A large part of the questionnaire is based on their human capital surveys. In the questionnaire there are a certain number of statements in the six areas as presented below, the answers to which make up the foundation for GAP (Analysis of difference between goal and present situation) and correlation analysis:

- workload
- demands
- recuperation
- worries
- work satisfaction
- well-being

and finally

- "Generally I feel fine."

The finishing statement is used as a summarizing index for well-being. Statistical analyses have shown that this question has a strong correlation with the above-mentioned areas. But obviously a coworker might answer positively on this question and still end up in the risk zone (e.g., because of a high workload).

The finished surveys are compiled centrally at the bank and are then addressed to the different levels of the bank. The manager at the lowest hierarchical level receives the results for his or her office. At all levels above the local manager, aggregated reports are compiled presenting the results of the city, region, and so on. The results are then debated and reacted upon in formal meetings held at each hierarchical level. Depending on the results of the surveys, a plan of action is developed. For example, if more then 20% of the employees at an office are found in the risk zone, a plan of action must be developed in order to handle the situation.

The Swedbank's surveys have gained strong acceptance among coworkers, with a response rate of about 90%. Much of this is thanks to the bank's regular surveys on HC and customer capital. Statistical measures made through correlation analysis indicate that there is no conflict between managing a profitable enterprise and a company where the coworkers have a high sense of well-being. On the contrary, there is palpable proof that vital elements (e.g., good structural support, effective routines, and strong leadership) in having a successful business favor customer satisfaction and profitability as well as the well-being of the employees. Other proven correlations are that those units that are not particularly successful also suffer higher sick-leave rates.

There has been a decrease in absenteeism since the start of the Swedbank surveys but there is no evidence indicating it is due to regular measurement. However, a representative of the Swedbank believes that measurement has led to a general improvement in preventive actions and rehabilitation planning, which hopefully will have a long-term effect.

7.9
Conclusion and Dilemmas

Present day accounting and management control models are deeply rooted in traditional accounting. This implies a focus on worth and costs derived from tangible resources whereas health, leadership, and competence aren't visible anywhere in the accounting documents. Even if a manager had, for example, knowledge of the profitability of health promotion, it wouldn't mean that the management of the organization was run with due respect for this fact. Management control and accounting models have a huge advantage compared to other factors in controlling the agenda and therefore the models and control systems may need to be changed. These changes, however, aren't quick fixes, assuming one doesn't settle for rough estimates as rehabilitation consultant Stig (Section 7.5) does. An altered use of management control systems will take time because it deals with the behavior of human beings and organizations that are mainly characterized by habits and routine actions.

The lost relevance of accounting [22] has promoted the idea of introducing a number of new accounting and management control models e.g., HRCA, balanced scorecard, intellectual capital, intangible assets monitoring, and most recently the HS. But the application of these models has faced a number of serious problems. These problems and future applicability vary between the models. The models can be classified into monetary (e.g., but not exclusively HRCA) and nonmonetary (e.g., but not exclusively IC (Intellectual Capital) and HS) models. All the models suggest that the employee and its intangible resources play a significant or even the most significant role in a firm's value creation. HRCA focuses solely on the person whereas IC and HS also emphasize other intangible resources. The general idea behind HRCA is that if the accounting *content* is changed i.e., by including HR issues, change will occur whereas IC propose a completely new and basically nonfinancial framework. HRCA has a strong focus on measurement and representation whereas mobilization is the key word connected to IC and HS. In the IC literature it is proposed that some intangible resources like organizational culture and above all the beneficial connectivity between different intangibles can never be subject to measurement in a justifiable way. The way of reporting on and demonstrating the importance of IC is preferably performed by means of using narratives [23].

The models discussed in this chapter have been successful in terms of attracting attention and expectation, but disappointments when applying the models have been numerous. What is the possible future for each model? Will it be possible to integrate health as an intangible resource in the formal management control by using the model?

We start by disposing of the balance sheet approach. A change in the current standards for what is allowed to be viewed upon as an asset in the balance sheet is not expected to come in the foreseeable future. Nothing stops organizations performing additional balance sheets in which health investments are considered; however, this additional balance sheet would probably be under the scrutiny of external accounting standards during the internal process, which would hinder the development of this kind of balance sheets.

The notion of bringing personnel-related issues into accounting routines by exposing the HR costs in the profit and loss account is compelling and comparably easy to achieve, but one disadvantage is the total focus on costs.

HR costings on health issues will always be done on paper (or in the head when needed), but a regular usage of HR costings is probably not something for the future. The usage of HR costings will continue to be used *ad hoc* for argumentation, learning or decision-making but scarcely for systematic management control. With costings the question, or rather the doubt, of the relationship between effort and effect is decisive for its credibility. That question will never be answered because the reality is far too complex for us to ever be able to isolate all causal connections when it comes to health-related issues in the workplace.

However, we are convinced that the creation of databases such as that of Swedbank might help to scatter the fogs of ignorance. Perhaps, or rather probably, there might be a connection between different subjective experiences of the reality benefiting costings, learning, decision-making, and even systematic management control.

In order to establish a connection between health issues and profitability there must be a profound integration of the treatment of health issues in management control. In the analysis of their experiences with HR, the Swedbank, other firms, and the HS projects in the seven municipalities might indicate a possible road forward. They might reveal where the mines are. We've already declared Swedbank a successful example and some of the municipalities will surely receive the same praise. We think that there is a possibility in following successful examples. However, changing management control systems and routines are complex processes that demand a long-lasting commitment.

One challenge is to find the appropriate balance between perfection with respect to representation and influence on action. From the HS project and from several other HR-related projects, it can be determined that too high demands of perfection might have a negative effect. If the demand for perfection concerns depicting a reality that isn't willing to be depicted, it becomes understandable that a project with the aim of developing new management control systems will not succeed. Within Swedbank, there are no restraining expectations on science ever delivering a perfect management control system. They *design* their own system and they use it, polish it, and continue to use it.

A question not yet discussed in this paper is of an ethical nature. What happens when we place numbers and monetary labels on health or when we use terms such as human capital [23, 24]? Does the usage of terms and the price-fixing of health create a risk of price-fixing human beings? Is there a future for models such as HR or the HS if the human being is depicted as an asset and therefore exchangeable for other types of asset? We may return to this issue in the future.

References

1 DWYER, T. (1991) *Life and Death at Work: Industrial Accidents as a Case of Socially Produced Error.* Plenum, New York.

2 JOHANSON, U., MÅRTENSSON, M., SKOOG, M. (2001) Measuring to understand intangible performance drivers. *Eur Accounting Rev* 10(3):1–31.

3 BRUMMET, R.L., FLAMHOLTZ, E.G., PYLE, W.C. (1968) Human resource measurement: a challenge for accountants. *Accounting Rev* 43:217–224.

4 FLAMHOLTZ, E (1987) Human Resource Accounting: Advances in Concepts, Methods and Applications, Jossey-Bass, San Francisco.

5 SACKMANN, S., FLAMHOLZ, E., BULLEN, M. (1989) Human resource accounting: a state of the art review. *J Accounting Lit* 8:235–264.

6 GRÖJER, J.E., JOHANSON, U. (1996) Human Resource Costing and Accounting. Personalekonomisk redovisning och kalkylering, Arbetarskyddsnämnden.

7 PELLETIER, K. (1993) A review and analysis of the health and cost-effective outcome studies of comprehensive health promotion and disease prevention programmes at the worksite. *Am J Health Promotion* 8(1):50–62.

8 OZMINKOWSKI, R., LING, D., GOETZEL, R., BRUNO, J., RUTTER, K., ISAAC, F., WANG, S. (2002) Long-term impact of Johnson & Johnson's Health & Wellness program on health care utilization and expenditures. *J Occup Environ Med* 44(1):21–29.

9 PELLETIER, K. (1999) A review and analysis of the clinical and cost-effectiveness studies of comprehensive health promotion and disease

management programs at worksites: 1995–1998 update. *Am J Health Promotion* 13:333–345.

10 GOETZEL, R., JUDAY, T., OZMINKOWSKI, R. (1999) What's the ROI? A systematic review of return-on-investment studies of corporate health and productivity management initiatives. *AWHP's Worksite Health* 6:12–21.

11 ALDANA, S. (2001) Financial impact of health promotion programs: a comprehensive review of the literature. *Am J Health Promotion* 15(5):296–320.

12 ANDERSON, D., SERXNER, S., GOLD, D. (2001) Conceptual framework, critical questions, and practical challenges in conducting research on the financial impact of worksite health promotion. *Am J Health Promotion* 15(5):281–288.

13 GOLASZEWSKI, T. (2001) Shining lights: studies that have most influenced the understanding of health promotion's financial impact. *Am J Health Promotion* 15(5):332–340.

14 RIEDEL, J.E., LYNCH, W., BAASE, C., HYMEL, P., PETERSON, K.W. (2001) The effect of disease prevention and health promotion on workplace productivity: a literature review. *Am J Health Promotion* 15(3):167–191.

15 JOHANSON, U. (1997) The profitability of investments in work life oriented rehabilitation: a measurement of perceptions. *Personnel Rev* 26(5):395–415.

16 JOHANSON, U. (2000) Human resource costing and accounting. In: BREWSTER, C., LARSEN, H.H. (eds.) *Human Resource Management in Northern Europe.* Blackwell, Oxford, Chapter 8:170–194.

17 JOHANSON, U. (1999) Why the concept of human resource costing and

accounting does not work. *Personnel Rev* 28(1/2):91–107.

18 BOUDREAU, J.W. (1996) The motivational impact of utility analysis and HR measurement. *J Hum Resource Costing Accounting* 1(2):73–84.

19 CASCIO, W.F. (1991) *Costing Human Resources: the Financial Impact of Behaviour in Organisations, 3rd Edn.* PWS-Kent, Boston.

20 MACAN, T.H., HIGHHOUSE, S. (1994) Communicating the utility of human resource activities: a survey of I/O and HR professionals. *J Business Psychol* 8(4):425–436.

21 WEICK, R., SWIERINGA, K. (1987) Management Accounting and Action, Accounting, Organization and Society 12(3):293–309.

22 JOHNSON, H.T., KAPLAN, R.S. (1987) *Relevance Lost the Rise and Fall of Management Accounting.* HBS, Massachusetts.

23 MOURITSEN, J., JOHANSON, U. (2005) Managing the person: human resource costing and accounting, intellectual capital and health statements. In: JÖNSSON, S., MOURITSEN, J. (eds.) *Northern Lights in Accounting.* NELSON, R., WINTER, S. (1982) An evolutionary theory of economic change, Harvard University Press, Cambridge.

24 JOHANSON, U. (2004) Human resource perspective on intellectual capital. In: MARR, B. (ed.) *Perspectives on Intellectual Capital: Multidisciplinary Insights Into Management, Measurement, And Reporting.* Butterworth Heinemann, Boston.

Stress and Brain Plasticity

8

The Neonatal and Pubertal Ontogeny of the Stress Response: Implications for Adult Physiology and Behavior

Russell D. Romeo and Bruce S. McEwen

8.1
Introduction

In response to challenges and stressors, animals release a series of neurochemical and hormonal signals into the brain and blood, allowing them to cope with the immediate internal and external demands imposed by the stressful event, while attempting to restore homeostasis. This active process is termed "allostasis" [1]. However, longer or more chronic exposures to stress and stress hormones can lead to "allostatic overload", resulting in a number of negative effects, particularly in regards to neurobiological function. As diagrammed in Fig. 8.1, the brain is the interpreter of what is threatening and therefore stressful and it determines the behavioral and physiological responses that enable the individual to cope with a challenge. Behavioral and physiological responses that are repeated or persistent, even in the absence of further external stressors, can lead to allostatic overload. Events in daily working and family life, major life events and trauma and abuse can all contribute to allostatic overload.

The magnitude and duration of the stress response changes dramatically throughout an animal's or person's lifespan. For instance, stress responses are difficult to elicit in neonatal animals, while aged animals show heightened and more prolonged stress responses compared to younger adults. Thus, parameters that change stress reactivity, such as development, may have profound consequences as to whether a stressor leads to an adaptive or maladaptive response.

In this chapter, we will focus on the neonatal and pubertal maturation of the hypothalamic–pituitary–adrenal (HPA) axis, the neuroendocrine axis that mediates the stress response, and how this maturation affects the development of stress reactivity. Particular attention will be given to how early life events can shape the neonatal maturation of the HPA axis and what lasting influences these earlier actions may have on the physiological and behavioral potentials of an organism upon reaching adulthood. We will also highlight some recent studies that have indicated that puberty serves as another significant period of HPA maturation and how this additional critical period of development could be a crucial time for interventions to reduce the negative effects induced by earlier challenges and perturbations. Fi-

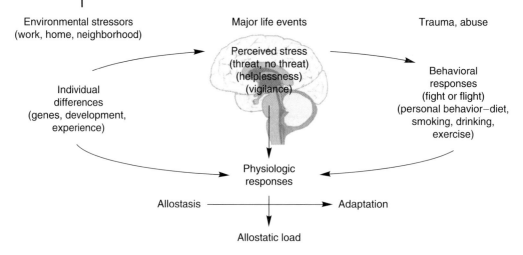

Fig. 8.1. Central role of the brain in appraising events as threatening and responding behaviorally and physiologically to them. Reprinted from McEwen (1998) by permission.

nally, we shall discuss possible implications for human health and development over a lifespan, as well as future directions for research concerning the neonatal and pubertal ontogeny of the stress response and HPA axis. However, we first shall consider the meaning of the word "stress" and some new terminology that helps to clarify ambiguities.

8.2
Stress, Homeostasis, Allostasis, and Allostatic Load

Stress is an overused word that means many things to different people. In biomedicine, stress refers to experiences that are novel and ego-involving and in which there is a perception of lack of control and the possibility of negative consequences. Mason is credited with having emphasized the importance of psychological factors in the stress response; however, it is Hans Selye (1907–1983) who is credited with introducing the concept of stress, albeit in the context of largely physical stressors, in his "General Adaptation Syndrome" paradigm [2].

A central construct in Selye's integrative model of stress was the notion of *homeostasis*, which refers to the stability of physiological systems that maintain life (e.g., body temperature, glucose levels), and are therefore maintained within a narrow range of a set-point. These set-points and other boundaries of control may change with environmental conditions, however, and these changes are not explained by the notion of homeostasis. We therefore introduced the concept of *allostasis* to refer to the superordinate system by which stability was achieved through change [1]. There are primary mediators of allostasis such as the hormones of the hypothalamo–pituitary–adrenal (HPA) axis (see Section 8.3). Allostasis also clarifies an inherent ambiguity in the term homeostasis and distinguishes between the systems that are essential for life (homeostasis) and those that maintain these systems in balance (allostasis).

When set-points or other boundaries of control vary beyond homeostatic mechanisms, these variables are referred to as *allostatic states*. An allostatic state results in an imbalance of the primary mediators reflecting excessive production of some and inadequate production of others. Allostatic states can produce wear and tear on the regulatory systems in the brain and body. Within limits, they are adaptive responses to challenges and demands. However, if one superimposes on this additional loads of unpredictable events in the environment, disease, human disturbance, and social interactions, then allostatic load can increase dramatically and becomes allostatic overload, serving no useful purpose and predisposing the individual to disease (Fig. 8.2).

Allostasis is a process occurring in every cell and tissue of the body when exposed to a change in the internal and/or external environment. One of the most important features of these processes is that they operate nonlinearly, that is, that there are reciprocal influences of many of these processes upon each other. The brain is the master controller of these processes, and is also a target, subject to both protection and damage. In the nervous system, neurochemical messengers

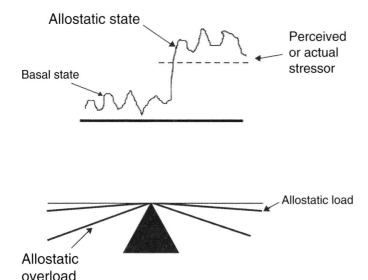

Fig. 8.2. A cartoon depicting allostatic state, allostatic load and allostatic overload. *Top* Perceived or actual stressors cause elevated activity of systems (e.g., cortisol, sympathetic and parasympathetic activity, cytokines) that promote adaptation. Sustained activity of such systems is referred to as an allostatic state (see text). *Bottom* Allostatic states lead over time to allostatic load but can also lead to allostatic overload.

are released by neuronal activity, and they produce effects locally to either propagate or inhibit further neural activity. Neurotransmitters and hormones are usually released during a discrete period of activation and then are shut off. However, if too much is released, not shut off efficiently, or not removed from the intracellular space by reuptake or metabolism, then allostatic overload may ensue, increasing the risk of damage to the nervous system and many other systems [3]. For example, in the brain, the secretion of stress hormones in response to an acutely threatening event promotes and improves memory for the situation so that the individual can stay out of trouble in the future, yet when the stress is repeated over many weeks, some neurons atrophy and memory is impaired, while other neurons grow and fear is enhanced. Similarly, in other systems such as the immune system, acute stress promotes immune function by enhancing movement of immune cells to places in the body where they are needed to defend against a pathogen, yet chronic stress suppresses immune function and uses the same hormonal mediators to suppress immune function. In the next sections, we shall briefly discuss one of the key systems in allostasis and allostatic load, namely, the hypothalamo–pituitary–adrenal (HPA) axis, and its development.

8.3
The Hypothalamic–Pituitary–Adrenal Axis

The release of stress hormones by the HPA axis is driven by the release of corticotropin-releasing hormone (CRH) from the medial parvocellular division of the paraventricular hypothalamic nucleus. CRH is released into the portal system of the pituitary, which in turn causes the release of adrenocorticotropic hormone (ACTH) from the anterior pituitary. ACTH then stimulates the secretion of the glucocorticoids (e.g., cortisol, corticosterone) from the adrenal cortex. The major stress steroid in primates is cortisol, while corticosterone is the major circulating stress steroid in most rodents. The stress hormones secreted by the HPA axis indirectly control their own secretion through a classic neuroendocrine negative feedback loop. That is, the glucocorticoids feedback on the paraventricular nucleus (PVN) and many other extrahypothalamic sites, in particular, the hippocampus, amygdala and prefrontal cortex, to inhibit the further release of CRH [4] (Fig. 8.3).

Two receptors mediate the actions of the glucocorticoids in the central nervous system, the mineralocorticoid receptor (MR) and the glucocorticoid receptor (GR). These steroid receptors are found in relatively high concentrations throughout the neural network that controls negative feedback and activation of the HPA axis. The high-affinity MR is typically saturated at basal glucocorticoid levels, while the low-affinity GR is primarily occupied only when relatively high concentrations of glucocorticoids are induced by challenges, such as stress. Thus, when glucocorticoid levels rise in response to stressors, the negative feedback on the HPA axis to reduce further increases in stress hormones is mediated by the low-affinity GR.

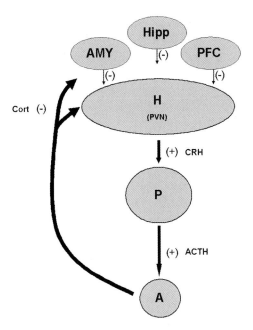

Fig. 8.3. A diagram of the hypothalamic–pituitary–adrenal (HPA) axis and various extrahypothalamic sites that play a role in glucocorticoid negative feedback. A Adrenal, ACTH adrenocorticotropic hormone, AMY amygdala, Cort corticosterone, CRH corticotropin-releasing hormone, Hipp hippocampus, H hypothalamus, P pituitary, PFC prefrontal cortex, PVN paraventricular nucleus, (+) positive drive, (−) negative feedback.

8.4
Neonatal Development of the HPA Axis

As early as during fetal development, the pituitary and adrenal glands are capable of secreting stress hormones under basal conditions and in response to stressors. However, corticosterone levels decrease shortly after birth and stay low during the first 2 weeks of life. In rats, basal corticosterone levels begin to increase at approximately postnatal day (PND) 15 in males and females, peaking around PND 24. In addition to these low basal levels of corticosterone from PND 1–14, stress responsiveness is also greatly reduced, such that stressors typically able to induce robust stress responses in adults fail to do so at this neonatal stage. This period of reduced HPA reactivity during neonatal development has been termed the stress hyporesponsive period (SHRP) [5].

At the level of the HPA axis, three mechanisms appear to mediate the reduced HPA activity during the neonatal SHRP. First, CRH and ACTH levels in the neonatal hypothalamus and anterior pituitary, respectively, are lower compared to those found in adult animals. Second, CRH-induced ACTH release from the neonatal pituitary is reduced compared to adults, in part due to enhanced corticosterone negative feedback on the pituitary in neonates. Finally, the neonatal adrenal cortex shows reduced glucocorticoid output compared to adults.

In addition to these changes at the level of the HPA axis during neonatal maturation, extrahypothalamic areas involved in negative feedback also change during this development stage. For instance, hippocampal GR levels increase during the first 2 weeks of life and stabilize at adult-like levels prior to puberty. The hippocampus has one of the highest concentration of GRs in the brain and plays a major role in glucocorticoid-induced negative feedback. Interestingly, in adulthood, GR levels are regulated by the glucocorticoids such that higher levels of glucocorticoids downregulate hippocampal GR expression. However, this autoregulation does not occur during neonatal development [6], presumably allowing GR levels to increase during later neonatal development independently of concomitantly increasing glucocorticoid levels during this time. Thus, changes in GR levels during development at key regulatory sites in the pituitary and brain contribute to the neonatal maturation of the HPA axis and the emergence of stress responsiveness in the pubertal and adult animal.

The neurophysiological implications and adaptive significance of the SHRP in animals during the neonatal period are presently unclear. Perhaps the reduced stress reactivity experienced by the neonate protects their developing nervous system from the negative influences of stress hormones. Indeed, neonatal animals administered high levels of corticosterone show reduced brain size with many fewer neurons. However, neonates exposed to corticosterone via the dam's milk show superior performance on the Morris water maze task, a test of spatial memory, yet also show heightened stress responsiveness at PND 30. Clearly, further research needs to be done to more fully understand and appreciate the significance of this hyporesponsive period in the neonate.

8.5
Early Life Events and the Shaping of the HPA Axis

Many internal and external factors experienced during neonatal development influence the maturation and future function of the HPA axis. During early neonatal life, the HPA axis is sensitive to the perinatal gonadal hormonal milieu. Indeed, the perinatal action of gonadal hormones on this developing neuroendocrine axis is, in part, responsible for the sex differences in stress responsiveness observed in adulthood. Furthermore, the HPA axis can be shaped by a variety of environmental and experimental manipulations during the neonatal stage that have long-lasting influences on basal and stress-induced activation of the HPA axis.

The perinatal hormonal environment has been shown to influence the neonatal maturation of the HPA axis such that males and females respond differently to stressors in adulthood. In fact, sex differences in HPA function begin to emerge in the first few weeks of life. For instance, although basal corticosterone levels begin to rise in both males and females around PND 15, this increase is greater in females. This sexually dimorphic pattern is maintained in adulthood, such that females typically have higher basal ACTH and corticosterone levels than males. Moreover, upon encountering a stressor in adulthood, females typically mount a greater hormonal stress response than do males.

The ovarian hormone estrogen appears to mediate this greater stress responsiveness, as adult females in the proestrous stage of their reproductive cycle (i.e., when estrogen levels are relatively high) show higher ACTH and corticosterone stress responses than females in the diestrous phase of their cycle (i.e., when estrogen levels are relatively low). Moreover, ovariectomized females treated with estrogen show greater stress reactivity than untreated, ovariectomized females [7]. In contrast to the stimulatory role of estrogen on the female HPA axis, testosterone appears to reduce stress responsiveness in males. For instance, castrated male rats demonstrate greater stress responsiveness than testosterone-treated castrates or intact males [7].

The studies reviewed above indicate that estrogen and testosterone have activational effects on the female and male HPA axes, respectively. However, the ability of the gonadal hormones to modulate stress responsiveness in adulthood appears to be "organized" during neonatal development. That is, the hormonal milieu experienced by the developing neonate shapes the HPA axis so the hormonal stimulation received in adulthood can modulate HPA activity and responsiveness in a sex-specific manner. Specifically, females that receive masculinizing doses of hormones during neonatal maturation show less stress-induced HPA activity in adulthood, similar to that displayed by males, suggesting a reversal of estrogen's stimulatory effects on the adult female stress response. Likewise, males that do not experience the normal increase in testosterone titers during neonatal development no longer experience the testosterone-reducing effects on HPA stress reactivity. Thus, the early hormonal stimulation experienced by neonates leads to profound and long-lasting changes in HPA function and is responsible for the sexually differentiated stress responses observed in adult males and females.

In addition to the internal hormonal environment, the external environment can also have profound influences on the maturation of the HPA axis. One area of research that has received considerable attention is the influence of maternal care on neonatal HPA development [8]. Naturally occurring variations in maternal care have been observed in rat dams, particularly in the amount of time dams spend licking and grooming their offspring. Interestingly, offspring that receive relatively high levels of licking and grooming during infancy show reduced HPA reactivity in adulthood compared to young that received relatively low levels of licking and grooming [9]. The reduced stress reactivity in animals derived from high licking and grooming mothers appears to be mediated by greater glucocorticoid-mediated negative feedback. Specifically, pups that receive high levels of licking grooming during infancy have increased hippocampal GR levels and reduced CRH levels in the PVN in adulthood [9].

Are offspring derived from high licking and grooming mothers less likely to suffer allostatic overload in adulthood? Interestingly, pups that received high levels of licking and grooming during infancy show reduced anxiety levels upon reaching adulthood, superior performance on a learning and memory task, and increased hippocampal neuronal survival during development. Whether these changes in emotionality, cognitive ability and hippocampal neuronal survival are caused by reduced HPA reactivity remains unclear. However, these studies suggest that offspring that receive greater levels of maternal care during neonatal development may be better able to cope with allostatic load in adulthood.

Experimental manipulations that directly alter dam–pup interactions have also been used to influence the neonatal development of the HPA axis. Two commonly used methods are neonatal handling and maternal separation. Neonatal handling involves daily separation of the pups from the mother for a brief period of time (3–15 min) during the first 2 weeks of life. Maternal separation is more extreme in that pups are separated daily from their mothers for much longer periods of time (3–4.5 h) during the first 2 weeks of life. Neonatal handling and maternal separation result in opposite effects on the developing HPA axis. Specifically, in mice and rats neonatal handling leads to reduced HPA responsiveness in adulthood [10], while maternal separation usually results in heightened HPA reactivity in adulthood [10].

Parallel to these changes in HPA responsiveness, anxiety behavior is also modulated by neonatal handling and maternal separation. Specifically, neonatally handled animals show reduced anxiety-related behaviors in adulthood [10], while maternally separated animals show an increase in anxiety in adulthood [10]. These maternally separated animals also show a greater sensitivity to cocaine-induced locomotor activity compared to neonatally handled or nonhandled animals.

The reduced stress reactivity of neonatally handled animals appears to be due to greater or more effective glucocorticoid negative feedback on the HPA axis. Indeed, these animals have higher hippocampal GR levels and less hypothalamic CRH compared to nonhandled animals [10]. Conversely, in maternally separated animals hippocampal GR levels are decreased and hypothalamic CRH content and mRNA are higher than that observed in nonmaternally separated animals [10]. Taken together, altering pup–dam interactions early in development can have long-lasting effects on HPA reactivity in adulthood and appears to be modulated by changes in glucocorticoid-mediated negative feedback and CRH hypothalamic content. Furthermore, while these early-life manipulations change the behavioral potential of these animals in adulthood, whether they are caused by the changes in HPA function remains to be elucidated.

The mechanisms that mediate the changes in HPA function in neonatally handled and maternally separated animals are not completely understood. However, the maternal care received by offspring experiencing these manipulations likely plays an important role [10]. For instance, it has been demonstrated that neonatal handling leads to increased licking and grooming behavior performed by the mother when the pups are returned to the nest, while maternal separation leads to less maternal care of offspring [10]. Thus, changes in the levels of licking and grooming received by offspring in response to these manipulations may mediate these effects. Interestingly, in the context of maternal separation, it appears that the separation adversely affects males more than females. For instance, male rats that experience maternal separation show heightened HPA reactivity while females do not. As dams spend more time licking and grooming male pups compared to females, any perturbation in the amount of licking and grooming provided by the mother would likely affect the males to a greater extent than the female offspring. This may explain why males are more affected by separation than females, and provides further support to the notion that alterations in maternal behavior, specifically licking and grooming, in response to these experimental manipulations may underlie the changes in HPA function upon reaching adulthood.

8.6
Pubertal Development of the HPA Axis

The maturation of the HPA axis does not end during neonatal development nor do environmental influences cease to affect HPA development after infancy (see Section 8.7). A number of both human and animal studies show increases in basal cortisol and corticosterone secretion during puberty, suggesting further changes in HPA function during pubertal maturation. Interestingly, little research has been done on the pubertal development of the HPA axis. However, if the HPA axis is still developing at this time, it is important to understand how prepubertal and adult animals may respond differently to stressors at the physiological, psychological and behavioral levels.

Studies that have examined stress responsiveness in juvenile animals have demonstrated that even though basal and stress-induced ACTH and corticosterone secretion are similar in prepubertal and adult animals, prepubertal animals have a much more prolonged stress response compared to adults (Fig. 8.4). For example, in males exposed to either intermittent foot shock [11], ether vapors [12], or restraint [13], corticosterone levels of prepubertal males take at least 45–60 min longer to return to baseline than adults. Similar to the extended corticosterone response, stress-induced ACTH responses are also more prolonged in prepubertal than in adult males [13] (Fig. 8.4).

As mentioned above, testosterone has been shown to reduce stress responsiveness in adult males such that castrated males demonstrate an extended stress response compared to testosterone-treated or intact adult males [7]. Therefore, the extended stress response exhibited by prepubertal males may be due to the relatively low levels of circulating testosterone normally experienced at this age. However, even when prepubertal males are supplemented with adult-like levels of testosterone, they continue to show an extended stress response compared to testosterone-treated adults [13]. Thus, as testosterone cannot activate an adult-like stress response prior to puberty, further development of the HPA axis must occur during pubertal maturation.

In addition to males, it was recently demonstrated that prepubertal females also display an extended stress response compared to adult females (Romeo, R. D., unpublished observation). Ovarian steroids have been shown to influence the stress

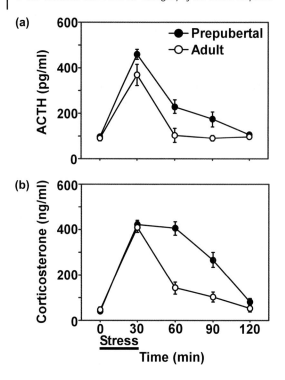

Fig. 8.4. Plasma ACTH and corticosterone concentrations in intact prepubertal and adult males before and after a 30-min session of restraint stress. Adapted from [13].

response of adult females [7]. However, the absence of gonadal hormones has no effect on this prolonged stress response in prepubertal females (Romeo, R. D., unpublished observation).

The prolonged stress response in prepubertal males and females suggests that glucocorticoid-induced negative feedback may be changing during this developmental stage. However, it is important to note that in addition to glucocorticoid negative feedback on the HPA axis, a stress response can also be terminated by central neural activity [14]. The PVN appears to mediate the central control of the HPA shut-off through GABAergic projections from various forebrain limbic areas (GABA = γ-aminobutyric acid) [14]. Therefore, differences in central control and/or glucocorticoid negative feedback may mediate the extended stress response exhibited by prepubertal males.

Although prepubertal and adult males have similar levels of GRs in the hippocampus [15], the levels of hippocampal GRs have not been assessed in response to a stressor. Thus, differences in GR levels and the influence of glucocorticoid-induced negative feedback in the prepubertal extended stress response needs to be addressed with future research. As the role of central control of the HPA axis in prepubertal males is presently unknown, research will need to focus on central mechanisms, such as differences in forebrain inputs to the PVN that may mediate differences in HPA inhibition before and after puberty. It is also possible that peripheral factors such as differential responsivity and sensitivity of the prepubertal and adult adrenal cortex to ACTH may play a role in the extended stress response observed in prepubertal males. Thus, a combination of central and peripheral mechanisms may mediate the extended stress response in prepubertal animals.

The abovementioned studies indicate that both prepubertal males and females exhibit a significantly extended stress response (i.e., approximately 60 min) compared to adults exposed to a similar stressor. Furthermore, gonadal steroids (e.g., testosterone, estrogen) cannot activate an adult-like stress response prior to puberty. Thus, in both sexes, the HPA axis undergoes further development during puberty that allows for a more quickly terminated stress response to emerge in adulthood. Stress hormones have been shown to alter the structure and function of many areas of the central nervous system in adulthood. These same areas show remarkable plasticity during puberty (e.g., hippocampus, prefrontal cortex, amygdala). Thus, further research will need to clarify what mechanisms are responsible for this shift in responsiveness during pubertal maturation and whether stressors encountered during pubertal development will have long-lasting effects on an individual's physiology, brain and behavior upon reaching adulthood.

8.7
Puberty as a Period of Intervention

Similar to neonatal maturation, the pubertal development of the HPA axis is sensitive to variety of environmental factors that have long-lasting effects on future HPA function. Recent research has focused on the role that environmental enrichment plays during puberty to reverse the effects of earlier experimental manipulations on HPA function in adulthood. For instance, animals that have undergone maternal separation during neonatal development, but raised in enriched environments (e.g., interconnected large burrow system, access to toys) during puberty, display less stress reactivity compared to maternally separated animals that did not experience an enriched environment during pubertal development [16]. In fact, the maternally separated animals that were raised in an enriched environment during puberty exhibited stress responses similar to those displayed by neonatally handled animals [16]. In addition to the change in HPA reactivity, maternally separated animals exposed to the enriched environment during puberty were less fearful and showed fewer anxiety-related behaviors than separated animals that had not experienced the enriched environment [16].

How exposure to enriched environments during pubertal maturation reverses the increased HPA reactivity and emotionality induced by earlier life manipulations is currently unknown. Furthermore, whether other environmental or pharmacological interventions during puberty would have similar effects has not been investigated. It is important to note that the nervous system, particularly the hypothalamus and amygdala, continues to develop into puberty [17]. Thus, puberty may represent a second developmental stage marked by distinctive sensitivity to internal and external factors that shape the future responsiveness of the HPA axis to stressors and challenges. Regardless of the mechanisms, the data on pubertal exposure to enriched environments indicate that although the influence of early life events on development of the HPA axis may be long-lasting, they are not permanent and can be reversed under certain conditions.

8.8
Implications for Human Health and Development

In humans, one of the most important factors affecting lifelong health is the stability of a child's early life and the powerful, long-term influences of stressors during childhood on physical and mental health. Early life experiences of abuse or family disruption can combine with genetic traits to influence adult patterns of behavior as well as mood [18], and lead to increases or decreases in allostatic overload (see Fig. 8.1).

Unstable parent–child relationships and outright abuse in childhood can lead to behavioral and physical problems in childhood that continue throughout adult life. Increased mortality and morbidity from a wide variety of common diseases are reported in individuals who were abused as children. Other, less extreme, characteristics of the family environment have also been shown to result in increased physical and mental health risks for children. As outlined in a recent review [19], families characterized by a lack of warmth and support, or by parental overregulation or underregulation of children's behavior, are also associated with increased physical and mental health risks for children.

In addition to the immediate health risks associated with such family environments, the physiological effects of such environments may have long-term effects on adult health and well-being, in the form of allostatic load. It is important to note that reactivity of cortisol secretion is very much dependent on attachment security. If these patterns continue into later life, they could contribute to allostatic load.

Experiences in childhood have other, deleterious consequences. For example, a history of abuse and neglect in childhood interferes with the normal functioning of the HPA axis, resulting in altered circadian rhythm or elevated baseline levels and reduced cerebral volume. The effects can be enduring, leading to exaggerated HPA response to challenges, hippocampal atrophy and cognitive impairment in adulthood. As noted above, there is new evidence from clinical studies for the consequences of child abuse and dysfunction of the family in early life leading to substantial increases in substance abuse, depression and suicide, as well as sexual promiscuity and increased incidences of heart disease, cancer, chronic lung disease, extreme obesity, skeletal fractures and liver disease.

Early life trauma and neglect both work on the background of the genotype of the individual. There is no longer a dichotomy between nature and nurture; rather, nature and nurture interact continuously over the lifespan. A recent study of alleles of monoamine oxidase A, an enzyme which inactivates catecholamines and serotonin in brain and other tissues, found that a more active allele of this enzyme was associated with a protection against the effects of early life abuse in producing patterns of abuse towards their own children later in life [20]. Thus the influences can be quite subtle and are only revealed when considering how a particular genetic trait increases or decreases the risk of a negative response to a stressful event.

It is important to note that problems that are caused by unstable or abusive caregiving in childhood are not necessarily irreversible. There is evidence that social support in the form of loving and caring relationships with a spouse or significant other appear to have powerful ameliorative effects to lower cumulative physiological burden and reduce allostatic load. Further studies of these protective effects are needed to determine their influence on the physiological, as well as the behavioral outcomes of individuals who have bad experiences in childhood.

8.9
Conclusions and Future Directions

The stress response is necessary and adaptive, allowing the organism to cope with the immediate internal and external demands imposed by the stressful event. However, longer or more chronic exposures to stress and stress hormones can increase allostatic load and lead to a number of negative outcomes. Thus, parameters that change stress responsiveness, such as development, may have profound consequences as to whether a stressor leads to an adaptive or maladaptive response. Stress responsiveness changes dramatically as an individual progresses through neonatal and pubertal development. Hormonally, neonatal development is marked by a period of hyporesponsiveness to stress, while puberty is associated with more prolonged stress responses. In addition to the developmental changes in HPA reactivity, the experiences and environment an individual encounters as a neonate or adolescent can shift their future stress responsiveness as an adult. This environmental shaping of the HPA axis may play an important role in the modulation and expression of behaviors, as well as pathophysiologies, in adulthood.

Although much work has been done to further our understanding of the neonatal and pubertal ontogeny of the HPA axis and stress responsiveness, many questions remain unanswered. For instance, what is the functional significance of the neonatal stress hyporesponsive period (SHRP) and the extended stress response exhibited prior to puberty? Do the changes in HPA reactivity induced by earlier neonatal handling and maternal separation mediate the changes in behavior observed in adulthood? Do these altered stress responses have an adaptive role? In the case of the extended stress response prior to puberty, does it result in enhanced memory, increased immune function and enhanced replenishment of energy stores in the aftermath of an acute challenge, as would be expected from the known effects of allostasis? Or, conversely, does the prolonged response confer the possibility of increased allostatic overload when these responses are overused due to traumatic events or to daily stressors? Do individuals who encounter acute or chronic stressors during puberty experience any delayed adverse effects in adulthood? Would environmental enrichment at times other than puberty be effective in mitigating the adverse consequences of early life neglect?

Clearly further research is needed to more fully appreciate and understand the neonatal and pubertal development of this complex neuroendocrine axis. Furthermore, as the link between stress and human health is becoming more apparent, understanding the interactions between stress and development, and the resulting impact on the physiology and behavior of an individual upon reaching adulthood, is a necessary and important objective.

References

1 McEwen, B. S., Stellar, E. (1993). Stress and the individual: mechanisms leading to disease. Arch Int Med, 153:2093–2101.

2 Selye, H. (1936). A syndrome produced by diverse nocuous agents. Nature, 138:32–35.

3 McEwen, B. S. (1998). Protective and damaging effects of stress mediators. New Eng J Med, 338:171–179.

4 Herman, J. P., Figueiredo, H., Mueller, N. K., Ulrich-Lai, Y., Ostander, M. M., Choi, D. C., et al. (2003). Central mechanisms of stress integration: hierarchical circuitry controlling hypothalamic-pituitary-adrenocortical responsiveness. Front Neuroendocrinol, 24:151–180.

5 Sapolsky, R. M., Meaney, M. J. (1986). Maturation of the adrenocortical stress response: neuroendocrine control mechanisms and the stress hyporesponsive period. Brain Res Rev, 396:64–76.

6 Meaney, M. J., Sapolsky, R. M., McEwen, B. S. (1985). The development of the glucocorticoid receptor system in the rat limbic brain. I. ontogeny and autoregulation. Dev Brain Res, 18:159–164.

7 Viau, V. (2002). Functional cross-talk between the hypothalamic-pituitary-gonadal and -adrenal axes. J Neuroendocrinol, 14:506–513.

8 Caldji, C., Diorio, J., Meaney, M. J. (2000). Variations in maternal care in infancy regulate the development of stress reactivity. Biol Psychiatry, 48:1164–1174.

9 Francis, D., Diorio, J., Lui, D.,

Meaney, M. J. (1999). Nongenomic transmission across generations of maternal behavior and stress responses in the rat. Science, 286:1155–1158.

10 Meaney, M. J. (2001). Maternal care, gene expression, and the transmission of individual differences in stress reactivity across generations. Ann Rev Neurosci, 24:1161–1192.

11 Goldman, L., Winget, C., Hollingshead, G. W., Levine, S. (1973). Postweaning development of negative feedback in the pituitary-adrenal system of the rat. Neuroendocrinology, 12:199–211.

12 Vazquez, D. M., Akil, H. (1993). Pituitary-adrenal response to ether vapor in the weanling animal: characterization of the inhibitory effect of glucocorticoids on adrenocorticotropin secretion. Pediatr Res, 34:646–653.

13 Romeo, R. D., Lee, S. J., Chhua, N., McPherson, C. R., McEwen, B. S. (2004). Testosterone cannot activate an adult-like stress response in prepubertal male rats. Neuroendocrinology, 79:125–132.

14 Herman, J. P., Cullinan, W. E. (1997). Neurocircuitry of stress: central control of the hypothalamo-pituitary-adrenocortical axis. Trend Neurosci, 20:78–84.

15 Vazquez, D. M. (1998). Stress and the developing limbic-hypothalamic-pituitary-adrenal axis. Psycho-neuroendocrinology, 23:663–700.

16 Francis, D. D., Diorio, J., Plotsky, P. M., Meaney, M. J. (2002).

Environmental enrichment reverses the effects of maternal separation on stress reactivity. J Neurosci, 22:7840–7843.

17 ROMEO, R. D. (2003). Puberty: a period of both organizational and activational effects of steroid hormones on neurobehavioral development. J Neuroendocrinol, 15:1185–1192.

18 HEIM, C., NEMEROFF, C. B. (2001). The role of childhood trauma in the neurobiology of mood and anxiety disorders: preclinical and clinical studies. Biol Psychiatry, 49:1023–1039.

19 REPETTI, R. L., TAYLOR, S. E., SEEMAN, T. E. (2002). Risky families: family social environments and the mental and physical health of offspring. Psych Bull, 128:330–366.

20 CASPI, A., McCLAY, J., MOFFITT, T. E., MILL, J., MARTIN, J., CRAIG, I. W., et al. (2002). Role of genotype in the cycle of violence in maltreated children. Science, 297:851–854.

9
Neurobiological and Behavioral Consequences of Exposure to Childhood Traumatic Stress

Martin H. Teicher, Jacqueline A. Samson, Akemi Tomoda,
Majed Ashy, and Susan L. Andersen

9.1
Introduction

The developing brain is a remarkably plastic and dynamic organ. Although the basic possibilities of what it has the potential to become appear to be set by genetic codes, the unique configuration that evolves for each human being is created though a complex process of communication with the environment. In the best circumstances, this ensures a maximal fit between the demands of the environment and the response possibilities available to the individual. However, under conditions of extreme stress, a cascade of events may be initiated that results in aberrations of brain development and subsequent vulnerability to psychopathology.

Our studies focus on the effects of early childhood maltreatment on the developing brain, and the implications for the emergence of psychiatric disorder. We have proposed that early maltreatment produces a cascade of physiological and neurohumoral responses built on the following five fundamental premises. First, that exposure to stress early in life activates stress response systems, and fundamentally alters their molecular organization to modify their sensitivity and response bias. Second, that exposure of the developing brain to stress hormones exerts consequences by affecting gene expression, myelination, neural morphology, neurogenesis and synaptogenesis. Third, that different brain regions vary in their sensitivity, which depends, in part, upon genetics, timing, rate of development, and density of glucocorticoid receptors. Fourth, that there are enduring functional consequences that include attenuated left hemisphere development, decreased right/left hemisphere integration, increased electrical irritability within the limbic system circuits, and diminished functional activity of the cerebellar vermis. Fifth, that there are associated neuropsychiatric consequences and vulnerabilities, which lead to an enhanced risk for the development of posttraumatic stress disorder (PTSD), depression, borderline personality disorder (BPD), dissociative identity disorder (DID), and substance abuse.

Stress in Health and Disease. Edited by Bengt B. Arnetz and Rolf Ekman
Copyright © 2006 WILEY-VCH Verlag GmbH & Co. KGaA, Weinheim
ISBN: 3-527-31221-8

9.2
Exposure to Stress in Early Life and Stress Response Systems

A series of seminal studies from the laboratories of Plotsky and Meaney have shown that early stress produces enduring changes in the molecular organization of stress response systems. In essence, stress response systems are programmed by experience to respond more drastically to events later in life. For instance, we are programmed by adverse early experience to have an enhanced cortisol and norepinephrine/adrenaline response to subsequent stressors. The positive aspect of enhanced stress responding is that it facilitates survival in the face of danger and acute injury. The negative effect is that it initiates a variety of processes that promote chronic pathology such as obesity, type II diabetes, cardiac disease, substance abuse, psychiatric illness and accelerated aging [1].

9.3
Gene Expression, Myelination, Neural Morphology, Neurogenesis and Synaptogenesis

Exposing the developing brain to heightened levels of glucocorticoids (such as cortisol) and stress-activated neurotransmitters (such as dopamine, norepinephrine,

---

Is It More Than Just Cortisol?

One puzzle in understanding the impact of stress hormones on human brain development is the absence of known neurodevelopmental consequences of childhood treatment with corticosteroids for asthma or arthritis. We suspect that the adverse effects of early stress on human brain development are not simply a consequence of increased exposure to corticosteroids. The suppressive effects of glucocorticoids on cell proliferation appear to occur indirectly via an N-methyl-D-aspartic acid (NMDA) receptor-dependent glutamate excitatory pathway. We hypothesize that stress affects brain development via the concerted activation of multiple pillars of the stress response. Norepinephrine, vasopressin and dopamine are released by stress and they synergistically potentiate the excitatory effects of glutamate on NMDA receptors. Hence, concerted activation of multiple systems may have far greater impact than exogenous administration of a single hormone.

This hypothesis is supported by a landmark study from Caspi et al. [2] who identified a very strong gene × environmental interaction mediating the effects of exposure to early abuse on development of aggressive behavior. Briefly, males with a functional polymorphism associated with low levels of monoamine oxidase-A (MAO-A) expression were more likely to develop antisocial behavior than abused males with a polymorphism associated with high levels of MAO-A expression. This research was based on the hypothesis that MAO-A develops before MAO-B, and serves during early life to buffer the stress-induced overactivation of monoamine systems. Hence, it is likely that stress-induced overactivation of monoamine systems is a key factor, acting alone or in concert with cortisol release, that links exposure to early trauma to enduring effects on brain or behavioral development.

and serotonin), affects crucial steps in postnatal brain development. For example, research in laboratory animals shows that excess exposure to glucocorticoids in early life is associated with reduced brain weight and DNA content, suppression of postnatal neural mitosis of granule cells in the cerebellum and dentate gyrus, alterations in patterns of myelination, and a reduction in dendritic spines in various brain regions. Animals exposed to excessive glucocorticoids also show social behavior changes and deficits in their ability to perform active avoidance tasks.

In normal development, there is a period characterized by reductions in basal corticosteroid levels called the "stress hyporesponsive period." This period likely exists to protect the developing brain from the effects of minor stressors. However, certain stressors such as maternal deprivation appear to override this effect.

9.4
Differential Sensitivity to the Effects of Stress in Various Brain Regions

In general, the regions of brain most vulnerable to the effects of early stress are those that develop slowly during the postnatal period and have a high density of glucocorticoid receptors. These include the hippocampus, the corpus callosum, the cerebellar vermis, and the cerebral cortex. Postnatal neurogenesis, evident in

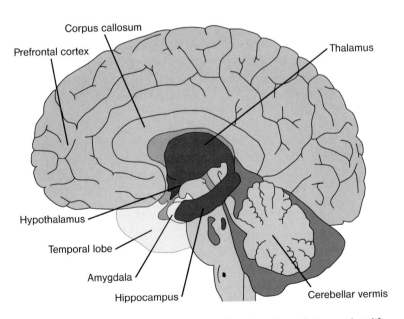

Fig. 9.1. The main regions of the brain vulnerable to the effects of stress early in life.

the human hippocampus, and debated in other brain regions, is an additional factor that may lead to stress-sensitivity (as illustrated in Figure 9.1).

9.4.1
Hippocampus

In preclinical studies of the hippocampus, exposure to stress or corticosteroids can suppress production of new granule cells, and can alter the morphology or even lead to the death of pyramidal cells. Stress also suppresses the production of new granule cells. Imaging studies of adults with a history of childhood abuse have consistently reported hippocampal volume reduction, particularly on the left side.

The hippocampus is known to be critical for memory storage and retrieval and is most likely critical for the generation of dissociative states. Both the hippocampus and the parahippocampal gyrus also appear to play a role in the pathophysiology of generalized anxiety and panic disorder, probably stimulated by noradrenergic activity originating in the locus coeruleus. Lastly, serotonergic projections from the median raphe nuclei to the hippocampus play an important role in establishing an individual's level of overall behavioral inhibition. Thus, alterations in hippocampal development may affect anxiogenic, dissociative, amnestic and disinhibitory aspects of the PTSD response.

The potential effect of childhood abuse on hippocampal volume has led to a consistent inconsistency in the imaging literature. Currently, there are four studies of hippocampal volume in adults with a history of childhood abuse with diagnoses of PTSD, DID, major depression, or BPD [3–6]. In all of these studies (total $n = 80$ abused and 73 healthy controls) there was a significant volume reduction in the hippocampus, which ranged from 5% to 16%, and was left-sided in three studies and bilateral in one. In contrast, there have been three separate studies of hippocampal volume in children with history of abuse and current symptoms of PTSD (total $n = 96$ abused and 153 healthy controls) [7–9]. In none of these studies was there a significant difference in hippocampal volume between abused and control children.

There are several possible explanations. One possibility is that PTSD exerts a very gradual effect on hippocampal morphology so that the adverse effects are not discernable in children or adolescents [10]. Another possibility is that reduced hippocampal size may be an artifact of the high levels of alcohol and substance abuse that often occurs in adults with PTSD. Indeed De Bellis et al. found that adolescent-onset alcohol abuse was associated with decreased hippocampal volume. Another intriguing possibility is that reduced hippocampal size may not be a result of childhood abuse or even a risk factor for the emergence of PTSD, but may be a risk factor for the persistence of PTSD into adulthood.

We have hypothesized that the effects of early experience on the hippocampus may be quite delayed and emerged as a consequence of neuromaturational changes [11] (see sidebar). This possibility was explored by performing volumetric analyses of the hippocampus in a group of 21 young adult (18–22 years of age) collegiate females with a history of repeated childhood sexual abuse (CSA) and 15 sociodemographically comparable healthy controls. None of the subjects had a history of substance abuse. CSA subjects were selected without regard to psychiatric diagnosis and most subjects did not have a current axis I diagnosis. Hence, this population was far healthier than previously reported abuse samples used in imaging studies. Overall, we found that there was an 8% reduction in hippocampal volume, bilaterally. Loss of hippocampal volume in CSA subjects was not related to past or current history of depression or PTSD. This supports the hypothesis that the effects of CSA on hippocampal volume become manifest by late adolescence or early adulthood, and are not an artifact of substance abuse, a gradual consequence of PTSD, or a preexisting abnormality increasing risk for the development or persistence of PTSD.

> Does Early Stress Exert a Delayed Effect on the Hippocampus?
>
> Using a rodent model, Andersen and Teicher [11] found that early stress prior to weaning (days 2–20) prevented the expected prepubertal overproduction of synapses in hippocampal regions CA1 and CA3, but did not prevent pruning. This combination of underproduction and normal pruning produced a net deficit in synaptic connections that was not apparent even at puberty (day 40), but was prominent by early adulthood (day 60). This suggests that early life stress may affect a brain region in a way that is not immediately apparent on a gross morphological level, but may become apparent with continued maturation.

9.4.2
Corpus Callosum

Myelinated regions, such as the corpus callosum, also appear to be vulnerable to the effects of early exposure to trauma. Elevated levels of stress hormones suppress the glial cell division critical for myelination. Monkeys reared in isolating environments show attenuation in development and diminished volume in the corpus callosum, which is associated with deficits in learning. In humans, Teicher and colleagues were the first to suggest that alterations in corpus callosum may be associated with exposure to early abuse after finding that the midsagittal area of the corpus callosum was reduced in psychiatrically ill children with a history of abuse or neglect relative to nonabused psychiatrically ill controls (see [12] for review). De Bellis et al. showed more definitively, in two separate studies, that corpus callosum area was reduced in abused children with PTSD relative to healthy controls [8, 9]. Indeed, reduced area of the midportions of the corpus callosum was the most prominent anatomical abnormality found in abused children suffering from PTSD. Subsequent work from our laboratory has shown that corpus callosum abnormalities in girls were more likely to be associated with a history of sexual abuse, whereas in boys, abnormalities were associated with neglect [13].

Reductions in size of corpus callosum appear to affect communications between cerebral hemispheres, possibly leading to an attenuated degree of integration. In adults with a history of trauma, Schiffer et al. [14] showed a marked suppression of electroencephalography (EEG) evoked potential response over the left hemisphere (indicative of left hemisphere processing) during recall of neutral memories, which shifted dramatically to a marked suppression of evoked responses over the right hemisphere (indicative of right hemisphere activation) during recall of traumatic memories. In adults with no trauma history, both hemispheres were equally involved in processing either type of memory. These results suggest that exposure to early trauma is associated with increased hemispheric laterality and decreased hemispheric integration.

9.4.3
Cerebral Cortex

Maturation in the neocortex occurs slowly, and the delayed myelination of the corpus callosum allows the two hemispheres to develop relatively independently. Language and motor lateralization is mostly set by the age of 5 years through a process that begins *in utero*. During the first few months of life, the right hemisphere shows more dendritic outgrowth than the left, and develops more rapidly. By 5 or 6 months of age, dendritic growth in the left hemisphere surpasses the right, which continues over the next 2 years. Between 3 and 6 years of age, growth in the right hemisphere speeds up and helps provide the components of prosody that peak between 5 and 6 years. Specialization for perception of human faces in the right hemisphere emerges between 8 and 13 years.

In the cortex, the two cerebral hemispheres are specialized to a great degree with respect to information processing. The left hemisphere is usually associated with the perception and expression of language, is logical and analytical, and is somewhat more intricate in its development than the right. The right hemisphere plays a central role in the perception and expression of emotion, particularly negative emotion. The two hemispheres are connected through the corpus callosum, and the anterior and posterior commissures. To ensure optimal functioning, the two hemispheres need to interact closely. Of importance is the fact that the normal bidirectional flow of information through the corpus callosum can be altered by early experience.

The prefrontal cortex has the most delayed ontogeny of any brain region. Myelination of major projections to the prefrontal cortex only begins in adolescence and then continues well into the third decade of life. The prefrontal cortex also has a relatively high density of glucocorticoid receptors. Dopamine projections to this area are specifically activated by stress. In turn, the prefrontal cortex exerts inhibitory effects on all of the major monoamine projections to subcortical regions and serves to limit their response to stress. While stress exerts a widespread effect on the brain regions early in development, we found that this response becomes more restricted as the prefrontal cortex matures. We have theorized that early exposure to stress may produce precocious maturation of the prefrontal cortex, leading to signs of early maturation (e.g., the "parentified child"), but may also arrest the development of this region and prevent it from reaching its full adult capacity.

Studies of cortical development in abused children with major psychopathology have reported: (a) increased levels of right hemisphere EEG coherence, indicative of delayed or attenuated maturation [15]; (b) loss of white matter volume and total volume of the prefrontal cortex [9]; (c) loss of normal left–right asymmetry in the frontal cortex [7]; (d) a reduction in the ratio of N-acetylaspartate to creatine in the anterior cingulate cortex, which is a marker for neuronal loss or dysfunction; and (e) alterations in gray matter volume of the superior temporal gyrus (see [12] for citations).

We have recently analyzed the effects of repeated exposure to sexual abuse on regional gray matter volume (GMV) in young adult females ($n = 23$ abused and 14 healthy controls) using voxel-based morphometry, and compared these results to a group of young adults with exposure to intense parental verbal abuse ($n = 10$ abused and 13 healthy controls). Young adults with a history of repeated sexual abuse had a highly significant and very selective reduction (17%) in GMV of the right visual cortex (Brodmann's Area 17 and 18). In contrast, young adults with exposure to severe parental verbal abuse had a significant and selective reduction (15%) of GMV in the right superior temporal gyrus (Brodmann's Area 42). The superior temporal gyrus is believed to be a key anatomical substrate for speech, language and communication. Together these studies strongly suggest that early maltreatment alters neuronal development of the neocortex, and may target primary sensory regions as well as prefrontal regions.

9.4.4
Cerebellar Vermis

The cerebellar vermis (also called *arbor vitae* or tree of life) is a midline structure that separates and connects the cerebellar hemispheres. It consists of a gray matter region with highly complex lobular architecture and a major white matter fiber tract. Also, residing in the vermis are the intrinsic fastigial nuclei, which provide output projections from the vermis.

Interestingly, the vermis increases in size to a greater degree during the postnatal period than any other brain region and, like the hippocampus, may continue to produce new granule cells after birth. Further, studies comparing brain regions in identical twins indicate that the vermis differs most between twins, suggesting that it may be most susceptible to the effects of early experience. During early postnatal development the vermis in rodents has a higher density of glucocorticoid receptors than the hippocampus, and some studies suggest that in primates it continues to have a higher density.

Studies from our group [16] have shown that increased basal cerebral blood volume in the vermis is associated with symptoms of limbic irritability in both healthy young adult controls and in individuals with abuse history. However, in individuals with an abuse history, there was an overall decrease in relative perfusion (see [12]). It is known that vermal stimulation can be used to suppress seizure activity. It is also known that the vermis is involved in regulation of affect, attention, eye-movement control, and components of sensorimotor integration and postural regulation. Thus, stress-induced functional abnormalities in the vermis may contribute to our understanding of the sequelae of exposure to early trauma.

New Insights into the Cerebellar Vermis as a Stress-Sensitive Region

Our interest in the vermis and its contribution to the effects of early stress followed, in part, from seminal studies conducted by Harlow, Mason and Prescott. Briefly, Harlow showed the critical importance of early experience in his studies in which monkeys were raised in isolation with wire-mesh- or terry-cloth-covered surrogate mothers. Isolation-reared monkeys were often violent and had highly deviant social relationships. Mason found that some of the effects of isolation rearing could be ameliorated if the surrogate mother was on a pivot that provided rocking motions. This led Prescott to write about the importance of the vestibular and proprioceptive systems to normal development, and to theorize about the importance of the cerebellar vermis, which receives major projections from these systems.

Rocking motion clearly has a dramatic effect on emotional state, and this is likely a consequence of vestibular projections to the vermis, which in turn has projections to the limbic system via the fastigial nucleus. Indeed, stimulation of this vermal–fastigial pathway can even suppress seizure activity within the limbic system. The vermis also plays an important role in regulating blood flow to the body and brain, which needs be constantly adjusted to cope with postural change, and this system has projections to the locus coeruleus, substantia nigra and ventral tegmental area, through which it modulates the release of dopamine and norepinephrine.

Abnormalities in the cerebellar vermis have recently been reported to be associated with various psychiatric disorders, including manic depressive illness, schizophrenia, autism and attention deficit/hyperactivity disorder (ADHD). These maladies emerge from genetic and prenatal factors, not childhood mistreatment, but the fact that vermal anomalies seem to sit at the core of so many psychiatric conditions suggests that this region plays a critical role in mental health. Lesions in the cerebellar vermis in childhood appear to be associated with mutism that can last from weeks to months, and sustained symptoms of affective instability.

The vermis appears to be affected by all known drugs of abuse, is also affected by anti-convulsants, mood-stabilizers and lithium, and may be the primary target of the putative antiaddictive drug ibogaine. Taken together, these results suggest that the vermis may mediate a variety of neurobehavioral consequences of early exposure to stress or trauma and that the vermis is an important region for regulation of emotional health.

9.5
Neuropsychiatric Consequences and Psychopathology

As outlined above, exposure to early trauma is associated with diminished development of the left hemisphere, including the neocortex and hippocampus, reduced size of the corpus callosum, and attenuated activity in the cerebellar vermis. These stress-induced alterations result from a cascade of physiological and neurohumoral responses, and then go on, in turn, to create vulnerabilities to a variety of emotional and behavioral pathologies. Included among these are depressive disorders, PTSD, DID, ADHD, BPD and substance abuse.

9.5.1
Depression

In our studies, 43% of young adults with a history of abuse had current or recurrent episodes of major depression. In addition to the psychosocial effects of childhood maltreatment, the cascade of neurobiological events described above is likely to shape brain development so as to create vulnerabilities to this disorder. Depression is known to be associated with alterations in the glucocorticoid system, and is often characterized by hypersecretion of corticotropin-releasing factor (CRF), hypercortisolemia, and diminished feedback regulation of cortisol. As described above, exposure to early trauma enhances CRF neuronal activity and sensitizes the brain to the effects of exposure to subsequent stressors. Moreover, exposure to chronic nonspecific stressors may result in downregulation of CRF receptors, dysregulation of cortisol rhythms and the emergence of symptoms of depression.

We have also found in animal studies that exposure to early stress is associated with an enduring reduction in serotonin turnover in the amygdala and nucleus accumbens, which may also predispose to the development of depression. Recently, there has been considerable interest in the possible role of hippocampal neurogenesis in the emergence of depression and response to antidepressants. Stress can markedly suppress hippocampal neurogenesis, and individuals exposed to early stress may be particularly vulnerable if their stress response systems become programmed to respond in an overly robust manner to subsequent stressors.

Caspi and colleagues [17] made the seminal finding that a functional polymorphism in the promoter region of the serotonin transporter (*5-HTT*) gene moderated the influence of stressful life events on risk of developing depression. Individuals with one or two copies of the short allele of the *5-HTT* promoter polymorphism, who were exposed to three or more adverse life events exhibited more depressive symptoms, diagnosable depression, and suicidality than individuals homozygous for the long allele. This study shows the potential importance of genetic factors in modulating vulnerability to the effects of stress.

Adults with major depression and history of childhood stress may respond differently to treatments than depressed adults with less stressful childhoods. Nemeroff and colleagues [18] found that depressed subjects with history of early abuse responded preferentially to the Cognitive Behavioral Analysis System of Psychotherapy (CBASP), a kind of cognitive–behavioral psychotherapy. Subjects with no early abuse history had a more favorable response to an antidepressant monotherapy, and had their best overall response to a combination of medication plus CBASP.

9.5.2
Posttraumatic Stress Disorder

Most children exposed to traumatic events never develop PTSD. Deblinger et al. [19] found that only 6.9% of psychiatrically hospitalized children with physical abuse and 20.7% with sexual abuse history met diagnostic criteria for PTSD.

Famularo and colleagues found that only 35% of severely maltreated and psychologically traumatized children who were removed from parental custody due to the trauma actually met strict criteria for PTSD. This is not necessarily a matter of resilience. Kiser et al. found that abused children and adolescents who did not develop PTSD actually exhibited more anxiety, depression, externalizing behaviors and more overall problems than children who did. Similarly, Glod et al. [20, 21] found that psychiatrically hospitalized abused children without PTSD had more agitated and disrupted sleep than abused children with PTSD. These findings suggest that the PTSD criteria formulated and validated in adults do not necessarily adequately describe the psychiatric impact of exposure to childhood trauma, and do not necessarily identify those children most adversely affected by trauma.

While exposure to early trauma does not necessarily produce disturbances that fit adult criteria for PTSD, early exposure to trauma primes the brain to be more susceptible to a PTSD response when later trauma strikes. Enhanced risk may be related to CRF neuronal overactivity. Molecular alterations within the amygdala and locus coeruleus may produce limbic irritability or kindling, induce sympa-

---

What Constitutes a Childhood Trauma?

Several investigators have recently reported surprisingly strong effects of emotional abuse or neglect on their measures of interest, often eclipsing the effects of sexual abuse. Bernet and colleagues [22] found that the severity of childhood trauma, most notably emotional abuse, was directly related to age of onset, course and severity of major depression in adulthood. DID, which includes multiple personality disorder and related conditions, is often assumed to result from childhood sexual trauma. However, recent studies show that neglect and exposure to emotional maltreatment are much stronger predictors than exposure to sexual abuse. We have recently analyzed results from a sample of 564 young adults (18–22 years of age) regarding childhood experiences and ratings of psychiatric symptoms. Across all of the measures of interest verbal abuse was associated with somewhat larger effect sizes (more deleterious outcomes) than witnessing domestic violence, and substantially greater effect sizes than familial physical abuse. However, witnessing of domestic violence and physical abuse can qualify in the Diagnostic and Statistical Manual of Mental Disorders, Fourth Edition, as a category A (1) traumatic event necessary for the diagnosis of PTSD, while exposure to verbal abuse cannot. The focus of the traumatic exposure criteria is on threats to the *physical* integrity of self or others. We wonder, particularly in children, if threats to ones *mental* integrity and sense of self can be equally traumatizing. Certainly, torture experts know the significance of verbal abuse and other forms of emotional abuse that threaten the mental integrity of an individual, rather than just their physical integrity as enshrined in the A (1) criteria.

Our results are consonant with the observations of Bremner and colleagues [23], who found that emotional abuse items, such as being often shouted at, appeared to substantially increase risk for PTSD. They suggest that the specific role of emotional abuse has yet to be determined, and, research is needed to evaluate if emotional abuse is causative, or if it contributes to the development of PTSD through association with other forms of abuse.

thetic hyperarousal, enhance fear or startle reactions, augment fight or flight responses, or promote the emergence of memories associated with the event. Dissociative and amnestic components of PTSD may be facilitated by stress-induced alterations in hippocampal functioning.

9.5.3
Attention-Deficit/Hyperactivity Disorder

At least three investigators have now reported that children with a history of abuse also show elevated rates of symptoms of ADHD. In our studies, about 30% of children with severe abuse histories meet criteria for ADHD. However, based on actigraph recording we found that children with classical ADHD were about 25% more active than controls while abused children meeting ADHD criteria were only 11% more active than controls [20]. This led us to hypothesize that early abuse can produce symptoms of overactivity and inattention that resemble ADHD, but that this is distinct from the actual disorder. Syndromic overlap may occur if early abuse affects functional activity of the cerebellar vermis, as a reduction in the size of the cerebellar vermis appears to be the most consistent anatomical abnormality found in ADHD. A second mechanism leading to syndromic overlap may be reduced size in the midportions of the corpus callosum, which occurs with early abuse or neglect and has been associated with increased rates of impulsive behavior.

9.5.4
Borderline Personality Disorder

Pioneering studies by Stone and by Herman and colleagues revealed a strong association between early abuse and the development of BPD. We have theorized at length about how different abuse-associated alterations in brain morphology or function can account for the diverse array of symptoms seen in subjects with BPD [24]. Our discoveries that abused patients show diminished right–left hemisphere integration and a smaller corpus callosum suggest a possible model for the emergence of borderline features in this population. This polarized hemispheric dominance could cause the rapid shifting of emotions from positive in one state to resoundingly negative in another. Further, limbic irritability could lead to increased aggression and, combined with the polarized hemispheric dominance, to an increased risk for suicide and self-destructive behavior. Previous research has shown higher rates of temporal lobe–limbic system dysfunction in borderline patients. Specifically, patients with BPD have been shown to have a higher incidence of EEG abnormalities (38% compared to 13% in dysthymic patients), and increased EEG sharp wave abnormalities (41% compared to 5% in unipolar depressed patients). We have found that children and adolescents with confirmed abuse histories have a markedly increased incidence of EEG abnormalities and symptoms suggestive of temporal lobe epilepsy. Self-destructive behavior, mood fluctuations, and susceptibility to brief psychotic states may also result from stress-induced alterations in dopamine and serotonin levels in the amygdala and nucleus accumbens.

9.5.5
Dissociative Identity Disorder

Another disorder sometimes reported both by patients with a trauma history and by patients with borderline personality disorder is DID. In one report, 23% of subjects with DID showed grossly abnormal EEG results with paroxysmal spike and sharp waves, which is between five and ten times the average rate found in populations of psychiatric ill patients. Another study reported DID patients showed an extreme degree of left hemisphere activation. We propose that DID may arise from an extreme attenuation of hemispheric integration that results in abrupt changes in personality when activation is shifted from the left to the right hemisphere dominant mode. Abnormal hippocampal development may facilitate the generation of dissociative states, which may be triggered or exacerbated by the presence of temporal lobe epilepsy.

9.5.6
Substance Abuse

Individuals who have been exposed to childhood physical and sexual abuse are at risk for a wide range of adjustment difficulties including substance use and abuse, both during adolescence and in later life. Several studies have assessed the relative risk and have identified factors that may influence risk. The association between early maltreatment and alcohol or drug use may manifest at an alarmingly young age. In one study, abuse was associated with more than a 3-fold increase in the odds that alcohol/cigarette experimentation had occurred, and more than a 12-fold increase in the odds that marijuana use or regular drinking had occurred by 10 years of age. For eighth graders, combined sexual and physical abuse was associated with a twofold greater risk of light to moderate drinking and an almost eightfold increase in risk of heavy drinking. Holmes found that early sexual abuse increased by more than 12-fold the risk of early initiation of parenteral drug abuse. Fergussen et al. found that CSA involving attempted/completed intercourse was associated with 2.7-fold increased risk of alcohol abuse/dependence and a 6.6-fold increased risk of substance abuse/dependence.

In our survey of 537 college students, there was an association between limbic irritability ratings and the amount of substance abuse they reported. In fact, limbic irritability ratings correlated more strongly with self-reported rates of substance abuse than did ratings of depression, anxiety or anger–irritability. Limbic irritability ratings were markedly increased by exposure to childhood trauma, and correlated with measures of regional blood flow into the cerebellar vermis [16].

There are compelling reasons to hypothesize that the vermis plays a role in modulating response to addictive drugs. Through its fastigial projections to the ventral tegmental area and the locus coeruleus, the vermis exerts strong effects on the turnover of dopamine and norepinephrine in the caudate and nucleus accumbens. The vermis receives direct monoamine projections from the midbrain and has dopamine receptors and transporters. Moreover, virtually all drugs of abuse are known to affect the vermis, and the antiaddictive agent, ibogaine, exerts profound effects here. In addition, ADHD is a serious risk factor for the development of substance abuse disorders, and given that the most consistently reported anatomical abnormality in ADHD is reduced vermal size, the vermis is likely involved in regulating substance use and abuse. Together, these findings suggest that early traumatic stress may enhance risk for later substance abuse by fostering limbic irritability and inadequate vermal development. Early stress may also increase risk for substance abuse by sensitizing the dopamine system, and by programming stress response systems to overreact to exposure to subsequent stressors.

9.6
Perspectives

The brain is a very malleable organ engineered to be sculpted by experience. Exposure to severe stress during childhood has probably been a routine occurrence throughout the natural history of *Homo sapiens*. It seems unlikely that the changes we see in the brain that result from exposure to early stress are simply forms of damage to a brain that has never evolved to cope with early stress. Rather, we postulate exposure to early stress initiates a cascade of responses that cause the brain to follow an alternative developmental pathway that molds the brain to be exquisitely suited to the demands of the environment in which it predicts it will find itself [15]. Hence, the neurobiological responses that we, and others, have observed may be perfectly natural and adaptive modifications in brain structure and functioned triggered by certain forms and levels of stress during key periods of development. In this way, the brain may match its wiring and configuration to the environment that it expects to survive and reproduce in.

If an individual is born into a harsh and aggressive environment, it will be crucial for him to maintain a heightened sense of vigilance that will alert him to the first signs of danger. It will be important for him to have the ability to mobilize an intense fight or flight response and to react quickly to environmental challenge with a strong aggressive response to facilitate survival. Alterations in the amygdala and limbic irritability may enhance the fight or flight response and aggression. Hippocampal alterations and changes in CRF receptor density and neuronal activity may augment corticosteroid responses. Further, hippocampal abnormalities may facilitate the emergence of dissociation as a psychic defensive maneuver against stress. Diminished left hemisphere maturation, reduced corpus callosum size and attenuated left hemisphere integration may substantially increase an individual's capacity to react rapidly and shift into an angry aggressive state when threatened with danger or loss. Diminished development of the cerebellar vermis may be essential for the maintenance of this state of limbic irritability, hyperarousal and sympathetic activation. Lastly, enduring alterations that occur in messenger RNA levels for vasopressin and oxytocin as a consequence of exposure to early stress may predispose to patterns of sexual behavioral and mating practices that foster reproductive success in a malevolent world [15].

However, these alterations may not be optimal for survival in a more benign environment, where impulsive responses, aggressive actions or dissociative states put the individual at a disadvantage in settings where cooperative problem-solving responses are needed. Moreover, the mismatch between brain responsiveness and environmental demands may lead to psychiatric conditions such as depression, PTSD, ADHD, BPD, DID, or problems with substance abuse.

What if the individual were to continue to exist in a hostile, aggressive environment to which his brain is optimally suited? It appears that this alternative developmental pathway would likely permit the individual to survive longer and to compete more successfully than would be possible without these adaptations. However, as McEwen [1] has reported, repeated glucocorticoid and catecholamine mobilization comes with a severe physical cost. Over time, these stress-induced responses create an "allostatic load" that further stresses the system and can accelerate physical disease processes, such as cardiovascular disease, diabetes and obesity. Thus, eventually, the alternative developmental pathway would probably lead to chronic illness and premature death. However, these disease processes emerge slowly, usually long after we have passed though our primary reproductive stage (which is what matters from an evolutionary perspective), and may go unnoticed in circumstances where life expectancies are relatively short.

Thus, although we are exquisitely created to be maximally adapted to the world into which we are born, the fact that we are mobile and that life circumstances may change means that many individuals struggle with neurobiological coping responses that are ill-suited to their realities. For these individuals optimal mental and physical health may require a dramatic change in our neurobiology. To what degree can we achieve this? Efforts to reduce exposure to stressors early in life are one preventative approach. Efforts to attenuate or modulate stress responses following early life exposure to trauma may be another. What remains to be determined is the degree to which early stress-associated alterations in brain structure or function can be reversed, and if so, by what means. It is our next challenge to seek answers to this question.

Acknowledgements

This study was supported by RO1 awards from the National Institute of Mental Health USA (MH-66222) and National Institute of Drug Abuse USA (DA-016934, DA-017846) to MHT. Drs. Carl M. Anderson, Dennis Kim, Carryl P. Navalta, Ann Polcari and Fred Schiffer are integral members of our scientific team, and have made major contributions to the findings and concepts put forth in this chapter.

References

1 McEwen BS. Allostasis and allostatic load: implications for neuropsychopharmacology. Neuropsychopharmacology. 2000; 22(2):108–124.

2 Caspi A, McClay J, Moffitt TE, Mill J, Martin J, Craig IW, Taylor A, Poulton R. Role of genotype in the cycle of violence in maltreated children. Science. 2002; 297(5582):851–854.

3 Bremner JD, Randall P, Vermetten E, Staib L, Bronen RA, Mazure C, Capelli S, McCarthy G, Innis RB, Charney DS. Magnetic resonance imaging-based measurement of hippocampal volume in posttraumatic stress disorder related to childhood physical and sexual abuse – a preliminary report. Biol Psychiatry. 1997; 41(1):23–32.

4 Driessen M, Herrmann J, Stahl K, Zwaan M, Meier S, Hill A, Osterheider M, Petersen D. Magnetic resonance imaging volumes of the hippocampus and the amygdala in women with borderline personality disorder and early traumatization. Arch Gen Psychiatry. 2000; 57(12):1115–1122.

5 Stein MB. Hippocampal volume in women victimized by childhood sexual abuse. Psychol Med. 1997; 27(4):951–959.

6 Vythilingam M, Heim C, Newport J, Miller AH, Anderson E, Bronen R, Brummer M, Staib L, Vermetten E, Charney DS, Nemeroff CB, Bremner JD. Childhood trauma associated with smaller hippocampal volume in women with major depression. Am J Psychiatry. 2002; 159(12):2072–2080.

7 Carrion VG, Weems CF, Eliez S, Patwardhan A, Brown W, Ray RD, Reiss AL. Attenuation of frontal asymmetry in pediatric posttraumatic stress disorder. Biol Psychiatry. 2001; 50(12):943–951.

8 De Bellis MD, Keshavan MS, Clark DB, Casey BJ, Giedd JN, Boring AM, Frustaci K, Ryan ND. Developmental traumatology. Part II: Brain development. Biol Psychiatry. 1999; 45(10):1271–1284.

9 De Bellis MD, Keshavan MS, Shifflett H, Iyengar S, Beers SR, Hall J, Moritz G. Brain structures in pediatric maltreatment-related posttraumatic stress disorder: a sociodemographically matched study. Biol Psychiatry. 2002; 52(11):1066–1078.

10 Sapolsky RM, Krey LC, McEwen BS. Prolonged glucocorticoid exposure reduces hippocampal neuron number: implications for aging. J Neurosci. 1985; 5(5):1222–1227.

11 Andersen SL, Teicher MH. Delayed effects of early stress on hippocampal development. Neuropsychopharmacology. 2004; 29(11):1988–1993.

12 Teicher MH, Andersen SL, Polcari A, Anderson CM, Navalta CP, Kim DM. The neurobiological consequences of early stress and childhood maltreatment. Neurosci Biobehav Rev. 2003; 27(1–2):33–44.

13 Teicher MH, Dumont NL, Ito Y, Vaituzis C, Giedd JN, Andersen SL. Childhood neglect is associated with reduced corpus callosum area. Biol Psychiatry. 2004; 56(2):80–85.

14 Schiffer F, Teicher MH, Papanicolaou AC. Evoked potential evidence for right brain activity during the recall of traumatic memories. J Neuropsychiatry Clin Neurosci. 1995; 7:169–175.

15 Teicher MH. Scars that won't heal: the neurobiology of child abuse. Sci Am. 2002; 286(3):68–75.

16 Anderson CM, Teicher MH, Polcari A, Renshaw PF. Abnormal T2 relaxation time in the cerebellar vermis of adults sexually abused in childhood: potential role of the vermis in stress-enhanced risk for drug abuse. Psychoneuroendocrinology. 2002; 27(1–2):231–244.

17 Caspi A, Sugden K, Moffitt TE, Taylor A, Craig IW, Harrington H, McClay J, Mill J, Martin J,

Braithwaite A, Poulton R. Influence of life stress on depression: moderation by a polymorphism in the 5-HTT gene. Science. 2003; 301(5631): 386–389.

18 Nemeroff CB, Heim CM, Thase ME, Klein DN, Rush AJ, Schatzberg AF, Ninan PT, McCullough JP Jr., Weiss PM, Dunner DL, Rothbaum BO, Kornstein S, Keitner G, Keller MB. Differential responses to psychotherapy versus pharmacotherapy in patients with chronic forms of major depression and childhood trauma. Proc Natl Acad Sci U S A. 2003; 100(24):14293–14296.

19 Deblinger E, McLeer SV, Atkins MS, Ralphe D, Fao E. Post-traumatic stress in sexually abused, physically abused, and nonabused children. Child Abuse Negl. 1989: 13(3): p. 403–408.

20 Glod CA, Teicher MH. Relationship between early abuse, posttraumatic stress disorder, and activity levels in prepubertal children. J Am Acad Child Adolesc Psychiatry. 1996; 35(10):1384–1393.

21 Glod CA, Teicher MH, Hartman CR, Harakal T. Increased nocturnal activity and impaired sleep maintenance in abused children. J Am Acad Child Adolesc Psychiatry. 1997; 36(9): p. 1236–1243.

22 Bernet CZ, Stein MB. Relationship of childhood maltreatment to the onset and course of major depression in adulthood. Depress Anxiety. 1999; 9(4): p. 169–174.

23 Bremner JD, Vermetten E, Mazure CM. Development and preliminary psychometric properties of an instrument for the measurement of childhood trauma: the Early Trauma Inventory. Depress Anxiety 2000; 12(1):1–12.

24 Teicher MH, Feldman R, Polcari A, Anderson CM, Andersen SL, Webster DM, Navalta CP. Early adverse experience and the neurobiology of borderline personality disorder: gender differences and implications for treatment. In: Pearson KH, Sonswalla SB, Rosenbaum JF (eds.) Women's Health and Psychiatry. Lipincott, Williams & Wilkins, New York. 2002; pp 9–26.

10

The Brain in Stress – Influence of Environment and Lifestyle on Stress-Related Disorders

Rolf Ekman and Bengt B. Arnetz

10.1
Background

The association between psychiatric disorders and the immune system was first observed as early as 1927 by Wagner-Jauregg, who noted that when his mentally disturbed patients developed fever, their mental status improved.

Owing to an increasing awareness of the brain immune system interactions, a number of papers have recently been published on the relationship between psychosocial stress and the inflammatory response system.

It is becoming more and more evident that diverse types of psychosocial stress episodes early in life can be related to diseases that appear later in life, and these stresses are recognized as contributing factors for the health problems of many of today's societies.

To introduce the reader to these concepts, we have selected the most pertinent background information as:

- Different aspects of the stress concept, such as an adaptive multimolecular neuroendocrine–immune process as a result of prolonged psychosocial strain, down to some kind of an unstable molecular adaptation, changing over time.
- The effects of prolonged psychosocial stressors, such as inflammatory like reactions as an overall response to the psychosocial strain, and the influence of various lifestyles producing different courses of metabolic perturbations appearing during the development of different stress-related disorders (SRDs).
- The brain and stress-related mental disorders, such as anxiety, depression, suicide, posttraumatic stress disorders (PTSDs), and dementia. All of these disturbances, in the long perspective, are activities that tear down the nervous tissue of the brain, linked to inflammatory-like reactions.

To make the message of this chapter comprehensible to any reader without a biomedical background, the ambition has been not to describe too much of the underlying molecular detail, but instead to explain it in more general language. We will, however, give examples of different molecular sequences and some mechanisms

Stress in Health and Disease. Edited by Bengt B. Arnetz and Rolf Ekman
Copyright © 2006 WILEY-VCH Verlag GmbH & Co. KGaA, Weinheim
ISBN: 3-527-31221-8

that are thought to be involved in the progression of different SRDs, in particular those related to inflammatory-like processes of the nervous systems and in particular the brain.

10.2
Introduction

Physiologically, stress triggered neuroendocrine–immune responses are beneficial in the short run. In the long run, however, it can be detrimental to the body's resistance to illness.

Evolution has produced a close molecular link between the central nervous, endocrine and immune systems, in order to maintain the integrity and safety of the body against both environmental and psychosocial threats. Almost any change at the cellular level that results from exogenous or endogenous imbalance will initiate complex cascades of stress-induced reactions in an attempt to reestablish cellular balance. Of course, it is the nature and quantity of stress that to some extent predicts the outcome of the cellular response. Cellular revitalization from stress is not achieved when the damage is too great, or when one or more of the molecules of the stress-activated cascades are impaired.

The way life sculptures our personality – unique and elusive – and how our molecules make us who we are – our memories, emotions, consciousness and ways of coping with life – is of basic importance for the health outcome of the individual.

Research into the molecular interactions in health and disease between the brain and the immune systems as well as the endocrine system begins to reflect several of the mechanisms that underlie the concept of hormonal programming, able to alter behavior, memory, and in its extension are linked to disorders and diseases such as anxiety, depression, dementia and PTSD, particularly in children exposed to maltreatment. This has attracted much attention from researchers as well as teachers as an upcoming field of interest.

Several lines of evidence have suggested that people with certain types of personality are at risk for developing SRD later in life due to problems related to how they manage to handle and cope with their psychosocial environment and circumvent the influences of unhealthy life styles [1, 2].

Little is known about the different mechanisms converting psychosocial stress into cellular dysfunction. But the challenge of tomorrow is really to understand the molecular mechanism underlying how ordinary and persistent psychosocial stressors such as poverty, unstable parent–child relationships, lack of support, insulting and prolonged extreme psychosocial stress influence the individual health profile.

A beginning is to learn more about the biochemistry, different molecular interactions of the neuroendocrine–immune axes, and the sympathoadrenal axis. Understanding the individual (phenotypic) molecular mechanisms underlying chronic SRDs and their links with each other and to diseases such as depression and dementia is a rapidly growing research field.

10.2.1
The Dynamic Brain

The brain develops due to changes and different challenges of the environment and the old dogma that our adult brains remains a stable, unchanging, hardwired black box has had to be revised. During the last 8 years, neuroscientists have discovered that the brain does indeed change throughout life. They are saying that the brain can be extensively remodeled throughout the course of a life: change a behavior, a physical skill, a mental exercise, or a psychosocial environment and the brain changes accordingly.

The brain helps us to interpret and respond to different potentially acute and/or chronic stressful events, and the brain is also the target for the actions of stress-related molecules from the endocrine and immune systems.

The response of the brain to both acute and chronic stress must be discussed in terms of its capacity to demonstrate its dynamic plasticity. The term plasticity describes virtually any change in the brain, from the chemical level to the formation of new neurons and synapses, the place where neurons communicate with one another by way of chemical signals, neurotransmitters [3]. Prolonged or chronic stress has specific effects on the function of the synapses, especially on cognitive functions, and the brain may show signs of atrophy, cell death, as a result of chronic psychosocial stress, as well as after severe, traumatic stress.

Recent evidence indicates that the region of the brain that is best studied is the hippocampal formation; involved in different forms of memory function, it is particularly sensitive to prolonged and frequently occurring stressful events. The most severely damaged stress victims have significantly smaller hippocampal volume than the least impaired. Other brain regions such as the prefrontal cortex, and amygdala have also been reported to atrophy as a result of severe or chronic stress events.

Individual differences in stress responsiveness may play a role in making some individuals more vulnerable to their own stress molecules than others. What makes this personality variation a real challenge is that we are ignorant of the effects of the early stress responses and which molecular changes occur with different traumatic emotional circumstances more than 20 years ago. Another interesting question is how these traumatic circumstances may underlie a progression of molecular and structural changes reflected in several SRDs. What is of particular importance is that you cannot turn off your brain, which creates dysfunctional circuits within regions of the brain such as the frontal cortex, hippocampus and amygdala, of relevance for various forms of PTSD.

10.2.2
The Hypothalamic–Pituitary–Adrenal Axis

Different components of the stress response include enhancement of central nervous system processes and the hypothalamic–pituitary–adrenocortical (HPA) axis (Fig. 10.1), in particular, is becoming more and more a focus not only as a major

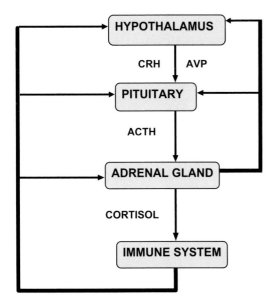

CYTOKINES, HORMONES, AND PEPTIDES

Fig. 10.1. A simplified diagram of the hypothalamic–pituitary–
adrenocortical (HPA) axis. *CRH* Corticotropin, *AVP* arginine
vasopressin, *ACTH* adrenocorticotropic hormone.

antiinflammatory actor, but more as a key link for the neurological, immunological
and endocrine systems [4].

During acute stress responses, different kinds of molecules, neurotransmitters
and hormones from the brain and endocrine system can improve immune function by informing the immune system about coming challenges and how to cope
with a specific situation. Even mental functions are improved during acute stress.

However, prolonged or chronic stress such as major life events, trauma, abuse,
or factors related to the environment in the home, school, workplace, family or
neighborhoods may have adverse effects on health, leading to exhaustion, distress
and disease. Both environmental, psychosocial and emotional stress activate the
production and release of the hormones corticotropin-releasing hormone (CRH)
and arginine vasopressin (AVP) from the hypothalamus. These hormones are
transported from the hypothalamus via the portal circulation to the pituitary where
they induce production of adrenocorticotropic hormone (ACTH), which enters the
blood circulation and cause the adrenal glands to release cortisol. When produced
in response to stress, cortisol has many different actions on several organs and systems of the body.

We may consider molecular components of the HPA axis, down- or upregulated
due to the effect of different particular circumstances, in several ways such as:

- a result of psychosocial stress in combination with an unhealthy lifestyle and/or the environment
- a primary defect, a genetic polymorphism, that reflects susceptibility for depression or other SRD
- intermediaries of biochemical and clinical expressions
- potential diagnostic and prognostic markers.

Classic endocrinology has taught us that the release of hormones from the pituitary is stimulated by hypothalamic releasing factors and downregulated by hormonal feedback from the adrenal gland and the immune system (see Fig. 10.1).

The result of increased or decreased release of CRH, AVP, and cytokines leads to health consequences relevant for:

- behavior changes such as depression, fatigue, pain, PTSD, and cognitive dysfunction
- neurobiologic changes such as modifications of the ratio of different neurotransmitters, the concentration and release of growth factors, protective molecules, brain function with cell loss, and in the long run, neurodegeneration
- several metabolic changes such as obesity, insulin resistance, osteoporosis
- immunological changes such as reduced immune responses, autoimmunity, different types of cancer.

10.2.3
Cytokines and Neuroendocrine–Immune Interactions

In general, cytokines are low molecular weight proteins that can be synthesized by a wide range of different cell types. They mediate cellular intercommunications through various mechanisms, operate within a complex network, and act either synergistically or antagonistically. As a result of their many modes of action, it is difficult to pinpoint the specific actions of individual cytokines at different cellular levels at different time intervals over a prolonged psychosocial stress experience.

Cytokines have three regulatory functions (a) within the cell; (b) on the cell membrane, such as signaling molecules, receptors; and (c) in the extracellular environment.

However, it soon became evident that cytokines are involved in key functions of the brain, such as the neuroendocrine regulation of: sleep, fever, food intake, memory and cognition. The cytokines can activate the brain in different ways: (a) several cytokines can be actively transported from blood to the brain; (b) the glia cells, the supporting cells to the neurons in the brain, secrete cytokines after antigenic activation; and (c) cytokine secretion in the brain can be stimulated by neurotransmitters such as noradrenaline. It is unclear if cytokines have different functional characteristics depending on whether they are released from the brain or other organs/tissues in the body. What is clear is that cytokines are central to several neurotransmitter and neuroendocrine responses that directly or indirectly contribute to a cognitive downturn such as general memory deficit and creativity, described among patients with mental disturbances.

It is now well-established that the nervous system is able to modulate immune activity, and on the other hand components of the immune system affect the function of the brain. The different actions of the cytokines within the brain have yet to be determined. Several studies have demonstrated an association between increased psychological stress with decreased immune function, mediated by altering the regulation of DNA and with consequences for the protein syntheses. Other relevant biological processes such as alterations in DNA repair, inhibition of programmed cell death e.g., apoptosis, might explain variance in disease outcome.

Different results have been reported in which DNA repair was positively associated with levels of perceived stress. These studies indicate that psychological factors have an effect on DNA repair.

Complex reactions have been described for peripheral cytokine actions, which are not necessarily translated directly to their action and regulation of the brain and the HPA axis.

However there are more and more indications that stress can induce inflammatory-like responses and that chronic stress may cause disorders and diseases in the endocrine, immune and nervous systems [5, 6].

Cytokines are the main inducers of an acute phase reaction and the major stress hormones, cortisol and adrenalin enhance this induction to a greater or lesser extent. It has been demonstrated in several studies that cytokine function within the pituitary regulates the synthesis and secretion of hormones.

A number of studies indicate that stress alone can induce a couple of reactions, characterized by fever, reduced social interaction, food intake and sexual activity, and increased sleep. The acute inflammatory response generally has a duration of about 24–48 h and thereafter the acute response turns down. At present it is difficult to describe the alterations from acute to chronic inflammation as a result of different psychosocial stressors and effects of disputable lifestyles, due to the lack of basic molecular knowledge.

If prolonged or chronic stress is important in the development of depression, we have to discuss the activity of the HPA axis and the HPA axis as part of important homeostatic mechanisms that regulate the degree of inflammation (Fig. 10.2), discussed later in this chapter (Section 10.4).

Cytokines induced by stress also cause increases in the concentrations of various lipids thought to participate particularly in the atherosclerotic inflammatory process. Studies of chronic job stress revealed increases of cholesterol. These changes were generally reversible in periods with reduced stress.

10.2.4
Psychoneuroimmunology

The introduction of the term psychoneuroimmunology, PNI, goes back to 1981 and is a field of research that deals with the complex interactions between the

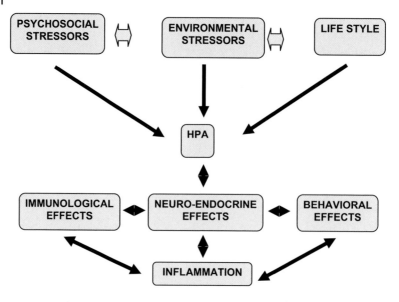

Fig. 10.2. Schematic representation of some of the inflammatory response.

brain, the endocrine and immune systems and how various forms of psychosocial stress can modify these interactions [7, 8].

Early PNI research focused on the suppressive effects of stress on the immune response. It later became clear that acute stressor exposure can enhance, as well as suppress, immune-mediated molecular interactions and direct reactions.

The existence of bidirectional pathways between the brain and the immune system could constitute mechanisms through which psychosocial factors influence the outcome of health. However, the association between stressful life experiences and susceptibility to diseases and the association between stressful life events does not establish a causal chain linking stress and immune function to various diseases. On the contrary, it is quite reasonable to suggest that environmental and psychosocial factors induce neuroendocrine changes capable of changing biologically relevant immune responses with clinical consequences.

A highly conserved and evolutionarily ancient cellular response can be engaged as a consequence of stress. Part of this response is mediated by heat shock or stress proteins. The heat shock proteins (Hsp) consist of several families of highly conserved proteins that play a role in a number of cellular functions and interact with molecules of signaling pathways that regulate growth and development [9, 10].

It is possible that during pathophysiological states such as atherosclerosis or dementia, likely candidates of SRDs, the Hsp proteins may exacerbate the chronic inflammatory processes that had started the atherosclerosis and dementia.

Indeed, there are growing numbers of indications that stress does not necessarily suppress the activity of the immune system, but may in fact enhance its activity.

What kind of activity that will occur is difficult to predict at any time because of the complexity of neuro–endocrine–immune systems interactions and the lack of a combination of biological and psychological research in this particular field.

Individuals who are stressed and depressed are more likely to have health habits that put them at a greater risk, including sleep problems, a tendency to alcohol and drug abuse, nutritional problems sometimes resulting in obesity and type 2 diabetes, and fewer exercise–health behaviors that have immunological and endocrinological consequences.

Future research in PNI will be needed to learn more about the molecular relationships and interactions between stress, psychological dysfunction, endocrine function, brain and immune functions and the interactions between these systems in order to get a better understanding of the function of the complex network to prevent us having different forms of SRD.

10.2.5
Is the Stress Response Comparable to an Inflammatory Reaction?

The immune system is regulated by sympathetic and parasympathetic nerves as well as by circulating neurotransmitters and hormones. As already mentioned, the available evidence suggests that diseases related to prolonged stress develop primarily as a consequence of long-term maladaptive changes in the brain–endocrine immune and sympathoadrenal axes of chemical modifications of the signaling molecules between these systems [11]. Thus the immune system may be able to display aspects of defense and damage highly relevant to many of the SRDs.

Current findings point to fundamental biological mechanisms in the molecular sensing of the psychosocial environment and the influence of the lifestyle. This particular molecular sensitivity changes the metabolic conditions and might generate the accumulation of proteins and other molecule complexes with abnormal structural conformation that are associated with the activation of inflammatory pathways.

Cortisol and monoamines, the major stress hormones, actually initiate a response characterized by production of cytokines, neuropeptides, and acute phase reactants as in an inflammatory reaction. Thus, the stress response evoked by psychosocial stimuli is similar to an inflammatory feedback.

A wide array of growth factors, proinflammatory molecules including cytokines, prostanoids, and neuropeptides contribute to the manifestation of inflammatory, neurodegenerative, and metabolic consequences, including increased risk for triggering cell-programmed cell death e.g., the apoptotic pathways, with influence on memory function, multiple subtypes of anxiety disorders, chronic fatigue syndrome, PTSDs, depressive illness sometimes together with chronic pain, early ageing, cancer and the metabolic syndrome (obesity, type 2 diabetes and high blood pressure) [12, 13].

It is probable that numerous mechanisms operate interactively in the setting of cytokine exposure. Cytokine-mediated inflammatory processes in the central nervous system involve a number of diverse reactions leading to different stages of neurodegeneration and changed synaptic transmission, and can also continue without neurodegeneration but will affect cognition to various degrees. As has been pointed out several times in this chapter this illustrates our lack of basic knowledge.

10.3
Relationship Between Chronic Stress and Stress-Related Disorders

Recently, a large number of studies reported that psychological stress and psychiatric illness reduce immune reactions. However, it turned out that the idea that stress reduces the immune feedback is an oversimplified statement, because the interactions between the neuroendocrine and immune systems can hardly be summarized in a few words, such is the molecular complexity of the interaction between the brain and the endocrine and immune systems *per se*.

Research and exploration of our basic molecular knowledge are now turning to the fascinating question of how a set of similar or even identical molecules is assembled in different ways in distinct cell types (organs, tissues) to control completely different biological processes and responses. That means that the individual molecules or clusters of molecules could act in several directions, and as cortisol, be the good or bad guy due to the actual circumstances.

The outcome of these interactions after various types of stressors depends on multiple variables; most important are the amount of stress, exposure time, coping behavior and strategies. What seems quite clear is that longer periods of mental stress or different forms of extreme stress have negative effects that may lead to loss of immune integrity.

Inflammation-like reactions might result from a number of causes: (a) protein structural changes, (b) protein aggregates or (c) accumulation of other abnormally modified cellular constituents. Most SRDs are associated with the accumulation of abnormal protein assemblies, and increasing evidence suggests that such protein assemblies can be components involved in the triggering mechanisms of cellular stress and the inflammation cascade of reactions.

It remains uncertain, however, to what extent the inflammatory changes associated with SRD explain why SRD are involved in the development and progression of several different diseases. Is it so that SRDs may hide elements of psychosocially triggered inflammatory-like reactions in the:

- nervous system, such as:
- mental disorders e.g., anxiety, depression, PTSDs, chronic fatigue syndrome, and schizophrenia
- neurodegenerative diseases e.g., dementia of the Alzheimer type, multiple sclerosis, amyotrophic lateral sclerosis and Parkinson's disease
- endocrine system, such as:

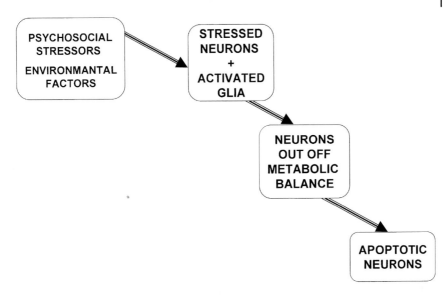

Fig. 10.3. A schematic representation of the neuronal and glial responses to prolonged psychosocial and environmental stressors.

- the metabolic syndrome including type 2 diabetes, obesity and high blood pressure
- immune system, such as:
- cancer and auto immune disorders.

Given the multiple functions of the many different inflammatory factors, it is often difficult to determine their roles in specific pathophysiological situations. Cytokines, chemokines, neuropeptides, and monoamines, as mentioned earlier, are among the key regulators of the inflammatory processes as a result of prolonged or chronic strains from the psychosocial environment. These different molecules regulate the activity and survival of inflammatory cells and mediate the communication of immune cells with each other and with other cells of the body. In fact, there is evidence for functional overlap between cytokines, chemokines and neuropeptides and their different target organs during extreme psychosocial stress.

These findings underline the importance of differentiating between the function(s) a molecule can fulfill and the specific role it plays in the progression of a SRD before manifestation in a specific disease. The associations between stress and diseases are based on a chain of different events such as; stressor(s), reaction to stress, and changes and abnormalities in the SRD regulation/response. Several studies have confirmed that not only the amount of hormone, neurotransmitter or cytokine is important in modulating a response, but that the prevailing molecular milieu of the cells e.g., for example in the brain, is crucial in determining whether there is an overall pro- or antiinflammatory effect and whether there will be a progression of various symptoms, turning into the development of some disorder, or later as a manifestation of disease (Fig. 10.3).

What is supported by several studies is that the outcome of chronic psychosocial inflammatory-like responses depends on the phenotype and on the specific environmental and psychosocial background interactions early in life, which may influence health outcome later.

That affective illness may be influenced by immunological processes and the production of cytokines is consistent with other evidence demonstrating that autoimmune reactivity is associated with enhanced emotionality.

10.4
The HPA Axis Out of Balance – a Link to Depression?

Stress and depression have significant impact on the quality of life for a majority of the inhabitants of modern societies.

Depression is described as a continuous course from a few symptoms over multiple subthreshold manifestations to the risk of later major depression. There are several risk factors and symptoms of depression signaling quite early in the process of developing a depression. Some important symptoms such as a lack of joy and interest, poor concentration, increased appetite, lack of energy and joint pain are early and prominent signs of an upcoming depressive illness. Many of the symptoms of depression appear behind different expressions, which often can be linked to stress, is generally described as a feeling of sadness, despair, and hopelessness as a result of resigned self-esteem. The neurophysiological alterations may be noticeable as disturbances in sleep, appetite, libido, energy.

Depression is one of the most common and perhaps most studied psychiatric SRD.

During an acute stress reaction the HPA axis and the sympathoadrenal system interact with other brain areas to enhance arousal and defense mechanisms. These reactions coordinate, interpreting information from different brain areas to ensure the survival of an animal or an individual. These responses are protective in acute situations.

However, in contrast to acute stress, prolonged, chronic stress gives the HPA axis a difficult and complex challenge, which may result in deregulations over long periods of time. Several observations indicate that it could result from an inability to make the appropriate adaptive responses from ongoing molecular perturbations as a result of a prolonged stress burden from an unhealthy psychosocial environment. Depression may result from a complex neural–endocrine–immune interaction triggered by prolonged stress situations and result in maladaptive changes in the HPA axis function [12–14].

Gender-specific aspects are important as female gonadal hormones modulate the HPA axis. There is also another issue to bear in mind: the variability of depression subtypes associated with differential HPA axis abnormalities. Results from studies done in younger populations are more heterogeneous than those done in adults.

There is a growing interest in perturbations of the neurological, endocrine and immune systems and how they may contribute to clinical depression and multiple subtypes of anxiety. However, there is a lack of information on how molecules of the immune system influence specific cellular components of the neuroendocrine systems and visa versa, in particular those molecules related to the development of different noticeable symptoms and the clinical progression of a depression.

Substantial evidence from many studies supports the early postnatal period being a critical time for the molecular programming of lifelong anxiety-related behavior that may predispose for depression later in life. Many clinical studies have demonstrated that divorce and bereavement increase susceptibility to anxiety and mood disorders in adulthood.

The mechanism linking stress with abnormal neuronal plastic events during brain development is thought to involve a specific serotonin receptor (5-HT1A) activity. Neuronal plasticity is the structural adaptation of neurons to functional requirements and plays an important role in brain development as well as learning and memory processes in the mature brain. Chronic stress has been shown to generate an explicit downregulation of these serotonin receptors in the hippocampus. This hippocampus insufficiency may partially explain the cognitive dysfunction observed in patients with depression. Of special interest are the interactions of immune system molecules with the adult brain neurogenesis, and that prolonged or chronic psychosocial stress causes a decrease in neurogenesis, which may be an important factor in the development of future episodes in the progression of a lifelong depressive illness [15].

Further understanding at the molecular level is likely to expand our ability to design future treatment strategies to control a progression of a depressive and inflammatory disease in which the neuroendocrine and immune axes as well as the sympathoadrenal axis play pivotal roles.

There is also growing evidence for an association between depression and later development of medical illnesses such as hypertension, type 2 diabetes, and decreased bone mineral density.

10.4.1
Cytokines and Depression

Several critical premises for a cytokine–neurogenesis interaction and its importance to different forms of depression appear to be more and more well-established.

As already mentioned, cytokines are a diverse group of small proteins that have been regarded first as a hormone of the immune system. However, it has now been demonstrated that a large part of the cytokines can be synthesized and released within the nervous system. The main part of the cytokines in the brain are secreted by the astrocytes and microglia, and only under certain conditions are produced by neurons. The glia cells have been compared with the immune system of the brain and have potential roles ranging from growth to protection.

As described in the previous section, depression is a recurrent disease; the interval between episodes tends to shorten while with each new episode there is increased risk for the occurrence of another. It is reported that the onset, recurrence and remission depend on harsh childhood conditions.

There is considerable individual variability in the immune response to prolonged stressful situations and the outcome of anxiety, and in particular depression. A depression may be associated with the enhancement of some of the components of the immune response, much like an infection, which eventually promotes suppression of other aspects of immune function.

Based on data from several studies it is quite conceivable that psychosocial stress is distinguished by the immune system and, through the secretion of proinflammatory cytokines, takes part in an integrated psycho–neuro–immune homeostatic response intended to prepare the individual to cope with the psychosocial strain of the lifestyle of our time and rapidly changing patterns into different habits such as the "now generation" of teenagers in the United States as well as the "Asian blues" among young people in Japan and China. The discovery that lifestyle and unhealthy societies can induce production of cytokines has important implications for human psychopathology, as there is now evidence of immune inflammatory responses in depression.

At present it looks like the cytokine hypothesis raises more questions than answers.

Depression may indeed be associated with impairment of some aspects of the immune system, and factors such as age-of-onset and psychosocial strain may be determining, as well as the loss of the ability to apprehend reality, so that after a while the individuals no longer seem to know why they are depressed.

10.4.2
Neuronal Atrophy and Loss in Response to Stress

It has been demonstrated in several recent preclinical and clinical studies that different categories of depression are accompanied by structural changes in the brain, including the prefrontal cortex and possibly other regions, and in particular by hippocampal atrophy. A reduction of brain volume of the hippocampal area has so far only been associated with hypersecretion of cortisol. Basic research studies have demonstrated that stress can result in atrophy and death of neurons in the hippocampus.

These data can provide an explanation for vulnerability to prolonged psychosocial stress and different types of depression e.g., the individual variation could result from (a) genetic or (b) problems with reestablishing a biochemical balance after different confrontations with the reality of life. Of course, these factors alone are not sufficient to cause neuronal damage and/or depression, but can create a state of increased vulnerability to subsequent exposure to psychosocial strain later in life.

Advances in molecular and cellular neuroscience have generated novel hypotheses to explain mechanisms behind the complex pathophysiology of different forms of depression. Several cellular signaling cascades and target genes have been identified, but a group of small proteins, the neurotrophic factors, has generated justified attention. Upregulation of neurotrophic factors could block or reverse the atrophy or cell loss resulting from prolonged psychosocial stress and depression. Measures of HPA axis activity should also be coupled with brain imaging studies and these studies will be helpful in investigating structure and function in different forms of mood disorders related to SRD.

10.5
Stress-Related Mental Disorders and Neurodegenerative Diseases

Neurodegeneration and stress seem to be connected with each other. Prolonged-to-chronic psychosocial stress has major functional influences at the cellular level of the brain, leading to biochemical, neurodegenerative, and structural abnormalities, with influences on learning and memory.

The reduction or loss of brain plasticity has been proposed as a common mechanism leading to the onset and progression of various neurodegenerative diseases.

As mentioned earlier, depression is a recurrent illness, the interval between episodes tending to shorten while each new episode increases risk for the occurrence of another. It has also been reported that the onset and reappearance depend on harsh childhood conditions.

Evidence from stress research for a connection between stress and neurodegenerative diseases as well as mental disorders begin to be more and more accepted [16].

Inflammation is an active defense reaction designed to remove or inactivate harmful components and to inhibit and reverse their negative effects. It typically can be triggered by invading microbes as well as by injurious chemicals or physical insults. Inflammation can also be triggered from within the organism by disorders affecting the immune system or the nervous system. When psychosocial stress continues over a period of time and become chronic, the immune system may be hyperactive and an increase of cytokines may occur together with acute phase proteins.

As earlier mentioned the cytokine–serotonin interaction plays an important role in the development of depression, and in some cases it shifts to neurodegeneration that disturbs all the coping strategies in the brain and may result in a treatment-resistant depression.

In neurodegenerative diseases, inflammation may be initiated by the accumulation of modified proteins by signals emanating from altered metabolism of cells in the brain or by accumulation of other abnormally modified cellular constituents, molecules from or associated with injured neurons or synapses an imbalance between pro- and antiinflammatory processes. Chronic inflammation might be maintained by cellular distress signals emanating from brain cells that survive for prolonged periods despite the accumulation of proteins. One of the outcomes of inflammation may relate closely to neurodegenerative diseases [17, 18].

Neurodegenerative disorders have been reported to be associated with accumulation of abnormal protein aggregates that may trigger the expression of different inflammatory-like responses. It is possible that the abnormal aggregates act as neuronal damaging agents in the brain and trigger inflammatory signals that increase the levels of inflammatory mediators such as cyclooxygenases and prostaglandin E2 seen in neurodegenerative disorders such as Alzheimer's disease, Parkinson's disease and amyotrophic lateral sclerosis. The mechanisms behind neurodegeneration are not well-defined. It has been demonstrated that exposure to the major brain prostaglandins can result in cellular events associated with neurodegeneration, as well as oxidative stress that hampers mitochondrial activity.

10.6
Unhealthy Environments; a Link to PTSD?

It is now widely accepted that a psychosocial environment including different types of psychological strain alters the internal homeostatic state of an individual. At first, different adaptive biochemical responses occur. These responses help the individual to cope with the situations, but may be damaging when experiences are extreme and prolonged, particularly if they occur early in life [19].

PTSD is a psychiatric disorder that can occur after confrontations with traumatic events. There is strict psychiatric definition of PTSD, but what is really understandable and the meaning of the word traumatic first referred to specific traumas such as; combat shock from war, physical attack, and later grew to include discussions of child physical maltreatment, and many more examples that are associated with a wider understanding of PTSD individual experiences [19].

The acute and prolonged effects of the related traumatic memories produced have complex molecular responses, which so far have not been characterized. Thus other types of psychosocial traumas will provide novel knowledge and information about the molecular relationships between stressful experiences and the neuro–endocrine–immune axes. Today we only have data indicating a HPA axis sensitization that results in increased HPA activity with every stressor, sooner or later leading to different symptoms of anxiety, depression and some of the other SRD-related problems. Again, it is important to underline the importance of analyzing subjects by gender, as male PTSD subjects have higher cortisol responses than females, indicating that studies on male subjects can not be generalized to female populations and vice versa.

Another aspect comes from recent research that indicates fundamental biological links between socioeconomic status, social relationships (including both social networks and social support), and health. We then shift gear to the aspect that some of the jobs that expose workers to unhealthy environments and boring repetitive tasks with a risk of increased stress levels are also obvious risk factors.

Studies have demonstrated that lack of control of one's life circumstances, increased social isolation and anxiety and depression can trigger neuro–endocrine–immune processes, which may be involved in inflammatory-like reactions that can weaken the body and predispose for some of the metabolic disturbances appearing early in SRDs.

Health differences in adult life have to reflect reciprocal interaction between the psychosocial environment, individual behavior, activities and social circumstances.

Since the beginning of 1990s employees are commonly faced with greater demands and less job security, both stressful events often followed by psychological disorders such as depression. Occupational stress is of increasing importance due to continuing structural changes in the workplace, with both increasing demands and insecurity imposed on employees.

However, there is a marked socioeconomic gradient in the number of disturbances of biological activities that contribute to disease risk. Recently differences in levels of circulating cytokines in groups with low socioeconomic status were described, interpreted as being due in part to chronic moderate inflammation and brain activation of stress pathways [20].

The literature is not univocal and it is possible that people with low income were more likely to be ill or infected, so it could be due to the different statuses of the subjects in different studies. There are methodological limitations to many of these studies. Thus, more extended monitoring might be required to demonstrate socioeconomic differences in cytokine responses to stress. It should also be emphasized that the lack of impact of socioeconomic status on cytokine response does not exclude other psychosocial factors from having influences. It was plausible that factors such as perceived stress, aggression, anxiety, and lack of social support might modulate the effect of socioeconomic status on cytokine responses.

10.7
Conclusions and Future Prospects

There is now accumulating evidence that there are many important interactions between the neuroendocrine and immune systems, which may explain, in part, some of the effects of mental dysfunctions which occur in the pathophysiology of acute and chronic psychosocial stress.

Studies are required to determine if "normalization" of brain, endocrine, immune, and sympathoadrenal axes (BEISA) dysfunction in animal models and in equivalent human states can restore aberrant signaling within such a complex system as BEISA. While fundamental molecular mechanisms help us identify the various elements of brain and immune system regulation, integrative studies allow us to analyze the complexities of these interactive systems in health and disease.

Future research in PNI will be needed to learn more about the molecular relations between stress, psychological dysfunction, endocrine function, brain and immune functions in order to get a better understanding of the function of the complex network that prevents us having different forms of SRDs.

If we want to convince people that there are important health benefits that could be gained by finding ways to reduce chronic stress and modifying poor health behaviors and thereby improve quality of life, we must all play our part and contribute to this challenging endeavor.

References

1 FRANCIS, D.D., CALDJI, C., CHAMPAGNE, F., PLOTSKY, P.M., MEANEY, M.J. 1999. The role of corticotropin-releasing factor-norepinephrine systems in mediating the effects of early experience on the development of behavioral and endocrine responses to stress. *Biol Psychiatry* 46:1153–1166.

2 HEIM, C., NEMEROFF, C.B. 2001. The role of childhood trauma in the neurobiology of mood and anxiety disorders: preclinical and clinical studies. *Biol Psychiatry* 48:1023–1039.

3 DUMAN, R.S. 2004. Role of neurotrophic factors in the etiology and treatment of mood disorders. *NeuroMol Med* 5:11–25.

4 HADDAD, J.J., SAADÉ, N.E., SAFIEH-GARABEDIAN, B. 2002. Cytokines and neuro-immune-endocrine interactions: a role for the Hypothalamic–pituitary–adrenal revolving axis. *J Neuroimmunol* 133:1–19.

5 MULLER, N., ACKENHEIL, M. 1998. Psychoneuroimmunology and the cytokine action in the CNS: implications for psychiatric disorders. *Prog NeuroPsychopharm Biol Psychiatry* 22:1–33.

6 KRONFOL, Z. 2002. Immune dysregulation in major depression: a critical review of existing evidence. *Int J Neuropsychopharmacol* 5:333–343.

7 IRWIN, M. 2002. Psychoneuro-immunology of depression: clinical implications. *Brain Behav Immunol* 16:1–16.

8 FLESHNER, M., LAUDENSLAGER, M.L.
2004. Psychoneuroimmunology: then and now. *Behav Cogn Neurosci Rev* 3:114–130.

9 LEWTHWAITE, J., OWEN, N., COATES, A., HENDERSON, B., STEPTOE, A. 2002. Circulating human heat shock protein 60 in the plasma of British civil servants relationship to physiological and psychosocial stress. *Circulation* 106:196–201.

10 PANAYI, G.S., CORRIGALL, V.M., HEDERSON, B. 2004. Stress cytokines: pivotal proteins in the immune regulatory networks. *Curr Opin Immunol* 16:531–534.

11 TSIGOS, C., CHROUSOS, G.P. 2002. Hypothalamic–pituitary–adrenal axis, neuro-endocrine factors and stress. *J Psychosom Res* 53:865–871.

12 TAFET, G.E., BERNARDINI, R. 2003. Psychoneuroendocrinological links between chronic stress and depression. *Prog NeuroPsychopharm Biol Psychiatry* 27:893–903.

13 MAIER, S.F. 2003. Bi-directional immune–brain communication: implications for understanding stress, pain, and cognition. *Brain Behav Immunol* 17:69–85.

14 RAISON, C.L., MILLER, A.H. 2003. When not enough is too much: the role of insufficient glucocorticoid signaling in the pathophysiology of stress-related disorders. *Am J Psychiatry* 157:683–694.

15 ANISMAN, H., MERALI, Z. 2003. Cytokines, stress and depressive illness: brain-immune interactions. *Ann Med* 35:2–11.

16 ESCH, T., STEFANO, G.B., FRICCHIONE, G.L., BENSON, H. 2002. The role of stress in neurodegenerative diseases and mental disorders. *Neuroendocrinol Lett* 23:199–208.

17 WYSS-CORAY, T., MUCKE, L. 2002. Inflammation in neurodegenerative disease – a double-edged sword. *Neuron* 35:419–432.

18 LI, Z., JANSEN, M., PIERRE, S.-R., FIGUEIREDO-PERERIA, M.E. 2003. Neurodegeneration: linking ubiquitin/proteasome pathway impairment with inflammation. *Int J Biochem Cell Biol* 35:547–552.

19 SHEA, A., WALSH, C., MacMILLAN, H., STEINER, M. 2004. Child maltreatment and HPA axis dysregulation: relationship to major depressive disorder and post traumatic stress disorders in females. *Psychoneuro-endocrinology* 30:162–178.

20 STEPTOE, A., OWEN, N., KUNZ-EBRECHT, S., MOHAMED-ALI, V. 2002. Inflammatory cytokines, socio-economic status, and acute stress responsivity. *Brain Behav Immunol* 16:774–784.

11
The Healthy Cortisol Response

Tommy Olsson and Robert Sapolsky

11.1
Introduction

A "stressor" can be defined as a challenge to homeostasis or, in more cognitively advanced species, the anticipation of such a challenge occurring. In response to stressors, a remarkably wide range of vertebrate species activates a fairly similar "stress response," an array of endocrine and neural adaptations. The most consistent features of the stress response involve the activation of the sympathetic nervous system (and its release of the catecholamines epinephrine and norepinephrine), and the secretion of glucocorticoids (GCs), which are adrenal steroid hormones. It is this class of hormones that is central to this review.

When released in response to an acute physical stressor (such as being chased by a predator, or the anticipation that this is about to occur), GCs are central to successfully surviving the stressor [1]. Coping with any acute physical stressor demands the transfer of energy from storage sites to exercising muscle, a key function of GCs. Moreover, such a transfer should be as rapid as possible, accomplished with increased blood pressure and heart rate, also an effect of GCs (although of smaller magnitude than the catecholamine role in this response). Furthermore, GCs help to defer long-term building projects that are unessential to immediate survival; this triaging includes inhibiting digestion, growth, tissue repair, and reproduction. Finally, GCs play a key role in enhancing cognition and sharpening sensory thresholds [2].

The importance of GC secretion during stress is best demonstrated by diseases in which it fails (e.g., Addison's Disease). Such maladies, if untreated, can prove fatal when an individual attempts something physically taxing.

Despite the adaptiveness of the stress response, chronic stress can be pathogenic. Originally, it was erroneously believed that chronic stress exhausts the capacity of the adrenals to secrete GCs. In fact, the pathologies of chronic stress emerge because the stress response, including the elevated GC secretion, if chronic, can become as damaging as the stressor itself.

Thus, if energy is constantly mobilized, it is never stored, producing muscle atrophy, fatigue, and an increased risk of insulin-resistant diabetes. Next, while

Stress in Health and Disease. Edited by Bengt B. Arnetz and Rolf Ekman
Copyright © 2006 WILEY-VCH Verlag GmbH & Co. KGaA, Weinheim
ISBN: 3-527-31221-8

hypertension is vital to sustaining a sprint from a predator, chronic hypertension damages blood vessels and, when combined with the metabolic stress response, predisposes towards atherosclerosis.

Deferring digestion, growth, repair and reproduction during an acute stressor is adaptive, but if chronic, increases risks of peptic ulcers, irritable bowel syndrome, impaired growth and tissue repair, irregular ovulatory cycles, and erectile dysfunction. Furthermore, the stimulation of immunity in response to stress (a short-term response to stress) soon gives way to immune suppression and impaired defenses against infectious disease, effects mediated by the GC excess. Finally, while short-term stress-induced GC secretion enhances cognition, chronic hypersecretion disrupts an array of aspects of neural function, the focus of this review.

These findings produce a double-edged sword. In the face of a typical mammalian stressor (i.e., a brief physical challenge), the elevated secretion of GCs is essential. However, during chronic stress, the hypersecretion can become pathogenic.

11.2
The Hippocampus as a GC Target

The most dramatic adverse effects of excessive GCs within the nervous system occur in the hippocampus, a brain region central to explicit learning and memory, and a primary GC target site (as illustrated in Figure 11.1). Two different classes of corticosteroid receptors exist which bind GCs, both of which occur in ample quantities in the hippocampus. A critical feature of GC action depends on this two-receptor system. The mineralocorticoid receptor (MR) is high affinity, and is normally nearly fully occupied under basal conditions, while the lower affinity glucocorticoid receptor (GR) is minimally occupied basally, and is only heavily occupied during major stressors. MR occupancy mediates a variety of salutary GC effects upon synaptic plasticity, cognition and neuronal survival, whereas it is heavy GR occupancy that mediates the adverse GC effects [3]. This produces an "inverse-U" pattern of GC actions in the hippocampus. Specifically, the transition from basal to mild or moderate stressors results in complete MR occupancy (with only a small increase in GR occupancy), producing salutary effects. In contrast, the transition to major stressors results in major GR occupancy, producing adverse GC effects. This makes intuitive sense; mild, transient stressors (i.e., stimulation) are typically beneficial and pleasurable. The forms of homeostatic challenge that we subjectively find to be aversive, and which carry pathogenic consequences, are typically ones that are severe and/or prolonged.

The adverse effects in the hippocampus of exposure to high levels of GCs include disruption of synaptic plasticity and of hippocampal-dependent cognition, atrophy of dendritic processes, inhibition of neurogenesis, overt neurotoxicity, and compromising of the ability of neurons to survive coincident insults. We now review the mechanisms underlying some of these GC actions.

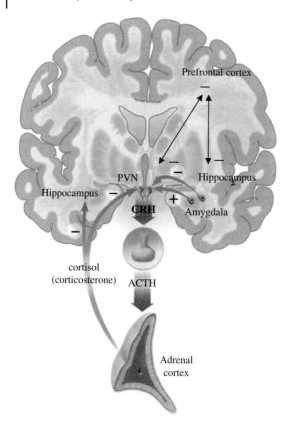

Fig. 11.1. The limbic-hypothalamic-pituitary-adrenal (LHPA) axis (modified from Nestler EJ et al, 2002). The LHPA axis forms a closed negative feedback loop. Corticotropin releasing hormone (CRH) from the paraventricular nuclei (PVN) in the hypothalamus stimulates release of adrenocorticotropin (ACTH) from the pituitary. ACTH mediates the release and synthesis of glucocorticoids (cortisol, corticosterone) from the adrenal glands. "Shutt-off" of stress responses are mediated by binding of glucocorticoids to receptors in the pituitary, hypothalamus and possibly the hippocampal formation and the prefrontal cortex. Note the inhibitory input from the prefrontal cortex and the hippocampus and the excitatory afferents from the amygdala on the hypothalamus.

11.3
Glucocorticoids, Stress and Synaptic Plasticity in the Hippocampus

GCs have varied effects on synaptic plasticity that readily fit into the inverse-U framework. Thus, in a low- or zero-GC environment, there is disruption of long-term potentiation (LTP) and primed-burst potentiation, two forms of synaptic plasticity that are thought to be central to, or at least good models for, learning and memory. However, exposure to GC levels at or above the upper physiological range disrupts such plasticity and strengthens the opposing phenomenon of long-term depression. While there is some disagreement as to which of these effects occurs in particular hippocampal cell fields, the broad features of the inverse-U pattern hold throughout the hippocampus.

Writ large, these findings suggest that synaptic plasticity in the hippocampus is optimal in the absence of stress and in the presence of mild stressors, but is impaired by more prolonged or severe stressors. This view is supported by studies involving stress, rather than GC manipulations.

The effects of GCs upon synaptic plasticity appear to be receptor-mediated genomic events, and fit within the two-receptor framework outlined above. Thus, the enhancing effects of low levels of GCs are mediated by MR, whereas the disruptive effects are mediated by GR.

A fair amount is understood about the mechanisms underlying these receptor-mediated effects. At the peak of an action potential, potassium channels open, allowing positively charged potassium to flow extracellularly. The prolonged opening of such channels produces the "afterhyperpolarization" (AHP), a period where the potential is even more negative than under resting conditions, transiently reducing neuronal excitability. The MR-mediated enhancing effects of stress and GCs involve reducing such potassium currents and shortening of the AHP. GCs, via GR, prolong AHPs, decreasing the likelihood that neurons will achieve the high firing rate needed for LTP or primed-burst potentiation [4].

Given these GC actions, it is not surprising that GCs should have disruptive effects upon hippocampal-dependent learning.

11.4
Glucocorticoids, Stress and Hippocampal-Dependent Cognition

An extensive literature now documents that GCs and stress regulate aspects of hippocampal-dependent learning and memory. The pattern of this regulation also forms an inverse-U; moreover, patterns of stress- or GC-exposure that enhance synaptic plasticity tend to enhance cognition, while those that disrupt plasticity disrupt cognition as well.

GCs are required for normal hippocampal-dependent cognition. Adrenalectomy impairs spatial memory performance and passive avoidance learning in adult rats (even under conditions in which there is no dentate gyrus neuron loss, a frequent consequence of adrenalectomy that will be discussed below), and such impairments are reversed by MR activation. Elevation of GC concentrations into the mild stress range enhances cognition. In contrast to the clear dichotomy established above regarding MR versus GR, in this case, these enhancing effects of mild GC elevations are mediated both by heavy MR occupancy, and by a mild, transient increase in GR occupancy. Supporting that involvement of GR, GR knockout mice are impaired in spatial learning.

Completing the inverse-U pattern, cognition is disrupted by severe or prolonged stressors, or by the GC levels commensurate with such stressors. In rodents, stress or the matching concentrations of GCs impair spatial discrimination learning and retrieval of long-term declarative memory. As expected, these effects are mediated by heavy and/or prolonged GR occupancy.

Thus, stress and GC levels in the stress range disrupt synaptic plasticity in the hippocampus, and hippocampal-dependent cognition.

11.5
Glucocorticoids, Stress and Neurogenesis

A revolutionary shift in neuroscience in recent years has been the extension of the pioneering work of Altman and colleagues, namely the recognition that there is ongoing, regulated neurogenesis in the adult hippocampus. Such neurogenesis is the focus of considerable current work, including some provocative, albeit as yet unreplicated, observations that such neurogenesis may be required for some types of learning [5].

Amid this work, it has become clear that GCs and stress modulate such neurogenesis, and in a manner commensurate with their other effects in the hippocampus. Stress and GCs inhibit hippocampal neurogenesis in rodents and nonhumans primates over the course of hours. Moreover, such effects are physiologically and etiologically relevant, in that exposure to predator odor is among the stressors that inhibit neurogenesis [6, 7].

At present, little is known about the mechanisms underlying such inhibition, beyond the fact that the phenomenon is N-methyl-D-aspartate (NMDA) receptor-dependent.

11.6
Glucocorticoids, Stress and Atrophy of Dendritic Processes

Arguably, the most distinctive feature of neurons is their heavily arborized dendrites; such processes make possible the vastly complex interconnections of neuronal networks. An extensive literature shows that a few days to weeks of stress causes retraction of dendritic processes in both the rodent and the nonhuman primate hippocampus [8]. Careful quantitative studies demonstrate that the atrophy arises from loss of apical dendritic branch points and decreased length of apical dendrites. Moreover, such effects of stress are mediated by GC secretion and subsequent activation of GR. Importantly, this atrophy is reversible; with the abatement of stress or GC exposure, processes slowly rearborize [9].

Some of the mechanisms underlying the dendritic atrophy are understood. The phenomenon is dependent upon activation of the NMDA subtype of glutamate receptor. Serotonin may also be involved, since the antidepressant tianeptine, which acts upon serotonergic synapses, blocks stress-induced dendritic atrophy [10].

Correlative data suggest that such stress-induced dendritic atrophy has adverse functional consequences. Specifically stress or GC paradigms that cause atrophy disrupt cognition as well, and pharmacological interventions that block the former also block the latter [9].

Thus, stress and GCs can disconnect neural networks in the hippocampus, with disruptive consequences. The recent literature shows, remarkably, that the opposite occurs in the basolateral amygdala and the bed nucleus of the stria terminalis, where sustained stress causes growth of dendritic processes [11]. This is thought to lead to enhanced amygdaloid excitability, and may be the cellular basis of stress-induced fear conditioning, a phenomenon dependent upon these brain regions.

11.7
Glucocorticoids, Stress and Neurotoxicity

Numerous studies indicate that GCs and stress can influence the survival of hippocampal neurons; as with many other realms of GC action in the hippocampus there is an inverse-U shape to such influences, but one of questionable physiological relevance. At one extreme, the pathological underexposure to GCs that occurs following adrenalectomy causes apoptotic death of neurons in the dentate gyrus. Low levels of occupancy of MR are sufficient to prevent such neurotoxicity; such occupancy induces expression of the key antiapoptotic protein bcl-2.

At the other end of the inverse-U, severe and prolonged exposure to stress or to high physiological concentrations of GCs can cause neuron death in the hippocampus. This was first observed in the 1960s in a little-appreciated report, and was subsequently replicated and expanded upon. Specifically, months (in a rodent) to years (in a nonhuman primate) of severe stress or GC exposure leads to loss of CA3 pyramidal neurons and, in some cases, CA1 neurons as well [12–14]. These early reports predated the use of unbiased stereology. With the introduction of stereology, a number of reports have failed to see hippocampal neurotoxicity following prolonged stress or GC exposure, amid a number continuing to report the phenomenon [4, 15]. As noted, some have questioned the physiological relevance of these reports. In the case of stress-induced neurotoxicity, this is because the regimes of prolonged, frequent and constantly shifting stressors needed to provoke such neuron loss are unlikely to occur in natural settings. In the case of GC treatment, while the concentrations utilized were typically in the (maximal) physiological range, the near constancy of exposure is not physiological.

Finally, heavy occupancy of only GR (by administration of a GR agonist such as dexamethasone) can kill neurons in the hippocampus, particularly in the dentate gyrus. Strikingly, such neuron death is apoptotic in nature, and can occur quite rapidly (over the course of hours or days). These studies are of obvious limited physiological relevance, given the artificiality of heavy occupancy of GR without saturation occupancy of MR (compounded by the use of dexamethasone concentrations, in some instances, that are sufficiently high to approach having nonspecific steroidal effects). However, they are certainly relevant to the clinical use of GR-specific agonists such as dexamethasone or prednisone, notably in situations with concomitant "endangerment" of neurons.

11.8
Glucocorticoids, Stress and the Endangerment of Hippocampal Neurons

The hippocampus is particularly vulnerable to necrotic insults such as seizure, hypoxia–ischemia, and hypoglycemia. Neuron death following such insults arises from excessive synaptic levels of excitatory amino acid (EAA) neurotransmitters such as glutamate and aspartate, resulting in excessive postsynaptic mobilization of free cytosolic calcium. Calcium excess causes promiscuous overactivation of calcium-dependent processes, leading to the generation of reactive oxygen species, cytoskeletal damage and DNA fragmentation that, collectively, lead to necrotic neuron death. It has recently come to be recognized that such necrosis triggers considerable inflammation, and that reactive inflammatory cells release sufficient amounts of cytokines and reactive oxygen species to damage bystander neurons that would have otherwise survived the insult. Finally, apoptosis is activated in a minority of moribund neurons. The advantage of this tightly regulated form of programmed cell death is that it is noninflammatory; the disadvantage (i.e., the factor which seemingly prevents it from occurring in all neurons destined to die after a necrotic insult) is that it is an energetically costly, active process. The severity and duration of the necrotic insult, the age of the cells, and the extent of energy availability all influence the likelihood of death by apoptosis, rather than by proinflammatory necrosis.

GCs and stress can impair the capacity of neurons to survive necrotic insults *in vivo*, including exposure to EAAs, global ischemia, hypoglycemia, antimetabolites, and cholinergic and serotonergic toxins [14]. These effects occur in all hippocampal cell fields, reflecting the high levels of GR expression throughout the rat hippocampus. The exacerbation of damage by GCs is apparent after a few days of GC exposure, can involve a tenfold increase in toxicity, and is steroid-specific and GR-mediated.

Insults such as seizure or cardiac arrest stimulate substantial GC secretion. Preventing such secretion (by adrenalectomy), or blocking GR decreases neurotoxicity. Thus, the typical extent of damage following an insult reflects, in part, GC-induced endangerment [4].

As reviewed, GCs have numerous peripheral actions that, theoretically, could be responsible for the endangering effects of the hormone. The GC actions, however, appear to arise at least partially through direct effects upon the nervous system. As evidence, GCs are endangering in primary neuronal cultures *in vitro*, and exacerbate the neuron loss caused by EAAs, hypoglycemia, cyanide, reactive oxygen species (ROS) the β-amyloid peptide, and gp120 (the glycoprotein of HIV). This endangerment also occurs in other brain regions, including the striatum, cortex and nucleus basalis, albeit less consistently or to a lesser extent than in the hippocampus. It should be noted that GCs do not worsen all insults. Exceptions include zinc neurotoxicity in hippocampal cultures and neonatal hypoxia–ischemia in rats. Moreover, GCs decrease damage caused by spinal cord trauma when used in supraphysiological megadoses, within a narrow time-window postinjury.

A number of mechanisms mediate the GC endangerment. These include the following.

11.8.1
Disruption of Neuronal Energetics

For most animals, stress is a physical challenge such as escaping a predator. At such times, GC adaptively divert energy to exercising muscle. This involves GCs inhibiting glucose uptake throughout the body. GCs do the same in the brain, inhibiting glucose uptake 15–25%, particularly in the hippocampus (or in hippocampal cultures).

These GC actions appear to have consequences during an insult. For example, GCs accelerate the decline in ATP levels in hippocampal neurons and glia during insults, and the endangering effects of GCs are lessened if neurons are supplemented with excess energy.

Necrotic insults such as stroke, global ischemia, hypoglycemia and seizure constitute energy crises (disrupting energy production or excessively consuming energy). In such crises, hippocampal neurons fail in the costly tasks of regulating EAA and calcium levels. GCs, by disrupting energetics, exacerbate the EAA and calcium accumulation during these insults; as evidence, energy supplementation can reverse these effects. While the source of the excess calcium influences the extent of damage at least as much as the absolute amount of calcium mobilized, a GC-induced increase in calcium load worsens the resulting ROS accumulation and cytoskeletal damage. GCs also decrease levels of reduced glutathione (the substrate for the antioxidant glutathione peroxidase), an effect secondary to the disruptive effects of GCs on energetics. These deleterious effects of GCs on various steps of this necrotic cascade are lessened when neurons are supplemented with excess energy substrates.

11.8.2
Endangering GC Actions that are Independent of Energetic Effects

There are also GC effects on EAAs, calcium and ROS that are likely to be nonenergetic, in that they occur in the absence of shifts in energetic profiles, or occur too quickly to be secondary to an energy deficit. For example, some GC actions on EAA or calcium trafficking are rapid. Moreover, in the absence of an insult, GCs rapidly increase voltage-dependent calcium conductance, calcium spike duration, and calcium-dependent AHPs in CA1 neurons. Within hours, GCs also decrease the expression of hippocampal PMCA-1 (plasma membrane calcium ATPase-1), which extrudes cytosolic calcium. Finally, GCs decrease the activity of catalase and glutathione peroxidase in the hippocampus in a manner that is at least partially energy-independent.

11.8.3
Disruption of Cellular Defenses

Neurons mobilize numerous defenses in response to insult. GCs impair some of these defenses. For example, the inhibition of synaptic glutamate removal or calcium extrusion by GCs can be viewed as impairments of defenses. Moreover, GCs block the defensive upregulation of glutathione peroxidase activity postinsult.

11.8.4
Glucocorticoid Endangerment and Apoptosis

As noted, following necrotic insults, a subset of hippocampal neurons die through the clean, tightly regulated pathway of programmed cell death called apoptosis.

GCs have long been recognized for their capacity to induce apoptosis in some immune cells. This has suggested to some that the endangering effects of GCs in the hippocampus are likely to involve increasing the number of neurons dying apoptotically. A pair of studies argue against this, reporting that GCs do not augment the apoptotic population of dead neurons, as assessed by a number of biochemical markers of apoptosis (cytochrome release from mitochondria, activation of caspases, internucleosomal cleavage of DNA). In contrast, one report suggests that GCs do indeed augment the apoptotic fraction (DeVries). This issue remains unresolved.

11.8.5
Glucocorticoid Endangerment and Inflammation

The preceding section reviews how GCs and stress can worsen the neurotoxicity of a variety of insults to the hippocampus. These findings, which have emerged over the last two decades, have always had to be counterbalanced in the context of the well-known antiinflammatory actions of GCs; such actions are not only exploited pharmacologically for a vast number of diseases outside the nervous system, but are also used heavily to decrease the inflammation associated with brain tumors. As noted, these insults cause considerable local inflammation, which adds to the eventual neuron death. Thus, following a necrotic insult, GCs seemingly have two opposing set of effects, namely their endangering actions at neurons themselves, and the protective antiinflammatory actions [14]. If the net result is for high-level GC exposure to worsen neurotoxicity, this implies that the endangering effects are more potent than the protective antiinflammatory effects.

This scenario has been called into question recently by the growing literature demonstrating that within the necrotically damaged nervous system, GCs often are not antiinflammatory and can, in fact, be proinflammatory [16]. For example, in rats undergoing sustained excitotoxic seizures, high stress levels of GCs augment the infiltration of inflammatory cells into the hippocampus and augment expression of proinflammatory cytokines; the magnitude of the GC effect on infiltration is sufficient to enhance neurotoxicity. Similarly, high levels of GCs potentiate expression of proinflammatory cytokines in cultured hippocampal neurons exposed to EAAs. Moreover, stress and stress levels of GCs exacerbate the hippocampal activation of the proinflammatory transcription factor NFkB following treatment with lipopolysaccharides. Thus, the endangering effects of GCs upon neurons may well be occurring in concert with, rather than in contrast to, the effects of GCs upon inflammation.

11.9
Clinical Implications

What, then, are the clinical implications of the data achieved in experimental settings? A clear excess in GCs, as in patients with Cushing's syndrome (due to an adrenocorticotropic hormone (ACTH) or cortisol-producing tumor) can lead to profound neuropsychiatric dysfunction. It is thus very common with increased irritability, sleep disturbances and anxiety in patients with Cushing's syndrome and a majority of patients fulfill criteria for major affective disorder whilst a minority of patients are manic. Cognitive impairment is distinctly common in these patients. This impairment can have a multifactorial background, as the often coexisting hypogonadism in this disease may contribute to neuronal dysfunction. Not unexpected, hippocampal-dependent tasks such as trace eyeblink conditioning are impaired in Cushing's syndrome and cognitive dysfunction links to hippocampal volume decrease. In addition, frontal-lobe-based working memory impairments, and widespread changes in brain metabolites have been found. Interestingly, cortisol levels associate negatively to hippocampal volume and this volume decrease seems at least partly reversible [17]. It is however possible that long-term cognitive dysfunction is not uncommon in this patient group.

Similar deficits are observed in patients given long-term GCs because of autoimmune or inflammatory disorders. In addition, healthy volunteers exposed for a number of days to GCs, or GR-specific agonists, show impaired declarative memory; this can be induced by pharmacological hormone levels and, even more importantly, by physiological levels.

Interestingly, increasing GC levels in some healthy humans predict poor hippocampal-dependent cognition and hippocampal volume loss [18].

Of note, there is disagreement as to which neuropsychological domains are disrupted by GCs. Some have interpreted GC actions as increasing nonspecific arousal, resulting in subjects paying less attention to relevant cues. Others suggest that GCs do indeed cause a direct impairment of cognition, rather than alter arousal state. In another view, GC actions are interpreted as representing a shift in attention during consolidation. Despite these different interpretations, there is agreement that it is hippocampal-dependent, declarative memory which is most impaired, and hippocampal-independent implicit memory tasks which are preserved.

Patients with Cushing's syndrome have profound changes in mood with sometimes a severe depressive state, as noted above. In non-Cushing patients with major depression, increased cortisol production and increased circulating levels of GCs have been linked to cognitive impairment as well as a decrement in hippocampal and prefrontal brain volumes. The reason for the volume loss in human hippocampi is not clear, but may relate to loss of neurons or glia cells, reductions in soma size of neurons and biochemical alterations linked to differential water content – as found in postmortem hippocampi in major depression [19].

Alzheimer's disease is a neurodegenerative disease that affects the hippocampal formation during the early phase of the disease [20]. A decreased sensitivity in hypothalamic–pituitary–adrenocortical (HPA) axis feedback, linked to increased GC production, is present in the earlier stages of this disease. Notably, the hippocampal formation has been suggested to be important for normal feedback function in the HPA axis, mainly based on rodent data. Interestingly, recent studies in humans link subtle alterations in negative feedback of the cortisol axis to cognitive dysfunction and loss of CA1 hippocampal volume. A vicious circle may thus ensue in this disease; increasing cortisol levels may accelerate neuron death through an endangering effect acting in concert with the (neurotoxic) degenerative process.

In stroke victims, increased cortisol production associated with multiple abnormalities in HPA axis regulation – notably decreased negative feedback and increased adrenal cortex sensitivity to ACTH stimulation – is linked to cognitive impairment and frontal brain damage. Exogenous glucocorticoids have been tried as adjunct therapy to other treatments in order to reduce the sequelae of the ischemic neurotoxic cascade that develops after critical brain ischemia. However, recent metaanalyses show that glucocorticoids in this setting have adverse effects on outcome. Of further interest is that endogenous cortisol levels at the extremes, i.e., abnormally low and high serum cortisol levels relative to the acute stress situation, during the acute phase links to increased mortality in these patients. Later, persistent hypercortisolism predicts the development of major depression, independent of other confounding factors; this is a major factor impeding stroke rehabilitation [21]. These study results are of obvious interest, relating glucocorticoids *per se* to mood changes.

11.10
Main Points

GCs are key to an adequate stress response, with effects on, in principle, every single cell in the body. However, adverse effects on the brain by long-term stress may to a major extent be mediated through increased GC exposure. The hippocampal formation is a main target for GCs, mediated by ligand activation of MRs and GRs. This may influence neuronal plasticity including neurophysiological signalling, neurogenesis and dendritic arborizing. Furthermore, neuronal death may ensue if excessive GC exposure and/or stress is present concomitant with brain insults such as ischemia and neurodegenerative disease. Clear links have been found in humans between increased circulating cortisol levels, decreased hippocampal volumes, mood and memory dysfunction. These alterations may form vicious circles and interrupting these chains of events by different means may be relevant for several diseases, including major depression, cognitive impairment and stroke.

11.11
Future

Further understanding of the initiating events during the development of brain dysfunction linked to HPA axis changes seems key in understanding putative treatment effects by influencing HPA axis regulation. It is possible that regulation of cortisol exposure to neurons in the hippocampus may be influenced by upregulation of receptor expression/function as well as by regimens aiming at reducing binding of cortisol to its receptors.

References

1 SAPOLSKY R, ROMERO M, MUNCK A. How do glucocorticoids influence the stress-response? Integrating permissive, suppressive, stimulatory, and preparative actions. Endocr Rev 2000; 21:55–89.

2 SAPOLSKY R. Stress and cognition. In: GAZZANIGA M, (ed.) The Cognitive Neurosciences, 3rd Edn. MIT Press, Cambridge, Mass., 2004; pp 1031–1042.

3 DE KLOET ER, OITZL MS, JOELS M. Stress and cognition: are corticosteroids good or bad guys? Trends Neurosci 1999; 22:422–426.

4 SAPOLSKY R. Stress, glucocorticoids and their adverse neurological effects: Relevance to aging. Exp Gerontol 1999; 34:721–732.

5 SHORS T, MIESEGAES G, BEYLIN A, ZHAO M, RYDEL T, GOULD E. Neurogenesis in the adult is involved in the formation of trace memories. Nature 2001; 410:372–376.

6 GOULD E, GROSS C. Neurogenesis in adult mammals: some progress and problems. J Neurosci 2002; 22:619–623.

7 KIM J, DIAMOND D. The stressed hippocampus, synaptic plasticity and lost memories. Nat Rev Neurosci 2002; 3:4534–4462.

8 MAGARINOS A, MCEWEN B, FLUGGE G, FUCHS E. Chronic psychosocial stress causes apical dendritic atrophy of hippocampal CA3 pyramidal neurons in subordinate tree shrews. J Neurosci 1996; 16:3534–3540.

9 MCEWEN B. Stress and hippocampal plasticity. Annu Rev Neurosci 1999; 22:105–122.

10 CZEH B, MICHAELIS T, WATANABE T, FRAHM J, DE BIURRUN G, VAN KAMPEN M, BARTOLOMUCCI A, FUCHS E. Stress-induced changes in cerebral metabolites, hippocampal volume, and cell proliferation are prevented by antidepressant treatment with tianeptine. Proc Natl Acad Sci U S A 2001; 98:12796–12801.

11 VYAS A, MITRA R, SHANKARANARAYANA RAO BS, CHATTARJI S. Chronic stress induces contrasting patterns of dendritic remodeling in hippocampal and amygdaloid neurons. J Neurosci 2002; 22:6810–6818.

12 KERR D, CAMPBELL L, HAO S, LAND-FIELD P. Corticosteroid modulation of hippocampal potentials: increased effect with aging. Science 1989; 245:1505–1509.

13 LANDFIELD P, BASKIN R, PITLER T. Brain-aging correlates: retardation by hormonal–pharmacological treatments. Science 1981; 214:581–584.

14 SAPOLSKY R, PULSINELLI W. Glucocorticoids potentiate ischemic injury to neurons: Therapeutic implications. Science 1985; 229:1397–1400.

15 SOUSA N, MADEIRA M, PAULA-BARBOSA M. Effects of corticosterone treatment and rehabilitation on the hippocampal formation of neonatal and adult rats. An unbiased stereological study. Brain Res 1998; 794:199.

16 DINKEL K, MACPHERSON A, SAPOLSKY R. Novel glucocorticoid effects on acute inflammation in the central nervous system. J Neurochem 2003; 84:705–716.

17 STARKMAN MN, GIORDANI B, GEBARSKI SS, SCHTEINGART DE. Improvement in learning associated with increase in hippocampal formation volume. Biol Psychiatry 2003; 53:233–238.

18 LUPIEN SJ, FIOCCO A, WAN N, MAHEU F, LORD C, SCHRAMEK T, TU MT. Stress hormones and human memory function across the lifespan. Psychoneuroendocrinology 2005; 30:225–242.

19 STOCKMEIER CA, MAHAJAN GJ, KONICK LC, OVERHOLSER JC, JURJUS GJ, MELTZER HY, UYLINGS HB, FRIEDMAN L, RAJKOWSKA G. Cellular changes in the postmortem hippocampus in major depression. Biol Psychiatry 2004; 56:640–650.

20 NÄSMAN B, OLSSON T, VIITANEN M, CARLSTRÖM K. A subtle disturbance in the feedback regulation of the hypothalamic–pituitary–adrenal axis in the early phase of Alzheimer's disease. Psychoneuroendocrinology 1995; 20:211–220.

21 ÅSTRÖM M, OLSSON T, ASPLUND K. Different linkage of major depression to hypercortisolism early versus late after stroke: results from a 3-year longitudinal study. Stroke 1993; 24:52–57.

12
Antistress, Well-Being, Empathy and Social Support

Kerstin Uvnäs Moberg and Maria Petersson

12.1
Introduction

Stress is a well-known physiological state. During normal circumstances, the stress and defense reactions are necessary for the ability of the organism to adapt to changes in its social or physiological environment. Continuous and strong activation of the stress system, however, leads in the long run to reduced well-being and also to physiological and psychological damage and even disease. The idea presented in this chapter is that the organism also contains powerful antistress systems. The antistress system does not only counteract the stress system, but it also increases tolerance of stress. Thus there is an active physiological antipole to stress. When the antistress system is activated, calm and relaxation prevails, and social interaction is stimulated, as well as processes that stimulate restoration, healing and growth of the body.

During the classical fight–flight reaction, some of the physiological mechanisms that are activated during stress are expressed. The activity of the cardiovascular system is increased to support the muscles with nutrients and oxygen. At the same time, the individual becomes wakeful, aggressive or afraid. The interpretation of environmental cues leads to a solution to the threat and may, depending on the circumstances, result in fight or flight.

When the state of antistress prevails the individual experiences calm and relaxation. Energy is used for anabolic purposes such as the storing of nutrients, growth and restoration, and not for catabolism as during the fight and flight reaction. In addition the state of antistress is linked to openness and positive social interaction. The antistress system which acts in part opposite to the fight and flight reaction might be named "calm and connection".

The stress and defense reactions are activated in response to harmful and painful (noxious) sensory stimulation, but also in response to other types of threats and dangers in the surrounding environment. Even internal threats and dangers such as unpleasant memories or the experience of being overstrained or unable to cope with a certain situation may activate the stress systems. In contrast, antistress reactions are activated in response to different types of harmless or pleasant (nonnoxious) sensory stimulation, such as touch, light pressure, warmth and closeness, but also in response to external factors of a calming, warming and supportive nature. In addition, positive memories and imaginations contribute to antistress.

A multitude of hormonal, neurogenic and complex neuroendocrine mechanisms in the peripheral and central nervous systems regulate and mediate the activity of the fight–flight or stress reactions. In a similar way the effects of the antistress system are mediated in a complicated interplay between nervous and endocrine mechanisms. Prolactin, enkephalin, beta-endorphin, GABA, serotonin, cholecystokinin and oxytocin are some of many hormones and neurotransmitters that participate in the antistress system.

In this chapter, we will describe how the neuropeptide oxytocin coordinates function in the antistress system. Oxytocin has the capacity to counteract stress reactions both as a hormone and as a neurotransmitter via a "micro nervous system" which originates from the hypothalamus and projects to other parts of the brain. For example, oxytocin counteracts or dampens the function of many of the mechanisms within the central nervous system (CNS) that coordinate and mediate the fight and flight reaction or stress reactions. At the same time, oxytocin stimulates the storing of nutrients, growth and healing through the activation of other mechanisms.

The role of oxytocin is unique in the sense that it mediates information from different parts of the body as well as from the environment to the brain. Different types of pleasant and positive experiences can, through our senses or through analogous psychological mechanisms, increase the release of oxytocin into the circulation and/or into the CNS. In this way pleasant or nonnoxious sensory stimulation will be transferred into a psychophysiological pattern consisting of mental calmness, physiological relaxation and positive social interaction, as well as stimulation of growth and healing.

12.2
Brief Overview of the Fight–Flight or Stress and Defense Mechanisms

The anatomy and the neurochemistry of the stress system are described in other chapters of this book. Only some fundamental data of relevance for the description and understanding of the function of the antistress system will be described here.

Important centers for coordination and regulation of the different factors in the stress system are located in the hypothalamus, the amygdala and the brainstem. Corticotrophin releasing hormone (CRH), which is produced in the amygdala and the paraventricular nucleus of the hypothalamus (PVN), holds a unique position as a main regulator and integrator of the stress system.

CRH containing neurons emanating from the amygdala project to and modulate the activity of the noradrenergic (NA) neurons, which originate from the locus coeruleus (LC) in the brainstem.

CRH produced in the PVN stimulates, together with the peptide vasopressin (also synthesized within the PVN), the release of Adreno corticotrophic hormones

ACTH from the adenohypophysis into the circulation, and thereby the release of cortisol from the adrenal gland. Both CRH and vasopressin are released from parvocellular neurons in the PVN e.g., into the hypothalamic–pituitary portal circulation to reach the adenohypophysis. CRH is in particular released in response to acute stress, whereas vasopressin plays a more important role during chronic stress.

CRH and vasopressin containing neurons in the hypothalamus also project to the brainstem, where they modulate the activity of the autonomic nervous system. CRH and vasopressin not only increase the activity of the sympathetic nervous system, but also reduce the activity of the parasympathetic nervous tone.

Thus, CRH and vasopressin can influence both the endocrine and the neurogenic aspects of the stress system. In addition, circulating vasopressin contributes to increased blood pressure through its contracting effects on the blood vessels (vasculature).

The NA system emanating from the brainstem, in particular the LC, is of great importance for stress and defense reactions. The level of arousal, wakefulness and aggression is enhanced when activity in the LC is increased. Moreover, the LC is connected to the autonomic nervous system and the sympathetic tone is increased. The stress related functions of the amygdala, hypothalamus and the brainstem are tightly linked to each other. For example, the NA input to the amygdala and hypothalamus increases the activity of the CRH- and vasopressin-containing neurons in these regions, just as the CRH neurons from the amygdala increase the activity in NA neurons emanating from the LC (see above).

The function in the stress system is influenced by many different levels of the nervous system. Noxious sensory stimulation from the skin activates the stress system of the hypothalamus. Environmental dangers and threats, experienced by more modern senses like vision and hearing, also activate defense reactions like the fight–flight reaction. The same type of reaction may be triggered by frightening memories or imaginations. The amygdala–hippocampus complex plays an important role in these mental reactions. The hypothalamic CRH neurons are under tonic inhibitory control from the hippocampus, and when this inhibitory pathway is disconnected, the hypothalamic stress axis becomes activated.

12.3
Deduction of Physiology of the Antistress Pattern from the Physiology of Breastfeeding

Both behavior and physiology are subject to changes in breastfeeding women. They become calmer and more socially interactive in connection with each breastfeeding episode. Simultaneously blood pressure and cortisol levels decrease. These changes may, after some time, become more or less permanent, i.e., changes in the personality profile towards increased calmness and social interaction occur. Further, a sustained decrease in blood pressure and cortisol levels is induced.

An important question to raise is how these breastfeeding-related effects are induced. During the breastfeeding period, estrogen and progesterone levels are low and therefore these hormones do not lie behind the antistress effects observed during breastfeeding. On the other hand, oxytocin and prolactin are released in connection to each breastfeeding episode to induce milk ejection and milk production, respectively. These hormones are both of importance for many of the physiological adaptations that occur during breastfeeding. Oxytocin is of particular interest since this substance, which is described more in detail below, is not only a hormone but also a neurotransmitter in an oxytocinergic micro nervous system in the brain. In addition, administration of oxytocin to animals mediates a pattern of effects reminiscent of the characteristics of the breastfeeding woman. Oxytocin induces calmness, stimulates social behavior and interaction and mediates a physiological antistress pattern. In support of a role for oxytocin behind the psychophysiological changes occurring during breastfeeding in women are the findings that the oxytocin levels measured during each breastfeeding session are related to the mental state of the women. The calmer and the more socially interactive the breastfeeding woman is, the higher and the more pulsatile her oxytocin levels are.

12.4
The Chemistry of Oxytocin

Oxytocin is a nonapeptide produced in the supraoptical (SON) and the paraventricular nuclei (PVN) in the hypothalamus. The chemical structure of oxytocin differs from that of vasopressin, the other neurohypophyseal hormone, by only two amino acids. Both peptides are produced in magnocellular neurons which project to the neurohypophysis, from where oxytocin and vasopressin are released into the circulation. Oxytocin and vasopressin are also synthesized in parvocellular neurons in the PVN. These neurons project to many different parts of the brain, including other parts of the hypothalamus, amygdala, hippocampus, periaqueductal grey (PAG), striatum, the raphe nuclei, LC, the dorsal vagal nucleus (DMX), the nucleus of the solitary tract (NTS) and the dorsal horn of the spinal cord. As a consequence, oxytocin may reach many important regulatory centers in the brain at the same time and thereby induce coordinated effect patterns. Oxytocin may, of course, also induce more specific neurogenic or endocrine effects. It is important to mention that oxytocin, like other peptides, does not easily pass the blood–brain barrier. Thus the circulating oxytocin and oxytocin derived from nerves in the brain constitute separate pools of oxytocin. However, the release of oxytocin into the brain and into the circulation is often activated simultaneously.

Only one oxytocin receptor, the uterine type of receptor, has been identified so far. The same type of oxytocin receptor has been demonstrated in the CNS, often in relation to oxytocin neurons. The distribution of oxytocin receptors varies between different species, and it is likely that additional subtypes of oxytocin receptors will be characterized. There are already data indicating that the antistress effects of oxytocin are linked to the C-terminal part of the oxytocin molecule, and that another receptor than the uterine type of oxytocin receptor is involved. Vasopressin, the sister molecule to oxytocin, has three types of receptors, V1a, V1b and V2, which mediate different effects in response to vasopressin.

The oxytocin molecule has some unusual properties, since it has the capacity to stimulate its own release, i.e., oxytocin has a positive feedforward mechanism. In contrast, C-terminal fragments of the oxytocin molecule seem to inhibit the release of oxytocin.

The distribution of oxytocin neurons in the brain is equal in males and females and plasma levels are almost the same. However, since estrogens increase the binding of oxytocin to the oxytocin receptors, some of the effects of oxytocin differ slightly between females and males. Estrogens may also increase oxytocin production and release. These latter effects are mediated through the estrogen beta receptor. In contrast, the related peptide vasopressin is modulated by testosterone. For example, testosterone increases the production of vasopressin in some parts of the brain.

12.5
Effects of Oxytocin

For a long time oxytocin was considered to be a female hormone that stimulated uterine contraction and milk ejection. However, during recent years oxytocin has been found to have many different behavioral and physiological effects.

12.5.1
Behavior and Social Interaction

Oxytocin, as well as some of its fragments, was quite early found to influence learning and behavior. The effects of oxytocin on learning and memory are complicated. Both improvement and impairment have been shown in different tests of learning. Oxytocin, however, always improves social learning, i.e., the ability to recognize other individuals.

One of the first behavioral of effects of oxytocin found was its ability to induce maternal behavior. Oxytocin administered intracerebroventricularly (ICV) induces maternal behavior in many mammals, even in female rats that have not given birth, if they have been pretreated with estrogens. With adequate sex steroid hormone levels oxytocin may also induce sexual behavior. It has recently been shown that social behavior is also stimulated by oxytocin. Rats, both males and females, treated with oxytocin increase their social interactions and grooming, both of themselves and also of other rats. The plasma levels and the pattern of sex steroid hormones are of importance for which of a wide spectrum of oxytocin-related effects will be induced.

As mentioned above, oxytocin administered to rats increases their ability to recognize other rats. In addition, the oxytocin-treated rat may often prefer the individual that was nearby when oxytocin was administered. Thus oxytocin can not only facilitate bonding or attachment for example between mother and child but also between female and male in monogamous animals, such as some species of voles. Interestingly the pattern of oxytocin receptors in the brain has been shown to differ between monogamous and nonmonogamous voles. The capacity of oxytocin to improve recognition of other individuals and to facilitate bonding or attachment is closely linked to the ability of oxytocin to stimulate social interaction. Experiments performed in sheep demonstrate that administration of an oxytocin antagonist or of peridural anesthesia to the ewe abolishes both maternal behavior and the bonding between mother and infant that normally follows parturition. It has also been shown that peridural anesthesia diminishes the release of oxytocin, which occurs in the brain in connection to parturition.

The important role of oxytocin for social behavior has recently been demonstrated in knockout mice that lack the oxytocin-producing gene. The knock out mice lose their ability to recognize other mice, and they lose their social competence. Note that this applies to both male and female mice.

In addition to the effects regarding social and interactive behavior, oxytocin has, in animal models, an antidepressive-like effect and oxytocin induces anxiolytic-like and sedative effects. The anxiolytic effect of oxytocin is exerted in the central amygdala, which is richly provided with oxytocin receptors. It has been demonstrated that oxytocin induces its anxiolytic effect by decreasing the production and the release of CRF in the amygdala. The recent finding that mice lacking the oxytocin gene are more anxious, afraid, stressed and have increased CRF levels in the amygdala compared to wild-type (normal) mice supports this assumption.

Oxytocin increases nociceptive thresholds, i.e., the oxytocin-treated rats are more tolerant to noxious stimuli. This effect is probably mediated at several sites in the CNS, for example in the PAG and the dorsal horn of the spinal cord.

12.5.2
Physiological Effects

Administration of oxytocin induces a whole spectrum of physiological effects. The acute pattern of effects is complex and sometimes difficult to interpret since different effects are induced depending on how and when oxytocin is administered and when the effects are studied. In rats, oxytocin may induce brief stress-like effects, such as a temporary rise in blood pressure and corticosterone levels when administered peripherally. Therefore oxytocin has sometimes been characterized as a stress hormone. However, these effects are never long-lasting and when the effects are observed over a longer period, they are converted into the opposite. These antistress effects become even more pronounced if oxytocin is administered repeatedly. As mentioned above, knockout mice lacking the oxytocin gene are more anxious and more easily stressed compared to their wild-type counterparts. In addition, they have higher levels of CRH in the amygdala. CRH levels also increase in the PVN, which is followed by higher cortisol levels and an increased tone in the sympathetic nervous system. Thus, studies of the oxytocin knockout mice demonstrate that the antistress effects in response to oxytocin dominate over the stress effects.

12.5.3
Long-Term Effects in Response to Repeatedly Given Oxytocin

The long-term and chronic effects induced in response to repeated oxytocin injections are of particular interest in this context. When oxytocin is administered repeatedly (one injection per day for 5 days), an obvious change of both behavior and physiology occurs. The rats become calmer, more socially interactive, have lower levels of cortisol, reduced blood pressure and increased nociceptive thresholds. Rats with difficulties in learning to avoid unpleasant stimuli improve their learning abilities when they are treated with oxytocin. These effects are sustained for approximately 10 days after the last oxytocin injection in males and for as long as 3 weeks in females. In addition, the oxytocin treatment changes the levels of some gastrointestinal hormones, as well as of insulin and insulin-like growth factor I. These changes facilitate digestion and storing of nutrients and female rats may even gain weight without an increase in food intake. Moreover, oxytocin improves wound healing and decreases inflammation.

Newborn rat pups treated with oxytocin in the postnatal period have lower blood pressure, decreased cortisol levels and increased nociceptive thresholds in adulthood. Some studies even indicate that these rats are larger as adults. Early administration of oxytocin may even induce an offspring which is calmer and less sensitive to stress throughout life. Oxytocin administered neonatally obviously induces the same pattern of effects as does oxytocin administered in adulthood, the difference being that the effects may become lifelong.

12.5.4
Mechanisms Involved in the Long-Term Effects of Oxytocin

The long-term effects in response to oxytocin are not related to the plasma levels of oxytocin. Since the half-life of oxytocin is only some minutes, the administered oxytocin disappears shortly after administration. Therefore it is likely that oxytocin activates secondary mechanisms, which mediate the long-term effects. A number of such oxytocin-induced secondary mechanisms have been identified.

The inhibitory effect of oxytocin on the stress system is not only mediated within the amygdala and the hypothalamus but also through the effects of oxytocin at several sites in the brain and in the periphery, which add to each other to induce the antistress effects.

The decrease in cortisol levels in response to oxytocin is caused by a change in the function of the hypothalamic–pituitary–adrenal (HPA) axis. The release of ACTH and CRH that normally occurs in response to decreased cortisol levels is lower than normal. At the same time, the pattern of glucocorticoid and mineralocorticoid receptors in the hippocampus – which is involved in the regulation of CRH release – is changed in a way that is consistent with antistress. In addition, the release, and probably also the production, of cortisol in the adrenal gland are decreased. Thus, the antistress effects in response to oxytocin are induced through counteracting the stress system both in the CNS and in other parts of the body.

Stroking of the ventral side of the rat induces similar effects as injections of oxytocin to the rat:

- Increased social interaction
- Sedative and anxiolytic-like effects
- Increased nociceptive thresholds
- Decreased heart rate and blood pressure
- Reduced corticosterone levels
- Modification of vagally controlled hormones
- Enhanced weight gain

Additional mechanisms behind the oxytocin-induced antistress effects have also been identified. A number of pharmacological studies have demonstrated that oxytocin treatment increases the function of alpha 2-adrenoreceptors within the brain. The activity of the alpha 2-adrenoreceptors has been linked to a basic physiological pattern of energy conservation.

Alpha 2-adrenoreceptors are situated both pre- and postsynaptically. Presynaptic alpha 2-adrenoreceptors inhibit the release of noradrenaline for example from neurons in the LC mediating lower arousal and vigilance etc. When noradrenaline and adrenaline activate the receptors that are situated postsynaptically, for example in the NTS, blood pressure and heart rate are decreased. This decrease is caused by inhibition of the sympathetic and stimulation of the parasympathetic nervous system which regulate the cardiovascular functions. Storing of nutrients is also stimulated, for example by stimulation of vagally controlled gastrointestinal hormones and insulin.

The fact that oxytocin induces this pattern of physiological effects in rats, for example decreased blood pressure, calm, and increased weight gain, is consistent with an increased alpha 2-adrenoreceptor function. In fact these effects in response to oxytocin are potentiated when the animals are treated with the alpha 2-adrenoreceptor agonist clonidine. For example, the decrease in blood pressure and the release of vagally controlled hormones such as insulin in response to clonidine are enhanced when rats are pretreated with oxytocin. Only half of a dose of clonidine is necessary to inhibit the activity of the noradrenergic LC neurons when the animals are pretreated with oxytocin. Studies by autoradiography show that the number or the function of the alpha 2-adrenoreceptors in areas where the oxytocin-induced antistress effects are meditated, for example in the amygdala, the NTS and the hypothalamus, is increased. In contrast alpha 2-adrenoreceptors in areas of the brain that do not contain oxytocin neurons or oxytocin receptors are not influenced by the oxytocin treatment. These studies support the assumption that there is a connection between the antistress and the growth-promoting effects of oxytocin and an increase in alpha 2-adrenoreceptor function.

A long-lasting increase in nociceptive thresholds is also mediated by repeatedly administered oxytocin. This long-lasting change in nociceptive thresholds seems to be caused by an increase in the activity of the endogenous opioids. The effect is probably mediated through my and kappa receptors, since the increase in nociceptive thresholds can be blocked temporarily by the opioid antagonist naloxone. The change in opioid activity is induced at several areas in the CNS, for example, the dorsal horn of the spinal cord and the PAG.

In a similar way, repeated oxytocin administration influences the activity of cholinergic and serotoninergic transmission and perhaps other signaling systems to cause long-term effects.

Oxytocin treatment of newborn rat pups induces similar, but even more long-lasting, effects as described above. These animals have an increased number of alpha 2-adrenoreceptors in the same areas of the brain as the adult animals treated with oxytocin. The postnatally treated rats also have a changed sensitivity in their dopaminergic receptors or the dopaminergic transmission. This is of particular interest since dopaminergic mechanisms are involved in bonding/attachment and social behavior.

In summary, repeatedly given oxytocin injections induces antistress effects, stimulates social behavior, as well as having restorative and growth-promoting effects. From a biological perspective the oxytocin-treated animals have a life strategy, which is opposite to that linked to the fight–flight and stress responses. It is extremely important to be able to defend oneself, but from an energy point of view it is expensive to mobilize energy for the muscles during the fight and flight reaction. Using oxytocin, attack and defense is substituted by calm and a positive interactive behavior. Energy is used for restoration and growth and in a more long-term perspective, for reproduction. This change of "biological principle" is based on a change in the function of other classical transmitter systems in a way that is consistent with this pattern. So far some of these functional adaptations have been described, but many more remain to be identified.

Some examples of signaling systems that can be modified by oxytocin is displayed in Fig. 12.1.

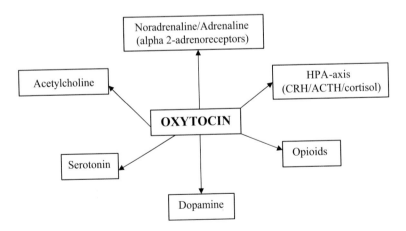

Fig. 12.1. Oxytocin induces long-term effects through influencing the activity in other classical hormone transmitter and receptor systems.

12.6
Release of Oxytocin in Response to Touch

It is well-known that oxytocin is released during parturition and in response to sucking during breastfeeding. Oxytocin can, however, also be released in response to other types of nonnoxious and pleasant sensory stimulation. Animal studies demonstrate that oxytocin is released in response to brushing, touch, stroking and warmth and in particular if these stimuli are applied on the ventral side of the body. The ventral side of the body is extra sensitive to this type of sensory stimulation.

Also data from humans show that oxytocin can be released in response to sensory stimulation. It is not only the baby's sucking, which stimulates oxytocin release, but also the sensory (skin-to-skin) contact between mother and infant. In addition the baby stimulates maternal oxytocin release by performing stroking like movements.

12.6.1
Sensory Nerves

Each sensory nerve contains several types of sensory fibers, which mediate different types of information. Touch is mediated via the thick, myelinated A-beta fibers. These fibers mediate the sensation of touch localized to specific areas in the sensory cortex of the brain. In addition, collaterals from these nerves reach more basal parts of the brain where they give rise to effects of physiological, behavioral and emotional natures. Recently it has been demonstrated that a subgroup of the thinner and more slowly conducting C-fibers can also be activated by touch. This finding is in contrast with what was previously assumed, i.e., that these types of fibers can only be activated by painful stimulation, and that they can in fact be activated by nonnoxious stimulation. The C fibers are, from an evolutionary perspective, older than the thicker and more rapidly conducting A and B fibers, and consequently these fibers are connected with older parts of the brain, where they influence emotions, physiology and behavior.

Painful and unpleasant experiences (such as toothache) do not only give rise to awareness as to from which part of the body the pain arises, but also to diffuse sensations of discomfort and even sickness. Analogously, fibers mediating the sensation of touch do not only give rise to the awareness of which part of the body that has been touched, but also to sensations of a calming, pleasant and relaxing nature.

Obviously these types of feelings and sensations have nothing to do with the sense of touch in the sensory cortex of the brain but are induced in older parts of the brain. They are not so distinctly localized from an anatomical perspective, but are diffuse and appear with a certain delay and may not even become conscious. The experiences can be compared with the feelings of well-being and relaxation that, after a while, follows ingestion of a good meal.

There is one more type of sensory nerve fiber that is worth mentioning in this context i.e., a special type of C-fiber that originates from the skin on the front side of the body. These fibers are linked to the CNS in a very special way, since they do not reach the CNS via the spinal cord, but instead follow the vagal nerves to the sensory areas in the brain stem. Thus the nuclei of these nerve cells are localized to the nodose ganglion and their axons terminate in the NTS. There is a direct NA connection from the NTS to the hypothalamus and the PVN and thereby to the oxytocin-producing neurons. The presence of these nerves may explain why more oxytocin is released, when the front side of a rat is stimulated by light stroking than with stimulation of the backside. Stimulation with this type of treatment (5 min at 40 strokes min^{-1}) also lowers pulse rate and blood pressure for several hours, elevates the pain threshold and makes the rats calmer. The effect on pulse and blood pressure in response to activation of these particular nerve fibers is probably in part exerted in the NTS via a change in the activity of the autonomic nervous system. By these "vagal reflexes" the sympathetic nervous tone is decreased and the parasympathetic tone increased, with consequent actions on cardiovascular function. The elevation of pain threshold and the calming and anxiolytic like effects are probably exerted higher up in the CNS, e.g., in the PAG, amygdala and LC by oxytocin released from oxytocinergic fibers originating in the PVN. Oxytocin released from such fibers projecting to the NTS probably reinforce the effects on pulse and blood pressure induced by the vagal type of sensory nerves mentioned above (Fig. 12.2). The connection between oxytocin and the massage-induced effects is supported by findings that some of the effects caused by this massage type of treatment are not induced if the animals are given an oxytocin antagonist. The oxytocin-like, massage-induced effects are summarized in Table 12.1.

12.6.2
Mother and Child Interaction

It is not, of course, possible to compare massage treatment of rats with interactions between humans. There are, however, certain similarities between the effects that are induced by massaging the front side of rats and the effects which are induced in response to the first meeting of all in humans, i.e., when the newborn infant is placed skin-to-skin on its mother's chest after birth.

In this situation the infant exhibits an inborn spontaneous behavior, i.e., the infant by itself moves to reach the mother's breast and start sucking. During this period maternal oxytocin levels rise. Before starting breastfeeding the infant massages the mothers' breast with its hands. Interestingly, the amount of oxytocin released in the mother is strongly related to the amount of hand movements performed by the baby, which supports the assumption that the release of oxytocin is triggered by the baby's hand movements. In this case mechanical energy has been transferred into an endocrine response.

When maternal oxytocin levels rise, milk is ejected and in addition the cutaneous blood vessels on the front side are dilated and skin temperature is increased. Obviously the mother does not only give milk, she also gives warmth to the baby.

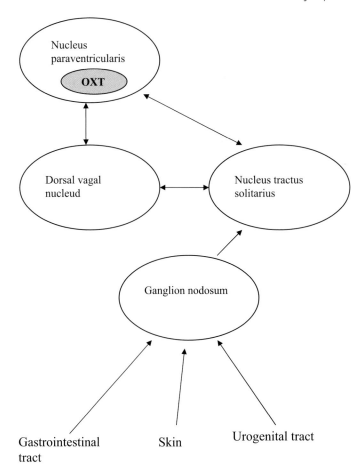

Fig. 12.2. Vagal afferents from different parts of the body stimulate the release of oxytocin from the paraventricular nucleus.

Tab. 12.1. Stroking of the ventral side of the rat induces similar effects as injections of oxytocin to the rat

---

- Increased social interaction
- Sedative and anxiolytic-like effects
- Increased nociceptive thresholds
- Decreased heart rate and blood pressure
- Reduced corticosterone levels
- Modification of vagally controlled hormones
- Enhanced weight gain

Since warmth also releases oxytocin a common feedforward process is initiated. At the same time cortisol levels and blood pressure decrease and the mother becomes calm and interactive. The pronounced release of oxytocin that is triggered by the interaction probably contributes to the relaxing effects in the mother, partly via an effect on the autonomic nervous system in the brainstem and partly via oxytocin which is released in other areas of the brain (just as in the rats receiving massage-like treatment).

The reactions taking place in the infants are not as well-known, but the temperature in the feet of the children rise immediately when the infant is placed in skin-to-skin contact on the mother's chest. The infants stop crying, which can be interpreted as an expression of calm. The sensitivity to pain also decreases. These changes do not occur if the infant is placed in a cot at the mother's side and, what is even more interesting, the changes occur at a much lower speed if the infant is dressed in clothes and held in the mother's arms. This finding demonstrates that the infant is influenced by the skin-to-skin contact, perhaps by activation of vagal reflexes and by oxytocin released in the brain when the sensory nerves, including the special vagal nerves on the chest side are being activated. The increased foot temperature is caused by a decreased activity in the sympathetic nervous system that ameliorates the cutaneous circulation in the feet. Oxytocin released in the brain may be related to the increased explorative behavior exhibited by the infant placed in the skin-to-skin position, and also to the calming effect and the fact that the infant becomes less sensitive to pain. In other words – the child staying with the mother is calmed and gets warm feet, whereas the infant that is separated from the mother becomes anxious and gets "cold feet".

12.6.3
The Same System is Activated in Connection with Sexual Activity

The pattern of effects induced by touch – which in part may involve oxytocin – during the mother–infant interaction is also activated in connection with other close relationships, not least in connection with sexuality. The increased circulation in the skin on the chest, the calm, the relaxation and the well-being, which is associated with sexuality, can in part be tied to a release of oxytocin in both men and women. Perhaps also the attachment, which may develop between the two individuals, is in part secondary to oxytocin.

12.6.4
Oxytocin Is Not Only Released by Stimulation of Sensory Nerves

Oxytocin is not only released in response to somatosensory stimulation, e.g., by touch, warmth and light pressure. Oxytocin-treated rats secrete a pheromone that makes rats in the close environment more socially interactive and calm. The effect of sound and light on oxytocin release has not yet been studied, but it is very likely that the oxytocin system can be activated by a multitude of calming stimuli irrespective of which type of sense is activated.

12.6.5
Conditioned Oxytocin Release

All mothers know that ejection of milk is facilitated after a period of breast-feeding.

The milk may start to flow when the mothers see their babies or when they hear them crying or even when they merely think of them. This also happens to the cow in the barn. The milk starts to flow as soon as the cow hears the sound of the milking machine or the person who is milking the cow. The oxytocin release that was originally triggered by a calf's suckling has developed into a conditioned reflex. This means that oxytocin release is triggered by a variety of stimuli or environmental factors that occurred at the same time as the original stimulation of oxytocin release. This is a clear example of classical Pavlovian conditioning. Pavlov demonstrated that the secretion of gastric juice or saliva, normally activated during ingestion of a meal, was after a while initiated when the dogs only saw or smelt the food. Even sounds that the dog heard and lights that the dog saw, when they received its food, could after a certain delay initiate the secretion of saliva and gastric juice even if the food was not presented to the dog. The difference between the example of the breastfeeding mother and the Pavlovian dog is that in the first case the release of oxytocin was conditioned and in the second case the secretion of saliva and gastric juice. It is very likely that oxytocin released by other stimuli than breastfeeding can also be conditioned in an analogous fashion.

12.6.6
Activation of Oxytocin Release via Psychological Mechanisms

As mentioned above, pain or damage to the body may induce defense and stress reactions. It is, however, more common that these systems are activated by mental activity in the sense that the brain, via more advanced mental processes, interprets the environment as dangerous or threatening. Such a comprehensive assessment is based on information obtained from the environment but also from previous experiences and memories, conscious or unconscious. By analogy, the brain may assess the environment in a way that results in an activation of the antistress system, which may involve oxytocin secretion. A safe, friendly and supportive environment informs the brain that the antistress pattern can be activated. Calm and relaxation is thereby induced and restorative processes and growth are promoted. Sensory stimulation, e.g., touch and warmth may serve as a prototype for the type of stimuli by which the antistress reactions are activated, but do not need to be present in the concrete sense. Instead mental stimuli of an analogous type may trigger these effects.

It is of importance to mention that oxytocin can also be triggered in response to certain types of stress and pain. Oxytocin may in these cases exert a stress-like effect pattern of short duration, but may above all serve as an endogenous stress or pain buffering system.

12.7
Health and Social Interaction

Many factors are well-known to exert negative effects on our health. Most people would agree that being substantially overweight and a smoker are important risk factors for the development of cardiovascular disease, and that it is possible to ameliorate your future health by reducing weight and by stopping smoking. It is also well-known that too much stress may facilitate the development of cardiovascular disease and that it is of importance to identify and remove unnecessary stressors and in order to decrease the risk for development of such disorders.

Knowledge about active and positive health-promoting mechanisms is more sparse. It has, however, become clear that good relationships and social support are related to a preventive effect against several types of disease, cardiovascular disease in particular. Obviously it is difficult to decide what is the hen and what is the egg in this context, but many epidemiological studies suggest that close positive relations, if they are experienced as good and supportive, do indeed have a true health-promoting effect, especially in men.

Positive relations can also be of a more down to earth type, i.e., to have a cat or a dog has also been shown to be good for your health, and in particular for your cardiovascular system and blood pressure.

12.7.1
How Does Closeness and Support Improve Health?

It has long been known that separations are related to stress and an increased risk for developing certain kinds of illness and disease. Separations not only lead to sadness and reduced well-being; they may also be followed by anxiety and depression and by an activation of the physiological stress systems. Data from animal as well as human physiology demonstrate that the activity in the sympathoadrenal system, as well as in the HPA axis, is enhanced with a consequent increase of pulse rate, blood pressure and cortisol levels. Obviously, loss and grief give rise to stress reactions, but it is of importance to ask the question whether something more happens when a close and beloved is lost? The fact is that the touch, warmth and support received in a close relationship also disappear as a consequence of separations. Perhaps the question that should be raised is whether warm and supportive relationships actively stimulate the bodies own antistress and healing systems and therefore have a positive and health-promoting effect?

12.7.2
Social Relationships

Data from animal experiments together with the oxytocin related adaptations shown to take place in breastfeeding women clearly show that oxytocin stimulates social interaction and also induces antistress-like effects. Touch and warmth are compulsory ingredients in positive, close relationships of all types. Since oxytocin is released in response to these stimuli, it follows that a long-term exposure to closeness in a relationship ought to result in physiological adaptations including relaxation and calm, an increased need for the receiving and giving aspect of social interaction. Obviously, other senses such as smell, vision and hearing as well as more advanced mental processes also contribute to this change.

If the organism is exposed to repeated sensory stimulation in close and positive relationships or if the brain interprets the surrounding world as good and support-ive the brain will be exposed to endogenous oxytocin. It is possible that as a con-sequence of this exposure to oxytocin, secondary biochemical effects are induced, e.g., a reduced activity in the HPA axis and an increased amount of alpha 2-adrenoreceptors. Such changes would make the organism less sensitive to stress and lead to stimulation of growth and restorative processes.

12.7.3
Lifestyle Without Closeness

The amount of interaction and closeness within the families has decreased as a consequence of changes in lifestyle. The microwave oven, the TV and the computer facilitate individual activities. The workload in our homes and in the working place steals time from social interaction with the other members of the family. In fact two major changes have occurred in parallel in our society, i.e., the amount of stress has increased and at the same time the natural input to the antistress sys-tems has decreased.

12.7.4
Touch Therapies

The strong link between stress on one hand and disease and illness on the other hand has increased the demand for and development of therapies that not only re-duce stress but also actively stimulate the antistress systems in the organism.

The increased use of touch therapies is an expression of this need. An increasing amount of investigations show that different types of massage, in particular those that focus on the effects of touch, not only release oxytocin, but also exert positive effects on body and soul which are in agreement with the antistress pattern. This fact may explain why a limited intervention consisting of 10 min of touch admin-istered when children in day care were resting, was shown to influence behavior of the children. With this type of treatment restless and aggressive boys became calmer and more socialized within a few months. This and many other studies demonstrate that extra massage and touch gives rise to positive effects and suggest that these types of interventions may serve as a partial substitute for the lack of physical contact that may have been received within the family setting.

The same type of effect can probably be achieved in response to several other types of therapy. Acupuncture has been shown to induce well-being, perhaps as a consequence of the touch and care received during the treatment. Relaxation and breathing therapies, meditation and some types of "energy" treatments may also give rise to antistress effects. Whether oxytocin is involved in these effects is very likely but remains to be demonstrated.

It is possible that also various types of psychological interventions or therapies just as a kind, caring and supportive treatment influence the same type of mechanisms. This type of positive influence does not occur only in therapeutic situations, but also in family life and in the workplace.

References

AMICO JA, MANTELLA RC, VOLLMER RR, LI X. Anxiety and stress responses in female oxytocin deficient mice. J Neuroendocrinol 16:319–324, 2004.

DIAZ-CABIALE Z, PETERSSON M, NARVAEZ JA, UVNÄS MOBERG K, FUXE K. Systemic oxytocin treatment modulates alpha 2 adrenoceptors in telencephalic and diencephalic regions of the rat. Brain Res 887:421–425, 2000.

ERIKSSON M, LINDH B, UVNÄS MOBERG K, HÖKFELT T. Distribution and origin of peptide-containing nerve fibers in the rat and human mammary gland. Neuroscience 70:227–245, 1996.

FOLKOW B, SCHMIDT T, UVNÄS MOBERG K (eds.) Stress and the environment. A commemorative issue for James P. Henry. Acta Physiol Scand 640, 1997.

KNOX S, UVNÄS MOBERG K. Social isolation and cardiovascular disease: an atherosclerotic connection. Psychoneuroendocrinol 23:877–890, 1988.

MATTHIESEN A-S, RANSJÖ-ARVIDSON A-B, NISSEN E, UVNÄS MOBERG K. Postpartum maternal oxytocin release by newborns: effects of infant handmassage and sucking. Birth 28:13–19, 2001.

OLAUSSON H, LAMARRE Y, BACKLUND H, MORIN C, WALLIN BG, STARCK G, EKHOLM S, STRIGO I, WORSLEY K, VALLBO AB, BUSHNELL MC. Unmyelinated tactile afferents signal touch and project to insular cortex. Nat Neurosci. 5(9):900–904, 2002.

PETERSSON M, ALSTER P, LUNDEBERG T, UVNÄS MOBERG K. Oxytocin causes a long-term decrease of blood pressure in female and male rats. Physiol Behav 60:311–315, 1996.

PETERSSON M, UVNAS MOBERG K. Systemic oxytocin treatment modulates glucocorticoid and mineralocorticoid receptor mRNA in the rat hippocampus. Neurosci Lett 343:97–100, 2003.

RYFF CD, SINGER B. Biopsychosocial challenges of the new millenium, Psychother Psychosom 2000 60:170–177.

UVNÄS MOBERG K. Oxytocin-linked antistress effects – the relaxation and growth response. Acta Physiol Scand 640, 38–42, 1997.

UVNÄS-MOBERG K. Oxytocin may mediate the benefits of positive social interaction and emotions. Psychoneuroendocrinol 23:819–835, 1999.

UVNÄS MOBERG K. The Oxytocin Factor. Tapping the Hormone of Calm, Love and Healing. Merloyd Lawrence, Boston, 2003.

UVNÄS MOBERG K, CARTER CS (eds.) Is there a neurobiology of love? Psychneuroendocrinology 23, 1998, 749–750.

WINSLOW JT, INSEL TR. Neuroendocrine basis of social recognition. Curr opin Neurobiol 14:248–253, 2004.

13
Stress, Sleep and Restitution

Torbjörn Åkerstedt

13.1
Introduction

Restitution is an important part of the body's response to stress. Sleep is particularly important in this context since it represents active restitution and seems to affect stress-related diseases. Unfortunately, the available knowledge is rather modest; we will examine what there is. In particular we will look at the direct relationship between stress and sleep, as well as at the more indirect evidence found in general sleep physiology, the effects of sleep loss on stress markers, and the role of sleep in stress-related diseases. First, however, a short introduction to the physiological description and measurement of sleep is necessary.

13.2
The Physiological Description of Sleep

Sleep is usually described using polysomnography, that is, a combination of different physiological measures. The electroencephalogram (EEG brainwaves) is the most important component, but eye movements [through the electroocculogram (EOG)] and electromyogram (EMG) (muscle tension measured from under the chin) adds to the information. The sleep EEG is measured and quantified in frequency and amplitude. The frequency is the number of waves per second and is measured in hertz (Hz). Amplitude is the size of the wave and is measured in microvolts (μV).

The polysomnography is then used to divide sleep into five stages depending on the EEG frequency and the amplitude.

- Stage 1 is a transitory phase from wakefulness to sleep and lacks restitution value. The EEG frequency is just below 8 Hz but has segments of faster activity. There are often slow, rolling eye movements and the EMG is slightly lowered. There should not be a total of more than 5% of stage 1 during the entire sleep.
- Stage 2 constitutes the "basal sleep", which takes up half of the sleep period.

Stress in Health and Disease. Edited by Bengt B. Arnetz and Rolf Ekman
Copyright © 2006 WILEY-VCH Verlag GmbH & Co. KGaA, Weinheim
ISBN: 3-527-31221-8

During this stage, the EEG has a frequency of 4–8 Hz with segments of short bursts, "spindles", with higher frequencies (4–16 Hz). Muscle tension is markedly reduced and the slow eye movements have ceased.

- Stages 3 and 4 constitute deep sleep, with what appears to be maximal restitution. The EEG frequency is lowered further and the pattern looks like rolling waves. The muscle tension is low; we are relaxed. During these stages we are very hard to awaken, and we are very confused when awoken. This deep sleep constitutes 15–20% of the total sleep period.
- Stage REM means "rapid eye movement sleep" (REM), and this is mainly where we dream (even if there are reports of dreams occurring in other stages as well). The EEG shows a high frequency and is similar to stage 1, while the rapid eye movements spatter in fast jerks on the EOG.

Sleep develops in cycles (Fig. 13.1) in which the sleep stages follow each other in a logical sequence. From the time of falling asleep the sleep stages appear in the order of 1 to 4 (together noted as nonREM or NREM), a process of about 20 min. After about 40–60 min in stage 4 there is a sudden appearance of REM sleep. After 5–10 min the REM sleep is over and transitions into stage 1 begin, and so on. This cycle is repeated four to six times per night (Fig. 13.2). Note that the deep sleep is always given priority and is allowed to dominate the first half of a sleep (Fig. 13.2).

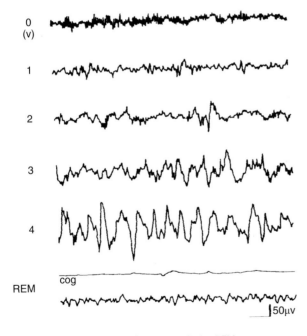

Fig. 13.1. EEG pattern for sleep stages 0–4 + REM.

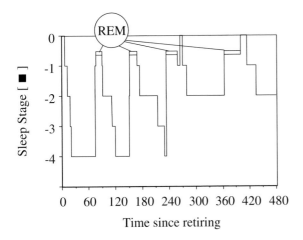

Fig. 13.2. Development of sleep from bedtime (0) across time.

At the beginning of the sleep, REM is compressed and is not allowed to develop to its fullest until the end of the sleep.

13.3
The Effects of Stress on Sleep

The first question is, of course, whether stress impairs sleep. We may here use two sources, human studies and animal studies.

13.3.1
Human Studies

Questionnaire studies of sleep usually show a close relationship between disturbed sleep and excessive work load. It is found, for example, that there are fewer sleep disturbances among individuals who are happy with their work and do not report any stress, and who have a good social support system at work. Not bringing work problems home appears to be especially important.

The number of physiological investigations of the effects of common life stress on sleep is surprisingly low. In addition, the stress levels that are used in such studies are fairly modest. Thus, there have been studies looking at students' sleep the night before a big exam, sleep before a day of skydiving, sleep when on call, or sleep before an early awakening. The results indicate a slightly negative effect on sleep efficiency and the amount of deep sleep. Other results suggest that it is the worrying and the tension before the following sleep or before the next day that are the most important factors. Sleep appears to contain less slow-wave sleep (SWS) under such circumstances. It has also been shown that sleep is disturbed under threats to national security, for example, after the nuclear accident at Three Mile Island and during the scud missiles attacks on Israel during the Gulf War. The effect of losing a life partner has been shown to have surprisingly modest effects – mainly an increase in REM intensity.

Posttraumatic stress (PTSD) is another well-established cause of disturbed sleep, even if many of the more common indicators of sleep quality (sleep latency, efficiency of sleep, total length of sleep, and amounts of stage 3 and 4) are relatively moderately affected. Instead it appears that the greatest part of the effect is connected to a disturbance of REM sleep, in particular in the form of increased or reduced amounts, or intensity, and a great number of awakenings. Unpleasant dreams also lead to a strong negative conditioning to the sleeping situation; one tends to avoid it.

If one turns the problem over and studies the physiology of insomniac patients (insomnia is assumed to result from stress exposure) one finds increased levels of stress parameters, such as cortisol levels, heart frequency, and body temperature. Today there is a tendency to see insomnia as a condition caused by increased physiological activation, probably as an effect of repeated stress. Repeated stress that occurs frequently prevents the normal development of sleep. This, in turn, gives rise to worrying about the next time one has to go to bed, which, in turn disrupts sleep, and so on. This vicious circle leads to an adjustment of the stress-regulating system and the establishment of a higher base level for physiological activation. This so-called allostatic regulation results in a relatively chronic sleep disturbance.

There also exists a number of laboratory studies of experimental stress (unpleasant films, etc.), but the results are inconclusive and suggest that laboratory stress may not be the right area to look for evidence.

13.3.2
Animal Studies on Stress

Over recent years, a series of animal studies have contributed to the understanding of the association between stress and sleep. An example of such knowledge is that during stress, through immobilization or "social degradation" in mice, SWS and REM decrease during exposure, but increase during recovery sleep. Exposure to stress that is terminated therefore leads to more and probably better sleep. The stress also changes the daily rhythm of corticosterone. Corticotropin-releasing hormone (CRH) [the releasing hormone of adrenocorticotropin (ACTH)] seems to mediate a part of the disruption of sleep due to stress. The stress-related increase of ACTH is linked to an increase in REM, and partly of SWS.

The effects of acute stress seem to be, in particular, centrally mediated since adrenalectomy does not modify it. It appears that CRH works as a neurotransmitter in the locus coeruleus and increases the activity in noradrenergic neurons, which increases REM. Different types of chronic stress (intermittent electric shocks, or learned helplessness) show increased REM during restitution. If the acute conditions of, for example, immobilization is prolonged, the increase of

SWS and REM disappears. Since adrenalectomized mice show a normal restitution of SWS and REM, and dexamethasone treatment recreates the stress effect, the peripheral corticosterone should be the mediating factor.

Both acute and chronic stress in rodents give a restitution of REM and SWS, which are both suppressed during the period of exposure. It is plausible that the effect is central and CRH-mediated since adrenalectomy does not influence the reactions. It appears, however, that chronic stress leads to disturbed sleep through increased levels of corticosterone.

13.4
Physiological Processes During Sleep

The normal physiological changes during sleep strongly suggest that sleep is a state of recovery. Sleep involves the entire central nervous system and indicates a dramatic physiological change. Metabolism and blood flow in most parts of the brain are lowered. The same happens to blood pressure, frequency of breathing, heart frequency, body temperature, and muscle tension.

On the other hand, sleep is a time of build-up through activation of the immune system and an increase in the internal secretion of, for example, growth hormone, testosterone, and much else. At the same time, there is a suppression of the internal secretion of hormones that raise the metabolism, such as cortisol or thyroid stimulating hormone. Thus, sleep appears to function as the opposite and the antagonist of stress.

Another interesting effect during sleep is that blood sugar remains at high levels instead of falling as it does during wakefulness. This effect is due to the effect of growth hormone (GH). The changes during sleep are of importance in relation to metabolism disorders (metabolic syndrome) that appear in connection with stress.

REM brings about a sudden increase in metabolism. Heart frequency, respiratory rate and blood pressure increase. In the brain, it is mainly the pons, hippocampus, amygdala, and the association cortex that are activated. The frontal lobes, which are important for planning, judgment etc., are not active.

REM plays an important role in learning, in particular for the consolidation of procedural memory. One of the main functions of sleep is probably to facilitate synaptic plasticity in the central nervous system's memory structures, that is, to create new connections between the brain's neurons. In addition, new research results indicate that even the deep sleep (SWS) can be related to the creation of new memories, but in particular declarative memories (e.g., years, names, etc.).

During REM, the muscle tension is also inhibited in all the positional muscles; it is not possible to sit or stand when dreaming. This means that REM provides an extreme form of relaxation. Whether this is of any long term importance in relation to stress is not understood. Furthermore, the hypothalamus stops regulating body temperature; even mammals become cold-blooded. The short duration of the REM periods counteract hypothermia.

13.5
Sleep and Stress Markers

Apart from the anabolic process during sleep and effects of stress on sleep one may gain information from the interaction between sleep stress markers. Apart from the suppression of cortisol during the early parts of sleep mentioned above, awakenings yield increased secretion of cortisol. Cortisol also appears to be negatively related to SWS, with a slight delay in that the decrease in cortisol precedes SWS by about 10 min.

The morning awakening is influenced by the rising ACTH levels. Thus, a subject who expects to be awakened unusually early will show an earlier peak of ACTH. If the predetermined awakening is set for a later time, the peak will occur later.

Infusing CRH reduces SWS during the sleep period, and REM during at least a part of the sleep. Infusion of ACTH results in an increased sleep latency, lowered SWS, and increased fragmentation. The effects of both CRH and ACTH are thus apparent sleep disturbances. Cortisol given during the day, however, results in increased SWS and decreased REM, probably through negative feedback via the hippocampus. Another interesting observation is that activation of mineralocorticoid receptors increases NREM sleep, while activation of glucocorticoid receptors increases wakefulness or REM.

The effects of stress on the immune system have been discussed in other chapters. However, several immune parameters also induce sleep, for example, interleukin-1β (IL-1β), tumor necrosis factor alpha (TNFa) and interferon Il-1β also contribute to the immune-regulating feedback that activates the hypothalamic–pituitary–adrenal (HPA) axis. IL-1β covaries with the sleep/wakefulness-cycle, and plasma TNFa increases during sleep deprivation. Disrupted sleep also worsens the natural killer cell (NK) functioning.

13.6
Sleep Loss

Another important aspect of the role of sleep in the regulation of stress is the effect of lack of sleep on stress markers. Thus, one night's sleep deprivation will result in increased cortisol levels the following night. It seems that the restitution from the high cortisol levels in the morning is slower after lack of sleep. It is possible that this can be interpreted as a disruption of the mediation of feedback of the hippocampus to the HPA system. This could have implications in connection with stress, and lead to raised cortisol levels, with additional effects on the hippocampus' HPA regulation. The latter can possibly also contribute to the cognitive problems (memory) that are associated with raised cortisol levels.

Another observation of metabolism and lack of sleep, is the lowered glucose tolerance: a slower elimination of glucose after a load, and a lowered insulin reaction. This can contribute to some of the negative metabolic effects that are associated with stress. Several researchers are currently working under the hypothesis that disrupted sleep could play a role in the connection with the development of age-related (type 2) diabetes.

Recently, is has also been shown that growth hormone, which plays an important part in glucose regulation during sleep, is decreased greatly with increased age. The level of growth hormone also seems to be directly related to a similar decrease of stages 3 and 4, and also an increase of the evening levels of cortisol. We do not yet know what this means, but these physiological age-effects resemble those of both a lack of sleep and the effects of stress.

13.7
Sleep Loss and Disease

Sleep is also related to several types of diseases that are considered to be stress-related. Thus, epidemiological cross-sectional studies have shown that depression in particular (and other psychological disorders), but also cardiovascular disorders are connected to severe sleep disturbances. In addition, cardiovascular disease and diabetes are predicted from prior sleep disturbances. In women, risks of reinfarction is increased in patients with sleep problems.

Sleep is also a predictor of overall mortality. Sleep durations deviating from 7 h per 24 h are associated with moderately increased risk, when controlling for a number of lifestyle factors.

We also know that sleep deprivation results in the immune system handling an influenza virus worse, and that many components in this system are weakened by sleep deprivation. Regulation of the immune system has been suggested as one of the main tasks of sleep.

13.8
Sleep Regulation

Finally, some of the understanding of the recuperative role of sleep may be gained from the way that sleep is regulated. Thus, the length of sleep, sleep efficiency (percentage of the time in bed spent asleep) and the amount of deep sleep (stages 3 and 4 or slow-wave sleep) increase with the time spent awake preceding sleep. Sleep becomes deeper than normal. Roughly, 1 h spent awake corresponds to 2–4 min of SWS. In addition, the awakening threshold is markedly increased; it becomes harder to wake up. Reduced sleep therefore leads to an increase in the need for sleep and to a shortened time to fall asleep (sleep latency).

Prolonged time awake leads to acute sleepiness and lowered levels of functioning, and also to a greater need for sleep and a shorter sleep latency. After the first 24-h period without sleep, performance may be lowered by 50%, and after two sleepless nights performance is at its lowest and there is a constant risk of falling asleep. After a day without sleep most people, however, can perform almost normally for one to a few minutes, but after only 3–4 min in a monotonous situation, the lack of sleep is clearly evident. Fragmentation of sleep gives similar results.

The amount of sleep that can be acutely lost without having any consequences on performance is 1–2 hours. If, instead, the sleep is reduced gradually with, for example, 15 min per week, the sleep pattern is changed so that the deep sleep takes over more and more from stage 2. The sleep is thus gradually becoming deeper and more efficient from a restitution point of view. Recently two studies have sought to determine what may be the minimum amount of sleep needed to prevent accumulation of sleepiness across several nights of sleep. Trying different daily sleep durations seem to arrive at 7 h. Below that level fatigue/performance impairment will start to increase over the days. This suggests that, at least under controlled laboratory conditions, 7 h may be a reasonable rule of thumb. Individual variation and contextual influences would have to be considered, however.

13.9
Final Comment

Apparently, stress influences a series of recovery processes during sleep and many of the processes during sleep involve the same physiological parameters as stress. However, there still remains a lack of detailed longitudinal/experimental studies of physiological changes during sleep in connection with naturally occurring stress.

References

ÅKERSTEDT, T., Sleep and stress. *Scand. J. Work. Environ. Health* (in press).

ÅKERSTEDT, T. and NILSSON, P. M., Sleep as restitution: an introduction. *J. Int. Med.* 2003, 254:6–12.

KRYGER, M. H., ROTH, T. and DEMENT, C. W. (Eds.), (2000). *Principles and Practice of Sleep Medicine* (3. ed.). Philadelphia.

RECHTSCHAFFEN, A. and KALES, A., *A manual of standardized terminology, techniques and scoring system for sleep stages of human subjects*. Bethesda, US Department of Health, Education and Welfare, Public Health Service, 1968.

SPIEGEL, K., LEPROULT, R. and VAN CAUTER, E., Impact of sleep debt on metabolic and endocrine function. *The Lancet* 1999, 354:1435–1439.

STICKGOLD, R., Sleep-dependent memory consolidation. *Nature* 2005, 437:1272–1278.

TONONI, G. and CIRELLI, C. Sleep function and synaptic homeostasis. *Sleep Med.* 2006, 10:49–62.

VGONTZAS, A. N., ZOUMAKIS, E., BIXLER, et al., Adverse effects of modest sleep restriction on sleepiness, performance, and inflammatory cytokines. *J. Clin. Endocrinol. Metab.* 2004, 89:2119–2126.

Stress and the Individual

14
Brain Mechanisms In Stress and Negative Affect

Mats Fredrikson and Tomas Furmark

14.1
Introduction

Brain mechanisms that regulate stress and negative affect have always attracted a lot of interest in the history of science. It is now even possible to study the brain mechanisms involved in affect regulation in humans *in vivo*. Early studies aiming at revealing neurophysiological mechanisms of importance for stress were predominantly restricted to lesion and stimulation studies in animals. Instead, stress responses measured in humans traditionally involved peripheral autonomic nervous system measures, endocrine parameters and other physiological alterations [1]. In particular, stress hormones such as cortisol, adrenaline and noradrenaline were sampled in studies aimed at determining stress-inducing and stress-reducing behaviors. Also in stress reactivity studies, measures of cardiovascular functions such as blood pressure and heart rate have been used extensively [2]. This approach has sought to characterize groups with given diseases like hypertension and myocardial infarction, to predict disease development from the nondisordered state and to evaluate the need for antihypertensive medication [3]. However, less is known about the brain mechanisms that govern the behavioral and bodily reactions associated with stress and negative affect. With the introduction of present-day brain-imaging techniques, that picture is rapidly changing.

14.2
Brain-Imaging Techniques and Paradigms

By use of noninvasive brain-imaging techniques it is possible to visualize structural, functional and neurochemical aspects of the living human brain. Since the introduction of these techniques some decades ago, there has been an increasing number of papers published using brain-imaging techniques. Recent reviews in Nature Neuroscience and Human Brain Mapping indicate that the number of published papers with brain-imaging techniques has shown an almost 100-fold increase in 10 years. In 2001, nearly 1000 papers on functional brain-imaging were

Stress in Health and Disease. Edited by Bengt B. Arnetz and Rolf Ekman
Copyright © 2006 WILEY-VCH Verlag GmbH & Co. KGaA, Weinheim
ISBN: 3-527-31221-8

published while in 1991 the number was less than 100. Even though the total number of papers published on emotion is lower than those on, for example, language and memory, there has been a steady increase in papers on stress and emotion over the years. Most published papers involve measures of neural activity using either positron emission tomography (PET) or functional magnetic resonance imaging (fMRI), which visualize brain hemodynamics. Most studies on emotive processes also involve activation studies, where one activated state is compared to a resting state or another activated state. Activation studies aim at localizing and isolating brain territories involved in certain mental processes. However, there are a number of different brain-imaging techniques that can visualize various other aspects of human brainwork [4]. These methods allow us to ask more complicated and specific questions on higher functions in the living human brain.

For example, in PET radioactive tracers are utilized to measure regional cerebral blood flow (rCBF) by means of ^{15}O-labeled water and glucose metabolism with ^{18}F-labeled fluorodeoxyglucose (FDG). PET may also be used to visualize neuroreceptor and transmitter characteristics in the brain. Examples of PET tracers used for this purpose are [^{11}C]WAY 100635 to characterize serotonin-1A receptor density and affinity, [^{11}C]-alpha-methyl-L-tryptophan and [^{11}C]-5-hydroxy-L-tryptophan to characterize presynaptic serotonin synthesis and [^{11}C]-3-amino-4-(2-dimethyl-aminomethylphenylthio)benzonitrile ^{11}C-labeled 3-amino-4-[2-(dimethylamino-methyl-phenylthio)]benzonitrile ([^{11}C]-DASB) that monitor reuptake functions within the serotonergic system. There are comparable tracers for other neurotransmitter systems. Single photon emission tomography (SPECT) is technically different but conceptually similar to PET, employing tracers such as 99mTechnetium-hexamethylpropylene amine oxime (TcHMPAO) that can measure cerebral blood flow and [^{18}F]-FDG for assessments of glucose metabolism. fMRI measures blood-oxygenation-level-dependent (BOLD) signal changes in the brain and is today probably the most common neuroimaging technique used in activation studies.

Maps that reflect regional brain activity during rest and in response to challenges may all be generated by means of PET, SPECT and fMRI. These techniques provide measures of subcortical as well as cortical neural alterations. Other imaging methods such as Xenon 133 inhalation, quantitative electroencephalography (EEG), and magnetoencephalography (MEG) can also generate functional brain maps, although these are more limited to cortical than subcortical areas. Besides functional neuroimaging, there are methods that permit measures of structural and other neurochemical characteristics of the brain. For example, computerized axial tomography (CT) and structural MRI enable volume calculations. Magnetic resonance spectroscopy (MRS) can be used to measure compounds like N-acetylaspartate (NAA), considered to be a marker of neuronal integrity and synaptic abundance. In sum, both brain structure and function may be revealed by neuroimaging tools that can provide measures of electrical, magnetic and metabolic changes, neuroreceptors and neurotransmitters as well as brain blood flow alterations. Even though most imaging methods yield maps of brain activity, they vary markedly e.g., with regard to spatial and temporal resolution. There are specific benefits and drawbacks associated with each imaging method that may affect the quality of the data obtained.

Functional imaging can be used to study brain activity, e.g., during cognitive activation, emotional experiences and perception [4, 5]. Particularly, PET- and fMRI-based measurements of blood flow alterations, expressed as rCBF or BOLD signal changes, in response to task activation have been used to reveal distributed neural representations of, for example, cognitive and emotional processes [6] and social cognition [7]. Activation studies frequently use subtractive designs in which a baseline condition (or reference task) is subtracted from the experimental condition of interest (the target task), resulting in regionally specific differences in brain activity corresponding to functionally specialized areas. For example, in studies of anxiety disorders induction of symptomatic anxiety states could be contrasted to a control condition, presumably revealing brain regions that are specifically engaged in the emotional response. In addition to subtractive analyses, event-related approaches as well as various forms of correlative and connectivity analyses exist, allowing more complex research designs to be used in neuroimaging. Also, functional and structural measures are sometimes combined, refining the understanding of their interplay.

14.3
Theories of Emotion and Neuroimaging Applications

The application of brain-imaging techniques in the areas of psychosomatic medicine, psychology and psychiatry has greatly expanded our knowledge of the functional anatomy mediating stress and negative affect [8]. In fact, the influence of those and other disciplines combined with modern brain-imaging methods has created a new area called affective neuroscience. Results from the emerging disciplines of affective and cognitive neuroscience have helped us to reorient or even redefine mind–body interactions in psychosomatic medicine as reflecting different aspects of brain activity. Imaging techniques have also been instrumental in tackling questions on the central nervous system architecture of emotions, and more generally on how emotions are organized and best described. For example, brain-imaging has been used to determine whether modular theories or circumplex models best describe emotions. Circumplex models presuppose that emotions vary across two dimensions, namely valence and arousal. The attempt then is to describe basic emotions, for example, fear, anger, disgust, sadness, surprise and happiness. This approach claims that basic emotions could be fully described by a given position in two-dimensional space [9]. An alternative perspective is offered by modular theories claiming that emotions are best described as distinct categories. The latter position maintains that emotions are evolutionarily shaped phenomena and that specific brain modules are designated to generate particular emotions. For example, the amygdala may be involved in detecting and generating the subjective experience of fear as well as regulating behavioral and physiological responses associated with this feeling state. Results from numerous animal lesion and stimulation as well as human neuroimaging studies have strongly implicated amygdala involvement in fear and negative affectivity in general [10]. A circumplex theory would then predict that certain areas in the brain would be specifically associated with valence and arousal respectively, and that different amounts of brain activity or certain patterns of activity in areas dedicated to valence and arousal would combine to produce a particular emotion. In contrast, a modular model would predict that different areas in the brain would be active during different emotions. Recently published studies suggest that rCBF during perception of emotional facial displays may be used to disentangle the two positions.

14.4
Dismantling Fear from Disgust: a Theory Test

Apart from fear, disgust is another negative emotion. When brain-imaging studies compared rCBF to pictures of fearful and disgusted faces different patterns emerged. While perception of fear predominantly seems to relate to amygdala activity, perceiving disgust involves activity in the insula cortex [9]. Thus, a modular rather than a circumplex theory of emotion best seems to accommodate the neurophysiological organization of emotional perception. Of course this does not mean that the experienced emotions could not be described as varying in valence and intensity, but the induction of emotions that differ in quality seems to rest on activity in separate brain territories. Also, even though modular processes specific to certain emotions may differentiate these from each other, there are also brain areas that are activated in response to emotional situations irrespective of emotional quality. For example, Lane and coworkers [11] have proposed, and provided data consistent with, a theory that part of the anterior cingulate cortex is activated during emotional experience regardless of hedonic tone. Naturally, the direction of causality between brain activity and emotional experience remains unclear, but data suggest that activity in certain brain areas segregate emotions with different quality from each other, while activity in other areas is common to different emotions.

14.5
Emotional Activation versus Emotional Control: Activating, Controlling and Modulating Brain Circuits

Imaging techniques have helped us to understand which brain areas are mainly involved in triggering emotions and which are the areas that predominantly seem to exert control over emotions. While the amygdala seems crucial in eliciting certain emotions, the prefrontal cortex is likely to be more involved in emotional control. Behavioral studies using neuropsychological tests have indicated that loss of prefrontal cortex is associated with diminished emotional control, and brain-imaging studies have particularly pointed out the anterior cingulate cortex as a regulatory node most likely affecting activity in the amygdala. This coupling provides a plausible mechanism for affect regulation in general, and raises the question of whether individuals having compromised affect regulation, ranging from poor impulsive control to disorders of mood and anxiety, display common and/or specific aberrant patterns of brain activity in emotive control areas of the brain, or if triggering areas are important. All of the areas mentioned so far, i.e., the amygdala and the insula, anterior cingulate and prefrontal cortices, have been suggested by a number of imaging studies [12] to form an important circuit for emotional control [8]. Thus, one would expect that problems of affect regulation observed in the anxiety disorders would involve altered activity in this emotional circuit of the human brain. Generally, this seems to be the case, and while patterns differ for different disorders there also seem to be some similarities.

14.6
Imaging Stress

14.6.1
Studies of Anxiety Disorders

Anxiety disorders are highly stressful syndromes and often involve an experience of loss of emotional control. For example, individuals with specific phobia for snakes or spiders consciously recognize that their fear is out of proportion to the situation. They may intellectually very well realize that a picture of a snake is only ink on a piece of paper but can not yet control their anxious emotional responses to the picture. Thus, phobic individuals are fearful against their better knowledge. This seems to be associated with an increased activity in the amygdala, but it declines rapidly with repeated presentations of the feared stimulus [13]. In addition, areas in the prefrontal cortex that seem to affect emotional control activate less when individuals with a specific phobia are fearful than when they are in a non-fearful state [14]. This supports that affect regulation is compromised either due to increased activity from triggering areas or as a result of decreased activity in control areas, corresponding to either bottom-up or top-down processes in the brain. Because symptom provocation with fearful stimulation activates the amygdala, but also at the same time deactivates the frontal cortex, it is hard to disentangle the effect of each process on the feeling state. Rauch, Whalen, Shin and coworkers have performed an elegant series of studies to separate these two putative mechanisms [15, 16].

14.6.2
Disentangling Studies

Posttraumatic stress disorder (PTSD) is characterized by profound anxiety reactions to cues associated with a previously experienced life-threatening trauma.

Symptom provocation with trauma-associated cues in PTSD has been reported to increase amygdala activity and diminish prefrontal cortical activity. To dissociate activity in one area from the other, probes that preferentially alter activity in one area but not in the other are needed. By backward masking techniques, where a brief stimulus (30 ms) is followed by stimulus of longer duration (500–1000 ms) it is possible to activate the amygdala without conscious knowledge of the masked stimulus pictures. Most often an angry or fearful face serves as the cue and a neutral face as the mask. Only the neutral face is consciously perceived. It has been demonstrated that backward masking procedures selectively activate the amygdala [17]. By using this technique in individuals with posttraumatic stress syndrome and by comparing activity in the amygdala with activity recorded from nonfearful individuals in response to the same stimuli, it is possible to determine whether the amygdala has an increased excitability in PTSD. This appears indeed to be the case. Rauch and coworkers demonstrated that the application of a backward masking protocol is associated with an increased rCBF response in the left amygdala of individuals with PTSD [15]. Thus, even in response to cues that are not directly associated with a traumatic event, individuals with PTSD overreact with amygdala activity suggesting a generally enhanced emotional reactivity.

In order to determine whether activity in the anterior cingulate that relates to emotional regulation is compromised in individuals with PTSD compared to in healthy volunteers, a probe that selectively activates the anterior cingulate is needed. One such task is the counting Stroop paradigm. In the counting Stroop, a varying number of words is presented and the subjects' task is to count and then to state the number of words. This response is delayed if the words contain threat, because threat automatically attracts attention and prolongs the reaction time of the subjects. Like the classic Stroop color conflict task and the emotional Stroop task, the counting Stroop also activates parts of the anterior cingulate [16]. By comparing individuals with and without PTSD in this protocol, it is possible to determine whether activity in the cingulate cortex is attenuated in PTSD patients. By demonstrating that the increase in rCBF during the Stroop task is lower in patients with PTSD than in controls, Rauch and coworkers were able to provide evidence that brain structures of relevance for emotional control seem to have a lower capacity in patients with PTSD. It is not clear whether those neural alterations are consequences of PTSD or if they constitute a vulnerability factor, but the results strongly suggest that emotion triggering is enhanced and emotional control is compromised in PTSD.

14.6.3
Function and Structure in Brain-Imaging

PTSD is associated not only with functional but also structural brain alterations [18]. A reduction in hippocampal volume has been found in several studies of individuals with PTSD using MR-techniques. In animal studies it has been observed that severe stress is associated with hippocampal atrophy (cf. Sapolsky and

McEwan, Chapter 12, this volume [19]). Stress is associated with a diminished hippocampal volume and when the stress ceases hippocampal volume is restored. Evidence suggests that increased cortisol levels may be a mediating mechanism accounting for this finding. Correlational data support this in humans as well, because patients with Huntington's disease having high cortisol levels show reductions in hippocampal size. The duration of depressive disorder is also a predictor of hippocampal volume, with more extensive periods being associated with more atrophy. Hippocampal volume is also associated with combat exposure in a dose–response-related fashion, with longer exposure being associated with smaller hippocampi. Based on the animal data, it is thus tempting to speculate that the smaller hippocampal volume in patients with PTSD results from combat exposure. This conclusion, however, is questioned by recent data from Pitman and colleagues [20]. They evaluated hippocampal size in monozygotic twins, where one but not the other twin had had combat experience in Vietnam. The relationship between PTSD severity and hippocampal size in the exposed twin replicated previous data with more severe symptomatology associated with smaller hippocampal volume. However, plotting the hippocampal volume of the nonexposed twin brother against the PTSD severity of the exposed brother yielded identical results. This pattern suggests that rather than being the result of combat exposure, hippocampal size may be a vulnerability factor. However, there was a long time lag between the return from Vietnam and present-day measurements of hippocampal volume and PTSD severity that may or may not introduce bias. For example, one could argue that the hippocampal volume might have been smaller on immediate return from the Vietnam War and that there might have been some cell growth thereafter. It is also possible that having a severely affected twin brother influences the mood and endocrinological status of the other brother and that cortisol-enhancing or cortisol-regulating mechanisms are activated, which in turn may influence hippocampal size. Thus, while the present data are intriguing, longitudinal prospective studies where hippocampal volume is used to predict the development of PTSD is needed to more firmly establish causality.

14.7
Relieving Stress: Treatment Studies

Additional support for the fact that the amygdala and the insula, anterior cingulate and prefrontal cortices are involved in emotional regulation would be provided if studies reducing anxiety and treating mood disorders were paralleled by an altered activity in emotional circuits. Generally, this seems to be the case, but successful treatment not only normalizes previously aberrant brain responses but also forms a more complex pattern of changes.

For example, Furmark and coworkers [21] studied the effect of the selective serotonin reuptake inhibitor (SSRI) citalopram and cognitive–behavioral group therapy

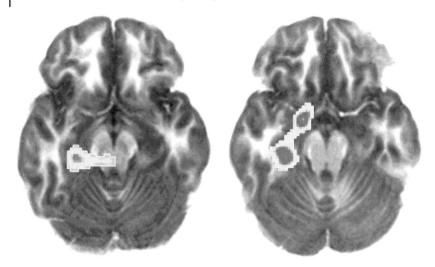

Fig. 14.1. Reduced activity [regional cerebral blood flow (rCBF)] in the medial temporal lobe in subjects with social anxiety disorder treated with cognitive–behavior therapy (*left*) or citalopram (*right*), as compared to waiting-list control subjects.

on rCBF during symptom provocation in social anxiety disorder (SAD). Subjects were scanned during an anxiety-provoking public speaking task before as well as after 9 weeks of treatment, and alterations in brain patterns were compared to a waiting-list control group. Both types of treatment were successful in alleviating social anxiety and it was noted that symptom improvement, regardless of treatment approach, was accompanied by a decreased neural response to public speaking in the medial temporal lobe, including the amygdala, the hippocampus, and the surrounding rhinal/parahippocampal cortical areas (see Fig. 14.1). Decreases were noted also in the anterior cingulate and prefrontal cortices. Before treatment, the amygdalo–hippocampal activity during public speaking stress was more elevated in patients with SAD than in normal healthy volunteers [22] (see Fig. 14.2), suggesting that effective treatments normalize hyperactivity in these brain areas. On the other hand, activity in widespread cortical areas in which abnormalities were noted when comparing untreated patients and controls were not affected by the therapies given. This suggests that treatments involve some normalization, but also other adaptive metabolic changes in the brain. As also noted in imaging studies of mood disorders [23], some brain anomalies may persist after therapy even though patients improve. The short-term and long-term effects of treatments may also correspond to different brain patterns [23]. However, at present only short-term responses have been thoroughly studied.

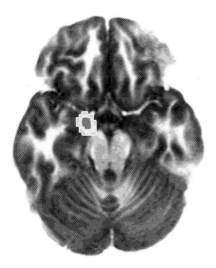

Fig. 14.2. Increased activation [regional cerebral blood flow (rCBF)] in the amygdaloid complex in subjects with social anxiety disorder ($n = 18$), as compared to healthy controls ($n = 6$), in response to a stressful public speaking task.

14.8
Genetic Influences on Stress and Brain Activity

It might be argued that the involvement of certain brain areas in regulating emotion and negative affect would be further strengthened if genes known to affect emotional behavior were also associated with activity in those areas. Genetically based predictions could be relatively fine-tuned because a number of mutations are functionally characterized. This means that it would be possible to predict in a more general fashion the brain areas that would alter as a consequence of genetic makeup, but also more specifically which neurotransmission system would be affected. For example, one of the most consistent findings relating genetic structure to negative affect is tied to a specific mutation in the serotonergic reuptake transporter gene [24]. This functional polymorphism in the serotonin reuptake transporter involves a short and a long repetition sequence. The short sequence is associated with more anxiety-related behavior and also with a compromised reuptake of serotonin, resulting in higher concentrations in the synaptic cleft in those with the allele having the short rather than the long repetition sequence [24]. The short allele is associated with an altered rCBF response to stress [25, 26].

There are several other lines of evidence to suggest that serotonergic activity is important both in normal anxiety and in anxiety-related disorders. First, in animals it has been demonstrated that perturbations of the serotonergic system are associated with alterations in emotional behavior [27]. Second, anxiety disorders including SAD, PTSD and also depression are responsive to SSRIs, implying that alterations in the serotonergic system affect anxiety and mood. The polymorphism in the serotonin transporter gene has been demonstrated to modulate the response to treatment with SSRIs [28].

Recently, it has been demonstrated that the short allele of the serotonin transporter is associated with enhanced fear conditionability, suggesting that its effect on anxiety-related behaviors may interact with environmental factors [29]. Similarly it was demonstrated that the short allele carries an increased risk for depression, but only in the presence of a number of severe life events like losing a loved one or being abused [30]. Those with the longer version of the gene were spared the adverse effect of exposure, but not those having short copies. Also, when viewing emotion-containing pictures those with a short allele activate the amygdala comparatively more than those having the long allele [25]. Conceptually, similar results have been obtained for patients with SAD. When the patients were studied during a stressful public speaking task, which resulted in anxious feelings and behaviors, those carrying a short allele showed more profound rCBF increases in the amygdala than individuals with long alleles [26]. Thus, at least emotion-triggering areas seem to activate more in those with the short than in those with the long variant of the allele. Whether this polymorphism also influences areas of relevance for emotion regulation is an interesting matter for future research.

14.9
Psychosomatic Stress and Emotional Brain Circuits

It is evident that several diverging lines of evidence strongly implicate the amygdala and the insula, anterior cingulate and prefrontal cortices being involved in the regulation of emotion. Studies of emotional activation in normal healthy volunteers, comparisons of disordered states with healthy controls, the effect of treatment responses as well as correlations with genetic markers of known behavioral and neurophysiological effects strengthen the importance of the emotional brain circuit previously outlined in regulating emotion and its behavior. To the extent that psychosomatic disorders reflect the interaction between central nervous system processes related to emotion and bodily responses, one would predict that known risk factors for psychosomatic disorders would be associated with activity in the emotional circuit of the brain. Without reviewing the literature exhaustively we will give a few examples where this seems to be the case. Anxiety, particularly panic disorder is associated with an increased risk for sudden cardiac death [31]. Sudden cardiac death is also associated with compromised heart rate variability, particularly a reduced respiratory sinus arrhythmia that mainly reflects vagal influence to the heart. In addition, reduced sinus arrhythmia is a known risk factor for cardiac deaths in the general population. Thus, if psychosomatic processes leading to premature cardiac death were key mechanisms mediating the effect of anxiety on cardiac death, one would suspect that emotional areas in the brain would be involved in the control of respiratory sinus arrhythmia. Supporting such a psychosomatic perspective a couple of recent studies [32, 33] have demonstrated that respiratory sinus arrhythmia and heart rate variability are related to activity in the subgenual part of the anterior cingulate cortex, particularly the so-called affective division of the cingulate cortex. This suggests that anterior cingulate functions may relate anxiety and cardiac death to each other via activity in a common brain network. In addition, the electrodermal system being highly responsive to arousing stimuli is also linked to activity in anterior cingulate cortex as well as the prefrontal cortex. Electrodermal activity has been frequently used to index arousal, habituation and fear conditioning [34]. Thus, converging lines of evidence suggest that physiological processes often studied in psychophysiology and psychosomatic medicine may be linked to activity in the emotional circuit of the brain.

In conclusion, brain circuitry of relevance for emotion and stress also seem to be implicated in processes involved in psychosomatic medicine and health mechanisms in behavioral medicine.

References

1 Selye H. *The Stress of Life*. McGraw-Hill; 1976.

2 Fredrikson M, Matthews KA. Cardiovascular responses to behavioral stress and hypertension: A meta-analytic review. *Ann Behav Med* 1990;12:30–39.

3 Tuomisto MT, Majahalme S, Kähönen M, Fredrikson M. Psychological stress tasks in the prediction of blood pressure level and need for antihypertensive medication: 9–12 years follow-up. *Health Psychol* 2005;24:77–87.

4 Fredrikson M, Furmark T. Brain-imaging studies in social anxiety disorder. In: Bandelow B, Stein DJ (eds.) *Social Anxiety Disorder*. New York: Marcel Dekker; 1994, pp. 215–233.

5 Illes J, Kirschen MP, Gabrieli JDE. From neuroimaging to neuroethics. *Nature Neurosci* 2003;3:205.

6 Rauch SL, Shin LM, Wright CI. Neuroimaging studies of amygdala function in anxiety disorders. *Ann N Y Acad Sci* 2003;985:389–410.

7 Adolphs R. Cognitive neuroscience of human social behaviour. *Nature Rev Neurosci* 2003;4:165–178.

8 Davidson RJ, Putnam KM, Larson CL. Dysfunction in the neural circuitry of emotion regulation – a possible prelude to violence. *Science* 2000;289:591–594.

9 Calder AJ, Lawrence AD, Young AW. Neuropsychology of fear and loathing. *Nature Rev Neurosci* 2001;2:352–363.

10 LeDoux JE. *The Emotional Brain: The Mysterious Underpinnings of Emotional Life*. New York: Simon & Schuster; 1996.

11 Lane RD, Reiman EM, Axelrod B, Yun LS, Holmes A, Schwartz GE. Neural correlates of levels of emotional awareness. Evidence of an interaction between emotion and attention in the anterior cingulate cortex. *J Cogn Neurosci* 1998;10:525–535.

12 Wager TD, Luan Phan K, Liberzon I, Taylor SF. Valence, gender, and lateralization of functional brain anatomy in emotion: a meta-analysis of findings from neuroimaging. *NeuroImage* 2002;19:513–531.

13 DILGER S, STRAUBE T, MENTZEL HJ, FITZEK C, REICHENBACH JR, HECHT H, KRIESCHEL S, GUTBERLET I, MILTNER WH. Brain activation to phobia-related pictures in spider phobic humans: an event-related functional magnetic resonance imaging study. *Neurosci Lett* 2003;348:29–32.

14 FREDRIKSON M, WIK G, ANNAS P, GREITZ T, ERICSSON C, STONE-ELANDER S. Functional neuroanatomy of fear: Additional data and theoretical analyses. *Psychophysiol* 1995;32:43–48.

15 RAUCH SL, WHALEN PJ, SHIN LM, MCINERNEY SC, MACKLIN ML, LASKO NB, ORR SP, PITMAN RK. Exaggerated amygdala response to masked facial stimuli in posttraumatic stress disorder: a functional MRI study. *Biol Psychiatry* 2000;47:769–776.

16 WHALEN PJ, BUSH G, MCNALLY RJ, WILHELM S, MCINERNEY SC, JENIKE MA, RAUCH SL. The emotional counting Stroop paradigm: A functional magnetic resonance imaging probe of the anterior cingulate affective division. *Biol Psychiatry* 1998;44:1219–1228.

17 WHALEN PJ, RAUCH SL, ETCOFF NL, MCINERNEY SC, LEE MB, JENIKE MA. Masked presentations of emotional facial expressions modulate amygdala activity without explicit knowledge. *J Neurosci* 1998;18:411–418.

18 NUTT DJ, MALIZIA AL. Structural and functional brain changes in posttraumatic stress disorder. *J Clin Psychiatry* 2004;65 Suppl 1:11–17.

19 OLSSON, SAPOLSKY. The Healthy Cortisol Response (in this volume). Weinheim: Wiley-VCH, 2006.

20 GILBERTSON MW, SHENTON ME, CISZEWSKI A, KASAI K, LASKO NB, ORR SP, PITMAN RK. Smaller hippocampal volume predicts pathologic vulnerability to psychological trauma. *Nat Neurosci* 2002;5:1242–1247.

21 FURMARK T, TILLFORS M, MARTEINSDOTTIR I, FISCHER H, PISSIOTA A, LANGSTROM B, FREDRIKSON M. Common changes in cerebral blood flow in patients with social phobia treated with citalopram or cognitive–behavioral therapy. *Arch Gen Psychiatry* 2002;59:425–433.

22 TILLFORS M, FURMARK T, MARTEINSDOTTIR I, FISCHER H, PISSIOTA A, LÅNGSTRÖM B, FREDRIKSON M. Cerebral blood flow in subjects with social phobia during stressful speaking tasks: A PET-study. *Am J Psychiatry* 2001;158:1220–1226.

23 MAYBERG HS, BRANNAN SK, TEKELL JL, SILVA JA, MAHURIN RK, MCGINNIS S, JERABEK PA. Regional metabolic effects of fluoxetine in major depression: serial changes and relationship to clinical response. *Biol Psychiatry* 2000;48:830–843.

24 LESCH KP, BENGEL D, HEILS A, SABOL SZ, GREENBERG BD, PETRI S, BENJAMIN J, MULLER CR, HAMER DH, MURPHY DL. Association of anxiety-related traits with a polymorphism in the serotonin transporter gene regulatory region. *Science* 1996;274:1527–1531.

25 HARIRI AR, MATTAY VS, TESSITORE A, KOLACHANA B, FERA F, GOLDMAN D, EGAN MF, WEINBERGER DR. Serotonin transporter genetic variation and the response of the human amygdala. *Science* 2002;297:400–403.

26 FURMARK T, TILLFORS M, GARPENSTRAND H, MARTEINSDOTTIR I, LANGSTROM B, ORELAND L, FREDRIKSON M. Serotonin transporter polymorphism related to amygdala excitability and symptom severity in patients with social phobia. *Neurosci Lett.* 2004; 362:189–192.

27 GRAEFF FG. On serotonin and experimental anxiety. *Psychopharmacol* 2002;163:467–476.

28 SERRETTI A, CUSIN C, ROSSINI D, ARTIOLI P, DOTOLI D, ZANARDI R. Further evidence of a combined effect of SERTPR and TPH on SSRIs response in mood disorders. *Am J Med Genet B Neuropsychiatr Genet* 2004;29:36–40.

29 GARPENSTRAND H, ANNAS P, EKBLOM J, ORELAND L, FREDRIKSON M, Human fear conditioning is related to dopaminergic and serotonergic

biological markers. *Behav Neurosci* 2001;115:358–364.

30 CASPI A, SUGDEN K, MOFFITT TE, TAYLOR A, CRAIG IW, HARRINGTON H, MCCLAY J, MILL J, MARTIN J, BRAITHWAITE A, POULTON R. Influence of life stress on depression: moderation by a polymorphism in the 5-HTT gene, *Science* 2003;301:386–389.

31 ESLER M, ALVARENGA M, LAMBERT G, KAYE D, HASTINGS J, JENNINGS G, MORRIS M, SCHWARTZ R, RICHARDS J. Cardiac sympathetic nerve biology and brain monoamine turnover in panic disorder. *Ann N Y Acad Sci* 2004;1018:505–514.

32 CRITCHLEY HD, MATHIAS CJ, JOSEPHS O, O'DOHERTY J, ZANINI S, DEWAR BK, CIPOLOTTI L, SHALLICE T, DOLAN RJ. Human cingulate cortex and autonomic control: converging neuroimaging and clinical evidence. *Brain* 2003;126:2139–2152.

33 MATTHEWS SC, PAULUS MP, SIMMONS AN, NELESEN RA, DIMSDALE JE. Functional subdivisions within anterior cingulate cortex and their relationship to autonomic nervous system function. *Neuroimage* 2004;22:1151–1156.

34 BOUCSEIN W. *Electrodermal Activity.* New York: Plenum Press; 1992.

15
Is It Dangerous To Be Afraid?

Markus Heilig

15.1
Introduction

An external danger that threatens the life or health of an organism is one of the most obvious reasons for the activation of the body's stress responses. Whether one is to fight the sabre-toothed tiger or flee from it, attention needs to be sharpened, the energy depots mobilized and the use of energy focused on functions essential to that particular emergency. This is the classic "fight or flight" response. It is intuitively easy to understand that it was developed early in evolution and has been conserved in a very similar kind of organization throughout the phylogenetic series. To safeguard ourselves and those closest to us against acute danger is a trait with obvious survival value, and thus one for which there is powerful selection pressure. Furthermore, dangers that have threatened survival on our globe have for millions of years and up until relatively recently been of a similar nature.

As fear and stress reactions are so highly conserved in phylogeny, it can be considered reasonable that we can learn a great deal about their organization from studies of lower species. This basic assumption also appears to be correct for the most part. At the same time it is just as apparent that humans, with their self-awareness and sophisticated cognitive functions, are unique in the phylogenetic series. One should not therefore be too sure that all the findings from animal experiments regarding fear and stress mechanisms can automatically be translated to human beings.

In order to better understand which similarities and differences that can be expected between us and lower species it may be useful to categorize the responses of the organism to dangerous situations into just a few main categories:

- Behavioral reactions. Run or fight belong here; in less drastic cases perhaps merely avoidance. The more pronounced reactions demand, in order to function effectively, not only that striated, will-governed muscles are activated, but that this is achieved in the form of ready-for-use, prepared behavior programmes that can be quickly activated in coordinated blocks and without time-consuming and advanced reflection. When the neighbor's angry Alsatian has broken loose it is not the moment to consciously begin thinking about which leg one should put forward first.

- Autonomic responses. These include the well-known signs of sympathetic nervous system activation: pupils that dilate in order to admit more light, increase in cardiac output, etc. These mechanisms naturally aim to mobilize the body's resources as quickly as possible to support the behavioral programmes.

- Endocrine responses. Most prominent amongst these is the well-known activation of the stress hormone axis, or hypothalamic–pituitary–adrenal (HPA) axis. The final link in this three-stage rocket, the release of glucocorticoids, has as its primary goal mobilization of the energy stores, in the form of both carbohydrates and free fatty acids, to put them at the disposal of the behavioral reactions. Other energy-demanding bodily functions that may be of long-term significance, but in the short-term can be spared, are dampened until the threat has passed. It is from this perspective one should, for example, regard the dampening effect of the glucocorticoids on a number of immunological functions. While one is running away from the angry watchdog the streptococci in one's throat can be allowed to grow undisturbed a while.

- The subjective feeling of being afraid. This part of the reaction is both the easiest and most difficult to explain. Easiest, because each of us reading these lines knows from our own experience how it feels. Most difficult, because this phenomenon is much harder to describe in mechanistic terms of the same type as the earlier three components, and can hardly be measured in laboratory animals.

15.2
Animal Models of Fear's Behavioral Component

It is of course impossible to know whether a laboratory animal experiences a feeling of fear. However, it is possible to observe behavior that is connected with the activation of this programme. An abundance of models using this as their point of departure have been developed and are used within research. An obvious function of these models is to chart the neural mechanisms of fear. Another important field of application is the development of drugs that can be useful in conditions involving a pathological activation of fear and stress reactions.

Now and then there is a lively debate about the validity of the laboratory animal models. Do they actually say anything meaningful? Can they be generalized to human beings? A whole body of literature has been devoted to the various types of validity that can be attributed to or challenged with regard to such models. "Face validity" is one aspect. This concerns the question of whether what the model purports to study is immediately and intuitively recognizable in it. This concept could be illustrated by filming a dog under attack from a superior opponent, showing the film to ten randomly selected laymen from the street and finding that they actually agree that the dog looks scared. This does not require the existence of any underlying theoretical model. Appealing as it may be at times, there are many examples in which this kind of face validity can be very deceptive, especially when it is a matter of interpreting and comparing behavior across species. Another concept that is discussed therefore is "construct validity", which focuses instead upon just the fact that there should be a meaningful theoretical model underlying what is observed.

However, in the end what most models tend to be based on is something much simpler and more robust. "Predictive validity" is based on whether the outcome in a behavioral model statistically speaking has a good predictive power regarding the situation we are ultimately interested in. An application of this is pharmacological validation. The latter is said to be present if, after introducing a pharmaceutical, a certain outcome in the model reliably predicts a desired effect in human beings. A number of well-known pharmaceuticals, e.g., benzodiazepines, have a known ability to dampen fear and stress in human beings. Others can, on the contrary, potentiate this state. Behavioral models that are selectively sensitive to these but not to other drugs therefore have an evident predictive validity, and have in fact provided us with extensive knowledge about the mechanisms underlying fear and stress.

There are many pharmacologically validated behavioral models of fear and stress reactions. The "elevated plus-maze" is perhaps the most common and can serve as an example. In this model an arrangement is used that consists of a plus-shaped maze, raised on a stand about half a meter over the ground. Two of its arms are open and exposed, whereas the other two are enclosed and thus protected. Everyone who has ever surprised a mouse in his/her cellar knows that small rodents spontaneously avoid open, exposed surfaces. There are good reasons for this: over time the individuals that did not do so were selected out of the gene pool by the hawks diving out of the sky. In the plus-maze the laboratory animals will therefore spontaneously explore the setup but in such a way as to spend more time in the protected arms than in the open ones. Compounds that in human beings have an antianxiety and antistress effect increase the animal's tendency to explore the exposed arms as well. Threat and stress have the reverse effect.

The effects of stress on behavior in this model have from the beginning been based on quite artificial stressors, e.g., restricted movement in a Plexiglas tube, "restraint stress". It has been questioned as to whether this provides meaningful information about reactions to more natural stressors. However, several laboratories have shown that, for example, confrontation with a dominant male in his own territory, an ethologically highly relevant stressor, has the same effect. Our own work has recently shown that an enforced longer exposure to the scent of a predator, e.g., fox, has the same effect.

15.3
Do You Run Because You Are Scared or Are You Scared Because You Run?

The emotional components of the fear programme can therefore be studied using objective measures, and it is even more apparent that the same thing applies to the autonomic and endocrine reactions. Accordingly, as stated, it has been possible to obtain much knowledge from animal experiment studies. But what about the subjective feeling of being afraid? This is not possible to measure objectively. And we can't ask experimental animals how they feel. Our understanding of the subjective feeling of fear, one of the most basic emotional states alongside joy, is therefore much more uncertain and debated.

A few fundamental conceptual models of fear as an emotional state have resurfaced in various shapes during the past 100 years or so in which the issue has been given any attention. Of these, the model that intuitively is embraced by those in the field of biomedicine can be traced in its original form to the renowned physiologist Walter Cannon. According to Cannon, environmental stimuli are registered by our sensory organs, conveyed to the cortex, and processed there by higher functions of the central nervous system (CNS). If this processesing results in a conclusion that danger is present, the cerebral cortex will initiate a response by activating lower brain centers, the activity of which turns on the various components of the fear programme.

Interestingly enough it was, however, a substantially different model that was first on the scene. The father of modern psychology, William James, wrote in 1884 a now-classic article entitled, "What is an emotion?" At that time little was known about the organization of the nervous system, which is why James did not specifically talk about the neural substrates of fear. However, he observed that fear principally appeared to be a physical state. It is not possible to conceive of the feeling of fear without the pounding heart and dry tongue. From this type of reasoning James formulated the following theory: one of the principal tasks of human consciousness – probably a uniquely human characteristic – is to continuously monitor the state of the body. Most, if not all, components of the fear reaction are triggered quite automatically and without the influence of consciousness and the higher brain functions. When, during the continuous monitoring of the body's condition, it is discovered that these activities are going on – that the heart is pounding, that the legs are running – the conclusion is drawn that there is reason to feel afraid.

This model is commonly perceived as somewhat counterintuitive. However, it is principally the one that has received support from more recent research that has rapidly developed our knowledge in this area over the past decade.

15.4
A Sketch of the Organization of Fear

Above all, it is two researchers who, through very systematic work, have provided us with a picture of how the neural substrates of fear are organized: Joseph LeDoux and Michael Davis. The picture that emerges is summarized in Fig. 15.1.

It has long been an established truth that sensory information reaches the cortex and thus consciousness in humans through a path that comprises three neurons:

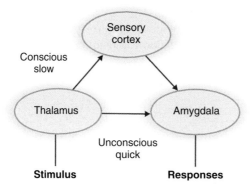

Fig. 15.1. Stimuli carrying information about possible dangers are processed along two parallel signal paths. The classic, thalamocortical path gives rise to sophisticated processing with high discriminatory ability, but is relatively slow. The projection from the thalamus to the amygdala creates the opportunity for a quicker, but crude integration, which when needed can lead to a rapid activation of the fear programme's various responses.

1. from the sensory "detector", whatever its type, to the dorsal horn of the spinal cord
2. from the dorsal horn to the relay station in the thalamus
3. from the thalamus to the sensory cortex.

According to this traditional view the information should only be able to lead to some form of behavioral or other functional result after it has reached the sensory cortex and been processed there. In a series of exceptionally elegant experiments, however, LeDoux was able to show that laboratory animals that had been taught to react with fear to an initially neutral tone still did so even if the third neuron in the classic chain, from the thalamus to the auditory cortex, was knocked out with selective lesions! Therefore another path for the sensory information must exist, and the information flowing along such an alternative path must be able to lead to an activation of the fear response. Many years of anatomical studies were finally able to prove that the sensory information that reaches the thalamus is not only sent on to the sensory cortex, but is also split off along a separate path. The target of this connection turned out to be the lateral and basolateral parts of the amygdala complex, situated subcortically in the temporal lobe.

This, together with, amongst others, Davis's result on the functional importance of the amygdala complex, provided a clearer picture. The amygdala complex is strategically localized specifically to activate behavioral, autonomic and endocrine stress and fear responses through both direct and indirect projections to the brain stem and hypothalamus (Fig. 15.2).

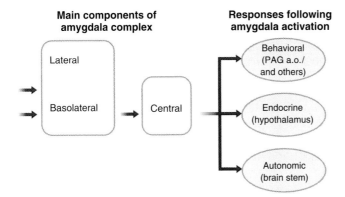

Fig. 15.2. Lateral and basolateral components of the amygdala complex are of cortical origin and form the receiver station of the complex. They also receive, apart from thalamic afferents, projections from the hippocampus and the cortex. An integration takes place here that in cases of danger gives rise to activation of the central nucleus of the amygdala, a structure that cytoarchitectonically belongs to the so-called extended amygdala, together with parts of the nucleus accumbens. From the central amygdala are sent both direct and indirect projections to a number of areas that permit activation of the various components of the fear programme. *PAG* Periaqueductal gray.

15.5
The Price of Being Conscious

Why is the processing of sensory information duplicated in this way? An indication of the answer is provided by an experiment that measures the speed with which the signals proceed along the two different paths. A sound signal that has been coupled with a fear-inducing feeling has already activated target neurons in the amygdala complex after 12 ms. Just as long then remains until nerve cells in the sensory cortex begin to be activated, and even longer before their activation leads to any output. The time issue thus rules out the possibility that the cortex and its activity govern the emotional responses. Furthermore, as impressions do not become conscious until they reach the cortex, the activation of the fear response is also most probably not a conscious process. This is well in accord with observations that Darwin had already made about the central signs for activation of fear: that it is rapid, appears outside consciousness and is difficult to control by will.

Why then does the cortex participate in the process at all? A clue is provided by another key experiment. If a laboratory animal is taught to associate a tone with a frequency of 1 000 Hz with a threat, the presentation of this particular tone will reliably lead to activation of both amygdala neurons as well as nerve cells in the sensory cortex, according to the time sequence described above. However, if a tone with a nearby but different frequency, e.g., 1 500 Hz, is presented to the animal, the situation becomes a completely different one. The nerve cells of the amygdala complex are still activated. The rapid system shows itself to be less sophisticated, and reacts more crudely and undifferentiatedly. However, activation in the cortex is not forthcoming; completely correct.

This is a very reasonable organization in the service of survival. It is expedient to have a rapid, unconscious processing that "just in case" sets in motion defensive reactions on the basis of what can be described as a crude preliminary assessment. One thus avoids getting into trouble while more sophisticated processing is being conducted. Should it turn out that the defense reactions have been started up unnecessarily or in an incorrect way, the cortex can always gradually shut them down or modulate them.

The cost of sophisticated, conscious processing is time. Sophisticated intellectual strategies are of no help in avoiding a dog bite when the neighbor's dog has broken loose. However, when one gradually realizes that a fence will prevent the dog from running out onto the street it is good to shut down one's fear system and stop running. Otherwise one would all too often squander one's energy resources without good reason.

These findings are very much in accord with the results from another prominent contemporary brain researcher, the neurologist Antonio Damasio, and his "somatic marker theory". Together these results provide support for the fact that James actually came quite close to the truth in his article of over 100 years ago: fear as a physical state appears to be a primary, rapid and unconscious event. Fear as a feeling is what arises when consciousness is reached by information that the body finds itself in this state. In the first case it is a question of "emotion" and in the second, one of "feeling".

15.6
Mediators of Emotions

Understanding the anatomic organization underlying emotional responses provides important insights, but has also major limitations. This is especially so if we want to find targets for drugs that can affect pathological activation of fear and stress reactions. We must then also identify the information-carrying molecules. Among these, the transmitters and their receptors are of particular interest. The past 20 years have yielded extensive knowledge in this area as well. Many systems are obviously involved in the complex processing of stress-related stimuli and responses. However, some of them, like gamma-amino butyric acid (GABA) and the glutamate system, are of a very general nature. Nevertheless, it has been possible to link some systems more specifically to stress and fear.

One of the most important internal stress signals is the corticotropin releasing hormone (CRH1). Its existence as a hypothalamic releasing factor for adrenocorticotropic hormone (ACTH) was postulated at an early stage by, among others, the Nobel laureate Roger Guillemin, codiscoverer of the other hypothalamic releasing factors. However, the releasing factor for ACTH in particular frustrated attempts at chemical isolation for a long time. It was in 1981, 4 years after Guillemin had received his Nobel Prize that his former co-worker Vale was first able to purify the substance to show that it is a peptide comprising 41 amino acids. CRH was located just where it should be, i.e., in the hypothalamic paraventricular nucleus, was released into the portal circulation and led to release of ACTH from pituicytes. Anatomical studies showed shortly after that CRH was also found in a number of extrahypothalamic brain areas. Among these, the CRH levels were highest in the central nucleus of the amygdala, an area of whose significance for activation of stress and fear responses we have already given an account.

The anatomical mapping was swiftly followed by a series of functional studies. These were able to show that CRH release in the amygdala entails activation of behavioral fear responses in a broad spectrum of situations, from confrontation with a hostile member of the same species to alcohol abstinence. This function of the peptide is independent of its ability, via stimulation of pituitary receptors, to release ACTH. Furthermore, it quickly became evident that the behavioral effects were not secondary to the endocrine ones but were mediated via direct effects within the CNS. Recently, two new subtypes of CRH receptors have been cloned as well as a related peptide ligand to these, urocortin (Ucn). Ucn has an important sequence homology with CRH and reproduces some, but not all, of these effects. An interesting finding that has recently come to light is the possibility of long-term regulation of the amygdala function. The final outflow from the amygdala nucleus is determined by a balance between glutamate-mediated excitation and GABA-mediated inhibition. It has recently been shown that a repeated administration of Ucn in the amygdala, in doses that in themselves did not have any acute effect, leads to significant permanent behavioral changes indicating a greatly increased level of fear/anxiety. This was accompanied by a long term shift of electrophysiological activity patterns. Under normal circumstances, appr. 70% of nerve impulses recorded in the amygdala are of the inhibitory kind. Following Ucn treatment, only about 30% of impulses fell in this category. Instead, excitatory signals dominated. This indicates that the amygdala had escaped from its normal, built in "break", and shifted into a higher level of activity.

On the basis of the functional studies, antagonists to CRH receptors constitute an attractive strategy for treatment of negative affective states. From this hypothesis, a preliminary study of such an antagonist has shown it to be active in depressed patients and, interestingly enough, has had good effects on the anxiety component of depression. Although that particular compound was pulled from development because of signs of some liver toxicity, the hunt is in on to produce clinically useful CRH receptor antagonists.

The neuropeptide Y (NPY) is another neuropeptide that, at the beginning of the 1980s, was isolated and demonstrated to be expressed in the CNS. In most contexts it appears to counteract the effects of CRH. In particular, it counteracts the effects of stress and fear. After a long series of pharmacological studies we were able, in a recently published study, to show that transgenic overexpression of NPY in rats leads to reduced measures of fear and complete absence of behavioral reactions to a stressor. Interestingly enough, NPY has an effect profile that over a broader spectrum is reminiscent of existing anxiolytic medications, e.g., benzodiazepines. Apart from dampening fear, NPY counteracts epileptic seizures, while also impairing memory function. However, an interesting difference is that NPY administration does not appear to lead to physical dependence, which makes pharmaceuticals that emulate NPY interesting prospects for development. The negative cognitive effects will probably not constitute any obstacle, as these seem to be mediated by NPY-Y2 receptors, whereas the antistress effects are conveyed by the Y1 receptor. Pharmaceutical development with this system as a target is currently in progress.

A more recently emerging aspect of NPY function is its role in the regulation of alcohol intake. Activation of Y1 receptors or blockade of presynaptic Y2 receptors (with increased release of the body's own NPY) lacks effect on basal alcohol consumption in nonaddicted animals. However, both these types of treatment completely block the powerful increase of alcohol intake that is caused by a history of dependence, or that exists spontaneously in animals that belong to strains selectively bred for high alcohol preference. This link is particularly interesting considering the well-known anxiety-dampening effects of alcohol. From a practical perspective, this is a very promising target for the development of clinical alcohol addiction treatment.

Finally, a third neuropeptide should be mentioned. Substance P (SP) was the very first neuropeptide to be isolated. It is the prototypical member of the tachykinin family and acts primarily by stimulating the NK-1 receptor. For many decades there have been hopes that it would be possible to develop SP antagonists into drugs against pain and/or inflammation, but these efforts have been to no avail. At the end of the 1990s, a research group at Merck was instead able to establish that SP is present in the amygdala and is released by stress, whilst blockade of these receptors in this region dampens signs of fear in laboratory animal models. A series of selective blockers of the NK-1-type of SP receptors was developed, and it was initially possible to show that one of these had good antidepressive effects, with particularly good effects against the anxiety component of the depressive symptomatology. Follow-up studies for depression had, however, varying results. Instead, NK-1 antagonists are presently being developed by several major pharmaceutical companies for use in anxiety disorders. In particular, a recent study has suggested this class of compounds to be effective in social anxiety, and to inhibit fear-induced amygdala activity in humans.

15.7
To Stop in Time

It is of course good to be able to be scared, otherwise evolution would not have equipped us with this ability. A very clear illustration of this is provided by a psychiatric condition that involves a systematic underrating of risks, probably to a great extent due to an inability to feel fear: the antisocial personality disorder. These individuals are able to unconcernedly carry out acts that the rest of us would not dare to try, and when their various stress responses in the face of threat are measured they are found to be greatly reduced. Functioning in this way can give short-term gains in the form of increased status in a gang or success as a criminal.

However, these persons are burdened, almost as a rule, by alcohol and drug abuse, accidents and other misfortunes, and have a greatly increased mortality rate.

However, it is equally obvious that fear can be unhealthy and contribute to a stress burden that finally gives rise to physical and mental illness. This is primarily connected with two factors: partly the type of danger that threatens us, partly the dynamics of the response.

As we have already noted the fear programme is strongly conserved by evolution. It did excellent service over the many millions of years that the fundamental threats were quite constant. However, this has radically changed, over a period of only a few hundred years, far too short a period for evolution to adapt our bodies and brains. Originally, threats were primarily of an acute nature and quickly passed: a predator that tried to devour one, or a fight with one of one's own species. Most of the threats that we now live with are infinitely more complex and prolonged: "Will I be able to keep my job after having failed to keep within the department's budget? Will the pension funds be enough? Will we survive the threat of nuclear weapons?" None of these threats can be very effectively managed by setting in motion the body's defensive reactions in the way we are made for and begin to fight or run, even if the members of a number of protest movements lack this insight. However, even if one succeeds in using the higher central nervous, cognitive functions in managing these complex threats, i.e., begin to keep the department's budget, save for your pension and support world peace by increased free trade, the old evolutionary reaction patterns remain within us, like the inner layers of an evolution-cultivated onion.

The question of the fear system's dynamics is central to understanding when the reactions risk passing from the adaptive to maladaptive. Every physiological system whose purpose is homeostatic regulation in the face of rapidly changing factors in the environment encounters the same problem: there is great value in a system that can be activated very rapidly when the environment changes, but at the same time the system must just as quickly be able to shut down in order to avoid unnecessarily taxing the body's resources. This is a classic control theory problem. Two standard ways of solving it are through negative feedback, or "feedback inhibition", and through the use of opposing forces, or "opposing process" organization. Both these mechanisms have proved useful with regard to the fear reactions, and the interaction between the CRH and NPY systems is an example of this in particular. However, too great a burdening of the system can lead to its adaptive capacity being overburdened, at which time a vicious circle can begin.

15.8
A Sea Horse that Bolts

As we have already mentioned, the release of glucocorticoids is one of the central components of the fear and stress response, which is initiated through a release of the corticotropin releasing hormone, CRH, which leads to secretion of ACTH, and ultimately cortisol. This system has precisely such a negative feedback regulation as indicated above. One of the more recent important discoveries in this field has been that glucocorticoid receptors, which mediate this negative feedback, are not only found at the pituitary and hypothalamic level, but also in the hippocampus. The hippocampal receptor population appears to be of major significance for negative feedback regulation.

There is a spontaneous individual variation in the strength of this feedback inhibition. It has recently been shown that this can be conditioned by early life experiences, both in the womb and after birth. Intrauterine exposure to glucocorticoids as a result of stress in the mother is something that the fetus is to a large extent protected from by a placenta barrier consisting of an active enzyme that breaks down the glucocorticoids. However, sufficiently powerful stressors can make this barrier temporarily break down and lead to exposure of the fetus. Both animal data and human results show that such an exposure can downregulate the number of glucocorticoid receptors in the hippocampus for life, thus turning down the sensitivity of feedback HPA axis inhibition.

Postnatal experience can have a similar effect. In a series of studies that has attracted a great deal of attention a Canadian research group has been able to show that at least the rodent mother's caring behavior towards her offspring regulates this parameter. The result is impaired feedback inhibition. This is not expressed through an increase in the amplitude of the glucocorticoid response. However, the ability to shut down this response in time is partly lost, with the consequence that our inner milieu bathes in raised levels of glucocorticoid. The Canadian research group was recently also able to identify a very interesting mechanism for this long-term regulation. Methylation of a DNA sequence has long been known as a mechanism for the long-term inactivation of the sequence in question. It is in this way that 100 or so genes are regulated so that we only express the maternal or paternal copy of the gene, but not both. Beyond that, however, methylation has not been known as a common regulatory mechanism in normal cells. In a 2004 study that attracted considerable attention, Meaney and coworkers were, however, able to show that the mother's caring behavior toward the offspring regulates the degree of methylation of the promoter region for the glucocorticoid receptor gene, and in this way governs its expression activity in the long-term.

Defective feedback control of cortisol release seems to set the scene for an unusually unpleasant vicious circle. It appears that transient high glucocorticoid levels are not particularly harmful. Long-term exposure has, on the other hand, such effects on several types of cell. One of these is the very hippocampus neuron that expresses the glucocorticoid receptors and that constitutes a central component of the feedback inhibition loop. The glucocorticoids are probably not toxic in themselves for these cells, but reduce their glucose uptake by inhibiting the glucose transporter and in this way make them more vulnerable to other damaging stimuli, e.g., excitotoxic effects of other transmitters. Furthermore, prolonged elevated glucocorticoid levels inhibit the new formation of nerve cells that is found in the hippocampus. This is probably the background to the important results of recent years that not only Cushing's disease – a hormone-producing tumor that leads to greatly raised levels of cortisol – but also depressive illnesses lead to a reduction in the volume of the hippocampus. In the latter case there is a further important lesson to be learned. The volume reduction of the hippocampus in depression has recently been shown to be in proportion to the length of time the patient has had depression and *not been treated for it with medication*. These observations provide a bit of perspective to the current debate about whether antidepressive medication is over prescribed.

That a stress-induced effect on the hippocampus leads to impaired feedback inhibition is obviously a disastrous scenario. A vulnerable individual, when challenged with a prolonged stressor, risks reacting with an extended stress response. This in turn contributes to breaking down the very feedback system whose function it is to help shut down the response. The scene is thus set for a further "full turnout" the next time the fear and stress reaction is activated, and thus the vicious circle is in motion. The increasing stress level also impairs the individual's cognitive functions, partly directly through the hippocampal effects, partly indirectly through dampening the activity of the frontal lobes. Through this cognitive impairment, the individual's chances of finding good coping strategies are also reduced.

It should be noted that not everything that looks like a stress effects on the hippocampus necessarily is one. Posttraumatic stress syndrome (PTSD) provides an instructive case. This is the psychiatric condition in which reduced hippocampal volumes were first reported. However, twin-study data have shown such a reduction also in identical healthy twins of patients with PTSD. Hippocampal volume reduction in this case might well be a preexisting vulnerability factor, rather than an effect of stress exposure. Interestingly, the activity of the stress–hormone axis in PTSD patients also appears to be abnormally low rather than raised.

15.9
Can a Vicious Circle Be Broken?

We cannot presently claim to fully understand the causes of depression and anxiety. It is also evident that genetic factors play a major role in these conditions. An increasing number of researchers are, however, persuaded that mechanisms of the type described here contribute to the emergence and/or maintenance of illnesses characterized by increased stress sensitivity, and negative affect. It is also possible that mechanisms of this type convey heritable vulnerability factors that must exist according to genetic studies. The picture thus becomes rather gloomy: with a very provocative formulation one could regard recurrent major depression as brain damage. Is it possible to make repairs?

The answer to this question is necessarily more speculative, as we now approach the current frontline of research. However, a series of recently published research reports indicate an interesting possibility. One factor that very clearly appears to be capable of stimulating neurogenesis in the hippocampus is the brain-derived neurotrophic factor (BDNF). It is well-established that most cases of depression can be very successfully treated with a number of different drugs. If these do not help, then electrotherapy does so in most cases. Virtually all clinically effective antidepressant drugs, as well as electrotherapy have recently been shown to stimulate production of BDNF and increase formation of new cells in the hippocampus in laboratory animals. In an exceptionally elegant article in Science (2003) a research group at Columbia University in New York was able to show that the formation of new cells in the hippocampus is in fact essential for the behavioral effects of anti-depressant medication in mice, believed to correspond to their clinical efficacy in humans. It is well-known that formation of new cells is inhibited by radiation. The "antidepressant" effects were blocked completely by selective irradiation of the hippocampus, using a lead cap that protected the rest of the brain. On the other hand, radiation through a lead cap that exposed the other brain area in which the formation of new cells takes place, the subventricular zone, was without effect.

If these effects are in accord with what happens in human beings it is a very at-tractive thought that this could be a central mechanism in successful treatment. By increasing the number of cells that express the glucocorticoid receptor in the hip-pocampus it would thus be possible to increase the sensitivity of the feedback inhi-bition and interrupt the vicious circle. If this really is the case, it becomes apparent that depression and anxiety should be treated very actively, a fact already known by every good psychiatrist, but all too often not fully appreciated by the public. If treat-ment is not forthcoming there is a great risk of a vicious circle with increasingly serious symptomatology that can finally end the patient's life through suicide.

References

BREMNER J.D., RANDALL P., SCOTT T.M., BRONEN R.A., SEIBYL J.P., SOUTHWICK S.M., DELANEY R.C., McCARTHY G., CHARNEY D.S., INNIS R.B. MRI-based measurement of hippocampal volume in patients with combat-related posttraumatic stress disorder. Am. J. Psychiatry 1995; 152(7):973–981.

GILBERTSON M.W., SHENTON M.E., CISZEWSKI A., KASAI K., LASKO N.B., ORR S.P., PITMAN R.K. Smaller hippocampal volume predicts pathologic vulnerability to psychological trauma. Nat. Neurosci 2002; 5(11):1242–1247.

HEILIG M., KOOB G.F., EKMAN R., BRITTON K.T. Corticotropin-releasing factor and neuropeptide Y: role in emotional integration. Trends Neurosci 1994; 17(2):80–85.

HEILIG M. The NPY system in stress, anxiety and depression. Neuropeptides 2004; 38:213–224.

HOLSBOER F. The corticosteroid receptor hypothesis of depression. Neuropsycho-pharmacology 2000; 23:477–501.

LADD C.O., HUOT R.L., THRIVIKRAMAN K.V., NEMEROFF C.B., MEANEY M.J., PLOTSKY P.M. Long-term behavioral and neuro-endocrine adaptations to adverse early experience. Prog Brain Res 2000; 122:81–103.

LEDOUX J. The Emotional Brain. Simon and Schuster, New York, 1996.

McEWEN B.S. Allostasis and allostatic load: implications for neuropsychopharmacology. Neuropsychopharmacology 2000; 22(2):108–24.

RAINNIE D.G., BERGERON R., SAJDYK T.J., PATIL M., GEHLERT D.R., SHEKHAR A. Corticotrophin releasing factor-induced synaptic plasticity in the amygdala translates stress into emotional disorders. J Neurosci 2004; 24:3471–3479.

SANTARELLI L., SAXE M., GROSS C., SURGET A., BATTAGLIA F., DULAWA S., WEISSTAUB N., LEE J., DUMAN R., ARANCIO O., BELZUNG C., HEN R. Requirement of hippocampal neurogenesis for the behavioral effects of antidepressants. Science 2003; 301:805–809.

SAPOLSKY R.M. Why zebras don't get ulcers: an updated guide to stress, stress-related diseases, and coping. Freeman, New York, 1998.

SHELINE Y.I., GADO M.H., KRAEMER H.C. Untreated depression and hippocampal volume loss. Am J Psychiatry 2003; 160(8):1516–1518.

THORSELL A., MICHALKIEWICZ M., DUMONT Y., QUIRION R., CABERLOTTO L., RIMONDINI R., MATHE A.A., HEILIG M. Behavioral insensitivity to restraint stress, absent fear suppression of behavior and impaired spatial learning in transgenic rats with hippocampal neuropeptide Y overexpression. Proc Natl Acad Sci U S A. 2000; 97(23):12852–12857.

WEAVER I.C., CERVONI N., CHAMPAGNE F.A., D'ALESSIO A.C., SHARMA S., SECKL J.R., DYMOV S., SZYF M., MEANEY M.J. Epigenetic programming by maternal behavior. NatNeurosci 2004; 7:847–854. A complete reference list is to be found at www.medicin.liber.se

16
Fatigue and Recovery

Bengt B. Arnetz and Rolf Ekman

16.1
Introduction

Fatigue is a common feature of a number of somatic and psychiatric diseases and disorders. Patients suffering from disorders and syndromes where fatigue is a major part of the condition often report that the fatigue has a major impact on their quality of life. Even though fatigue is a common characteristic of a number of disorders and often used for diagnostic purposes, it is not easily defined.

16.2
Fatigue – a Distinct Entity or Part of a Syndrome?

The current chapter will focus on fatigue as an entity by itself, in circumstances where it is not used a part of a syndrome. Fatigue is essentially a subjective experience. As stated by Dittner and coworkers, fatigue "has largely defied efforts to conceptualize or define it in a way that separates it from normal experiences such as tiredness and sleepiness." This chapter will look at fatigue in contrast to tiredness and sleepiness. Are these all concepts part of a continuum, differing only in the degree of symptoms?

In what way does fatigue differ from tiredness and sleepiness? Typically, fatigue is defined as extreme and persistent tiredness, weakness or exhaustion. Symptoms are mental, physical or both. However, there is no generally accepted definition of fatigue. Much of the debate has focused on whether fatigue is a discrete entity, a set of symptoms of unknown origin, or a specific form a psychological disturbance. Given the difficulties in conceptualizing and defining fatigue, it is no surprise that the prevalence of fatigue varies between studies. Nevertheless, fatigue is a common phenomenon in society. The reported prevalence rates range from under 10% to 45% or more. Studies carried out in primary health care settings and the general community have shown that fatigue is a continuously distributed variable, with some fatigue in all of the populations studied.

An important issue is whether tiredness, sleepiness and fatigue are part of a continuum or separate entities. For example, is there any association between the rather common reports of fatigue in community settings and the development of chronic fatigue syndrome (CFS), characterized by severe and disabling fatigue? Commonly, it is stated that tiredness, sleepiness and everyday-type fatigue is usually relieved by a period of rest, while prolonged and debilitating fatigue is not.

16.3
Fatigue-Dominating Syndromes

In the clinical setting, severe and disabling fatigue is a common cofactor in syndromes also characterized by self-reported impairments in concentration and short-term memory, sleep disturbances, and musculoskeletal pain. Patients suffering from fibromyalgic syndromes often say that even though the muscle pain is affecting them in their daily life, the consistent and severe fatigue is the symptom most severely impacting on their quality of life.

Patients diagnosed with CFS commonly report a combination of long-term disabling fatigue, self-reported impairment of short-term memory or concentration, and muscle pain.

Long-term or chronic stress has commonly been implicated in the etiology of fatigue conditions. There appears to be a temporal relationship between unexplained fatigue and depression. Thus, persons with a prior history of fatigue are more likely to develop depression in the future. Furthermore, patients with a prior history of depression appear to be at increased risk of developing fatiguing disorders.

The close link between unexplained fatigue, psychiatric states such as anxiety disorders, panic disorders and dysthymia as well as major depressive disorders necessitates careful selection and evaluation of participants in studies focusing on unexplained fatigue.

A study by Heim et al. is also of great interest concerning the importance of stress in the development of fatiguing illness. They interviewed a multigeographic random sample of people living in different regions of the United States before as well as after the terrorist attacks of September 11, 2001. In that study, the prevalence of prolonged fatigue, defined as those who reported that their fatigue had lasted between 1 and 6 months, was 5450 persons per 100 000 persons before the terrorist attacks of September 11, 2001, and 1530 per 100 000 persons after the attacks. The reason for the apparent decrease in the prevalence of prolonged fatigue is not known, but it does raise the possibility that at least short- to mid-term stressor exposure might actually decrease the prevalence of prolonged fatigue.

16.4
Fatigue Among the General Population

The Maastricht Cohort Study is a large prospective cohort study of the prevalence, incidence and natural course of prolonged fatigue in the working population as well as risk factors for the development of fatigue. A number of relevant exposure factors in the occupational and private arena as well as health outcome factors are studied. Prolonged fatigue is measured with the self-reported Checklist Individual Strengths (CIS). This scale was originally developed for the study of CFS. The CIS scale covers constructs such as severity of fatigue, concentration, motivation, and the level of physical activity. Thus, the scale measures fatigue in a more comprehensive fashion, also involving constructs that are part of anxiety as well as depressive disorders. The Maastricht Cohort Study involved over 12 000 employees from a broad range of Dutch companies and organizations. Employees scoring > 76 points on the CIS scale were defined as suffering from prolonged fatigue. The prevalence of fatigue differed markedly across different companies, between a low of 9.7% and a high of 28%.

There was a marked overlap or correlation between CIS scores and scores on the Maslach Burnout Inventory–General Survey, as well as the General Health Questionnaire and the Dutch version of the Perception and Judgment of Work scale – a scale assessing the need for recovery. These findings support the notion that the concept of prolonged fatigue is not easily delineated but shares common features with other concepts as well. Prolonged fatigue was found, as has been reported in a number of previous studies, to be associated with psychological distress. Even though prolonged fatigue and psychological distress did partly overlap, there is some support according to the Maastricht researchers that these are separate concepts.

16.5
Fatigue, Chronic Fatigue and Chronic Semantic Confusion

In an editorial in the *Journal of Psychosomatic Medicine* (Shapiro 2004) entitled "Chronic fatigue – chronically confusing but growing information," accompanying an issue entailing a large number of articles under the rubric of fatigue and sleepiness, Shapiro summarizes some of the major challenges in fatigue and sleepiness research. Of special interest is the reference to the need to focus on fatigue and sleepiness as "energy states." Neuropsychiatry as a field deals with some constructs, such as memory, but does not consider fatigue and sleepiness as a continuum on a scale assessing energy, ranging from none to completely energized. Energy as a concept is also controversial and hard to define, although a common complaint among patients: "I have no energy left." Self-rated energy states are closely related to tiredness and sleepiness ratings as well as classical psychiatric states, such as depression. Scales assessing chronic fatigue also include items assessing self-rated energy, but mostly from a static, and not dynamic, point of view.

Considering tiredness, sleepiness and fatigue as energy states allows for more dynamic studies of the interrelationships between these three concepts, as well as recovery. At what self-rated level of energy is there a risk that tiredness and sleepiness transforms into prolonged fatigue and an attenuated ability to recover? What are the physiological and molecular correlates, if any, to self-rated health and fatigue? By better defining energy and energy states, our ability to identify risk factors should improve. By developing better pathophysiological understanding of the biological and molecular bases of decreased energy states, we should be able to assess the efficacy of various pharmacological and nonpharmacological treatment methods.

In the following, we will review some possible physiological and molecular bases for decreased self-rated energy states. We will also report some preliminary results from prospective studies of self-rated energy, sleepiness and fatigue. In addition, we will present some data concerning the recovery phase from states of tiredness and fatigue.

16.6
Assessing Fatigue

At the Center for Environmental Illness and Stress (CEOS), we have followed over 300 media and information technology employees over a period of approximately 1 year. At the start of the study, at 6 and 12 months, respectively, the participants responded to a comprehensive web-based questionnaire. Questions concerned socioeconomics, stressors in their working life as well as in their social life outside work, health-promoting factors, lifestyle issues such as smoking and drinking habits. In addition, the respondents scored their current self-rated health, stress, cognitive functions, sleep and general well-being. The study was part of a larger study focusing on a prospective and controlled web-based intervention study assessing the feasibility of web-based, real-time stress and health assessments, as well as interventions. In addition to self-rated questionnaire-based data, we collected blood samples and analyzed for stress hormones, restorative/anabolic hormones, metabolic parameters as well as immune variables. As part of the study, we used a fatigue scale, prior validated using a Mental Energy scale, with the items listed in Table 16.1.

Tab. 16.1. Items in the Mental Energy scale. (Item scores).

Have you experienced any of the following during the past month?	Yes, daily (1)	Yes, several times (2)	Yes, once or twice (3)	No (4)
Restlessness	☐	☐	☐	☐
Irritation	☐	☐	☐	☐
Moodiness	☐	☐	☐	☐
Anxiety/Nervousness	☐	☐	☐	☐
Difficulty Concentrating	☐	☐	☐	☐

The Mental Energy scale has been validated in a serious of studies versus more comprehensive scales assessing mental well-being, sleep and general health. The Mental Energy scale has been applied to over 200 000 respondents, many followed over a long period of time. The scores of the individual Likert-type questions are summarized to a total score that is transformed into percentage, ranging from a theoretical low of 0% to a high of 100%. Prospective studies have identified scores 70% or higher as normal. Scores below 70% are considered to be representing fatigue, and scores below 50% represent severe fatigue.

16.7
Stress-Related Fatigue

Figure 16.1 depicts prospective self-rated data for a person who regularly monitored her stress and health indicators, using web-based visual analogue scales. The person was initially healthy, as indicated by acceptable ratings on the scale assessing sleep, value > 70%. Her self-rated energy, self-rated health as well as

The Stress – Health – Recovery Process

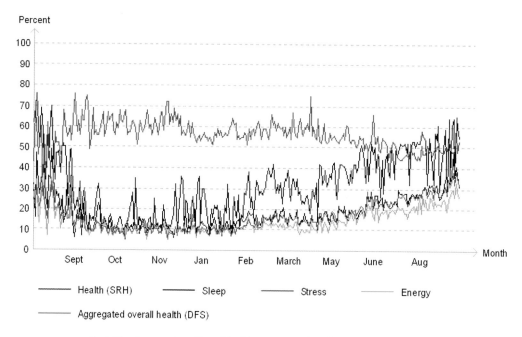

Fig. 16.1. A person's self-rated health, using visual analogue scales, before, during and following stress-related fatigue. *DFS* – an aggregate summary measure of various health and stress visual analogue scales, including self-rated health, sleep and energy level. Reprinted with the permission from the person.

her aggregate overall health were, however, already a bit low, although not low enough to be defined as exhaustion. However, after some months of high stressor exposure she developed severe sleep disturbance and loss of energy. At this point she was referred to our stress clinic. Following biological, psychosocial and somatic work-up as well as counseling, she regained most of her health and well-being over a period of months. Interestingly enough, she never recovered completely.

In the IT/media study, we included fatigue-relevant questions. We based the questions on a theoretical approach focusing on neurocognitive functions, self-rated health and energy. The fatigue-relevant areas we decided to include in exploratory and confirmatory factor analyses were: cognitive functions, measured by questions on ability to concentrate and memory, sleep quality, global health, and global energy. We asked the participants to score their current perceptions in these areas on visual analogue scales (VAS), with anchoring terms in both ends. The following questions were included: self-rated health (how do you feel right now, anchoring terms, very bad, very good), ability to concentrate (very bad, very good), memory (very bad, very good), sleep last night (very bad, very good), and energy level (no energy, high energy).

The scores on the individual VAS scales were reversed and summarized to create a global fatigue scale. The total scores were divided by 5, the number of items in the scale. The theoretical range on each scale was a low of 0 to a high of 100. Figure 16.2 depicts the distribution of mean scores of this fatigue scale.

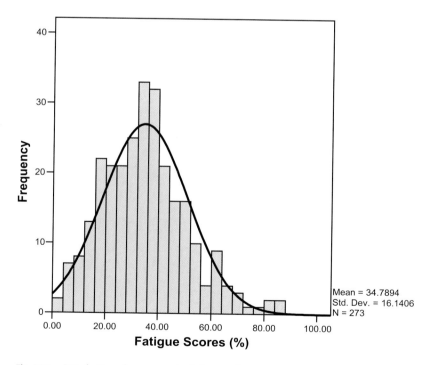

Fig. 16.2. Distribution of scores on the fatigue scale.

We validated the fatigue scale, both in repeated measures of the same participants in the previously described IT/media study as well as in a separate and independent study, carried out in collaboration with Dr. Jan Lisspers, focusing on the recovery process from fatigue-related health disorders. Participants in this latter study were 24 persons recovering from stress-related cardiovascular disorders, 17 being part of a lifestyle moderation program, and 21 healthy controls. The participants in both studies referred to here consisted of men as well as women.

Exploratory and confirmatory factor analysis confirmed that the scale consisted of one factor. The scale also had a high internal consistency (Cronbach's alpha 0.75 or higher).

Thus, the fatigue scale was used both in a sample of working subjects as well as in a sample recovering from stress-related disorders, where fatigue is a common problem.

The aggregated mean score for subjects in the two control groups was 36.11% (SD = 15.16) as compared to a 56.77% (21.43) aggregate score for the combined lifestyle modification and cardiovascular rehabilitation groups. There were no statistically significant differences in fatigue scores between the two reference groups. However, participants in the lifestyle modification group and the cardiovascular rehabilitation group differed significantly from the reference groups. Figure 16.3 depicts the differences in mean fatigue scores across the four groups studied.

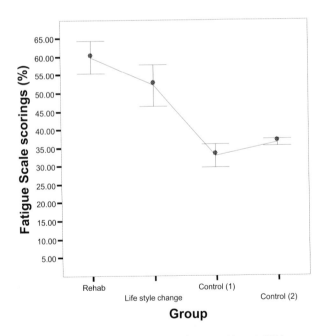

Fig. 16.3. Fatigue scale scores by study group. Mean ± SEM. *Rehab* Cardiovascular rehabilitation, *lifestyle change* lifestyle modification, *control (1)* reference group to the rehabilitation and cardiovascular rehabilitation groups, respectively, *control (2)* IT/media employees.

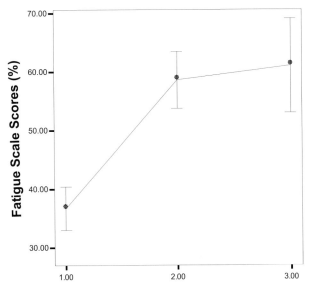

Fig. 16.4. Fatigue scale scorings by Shirom–Melamed burnout scale scores. *1* Healthy controls, scores < 2.75 points (on the Shirom–Melamed burnout scale); *2* intermediate between burnout and healthy (2.75–4.75 points); and *3* burnout (>4.75 points). MEAN ± SEM.

16.8
Fatigue Scale Versus Other Scales Assessing Fatigue-Related Conditions

The Shirom–Melamed burnout questionnaire was also used to validate the fatigue scale. Based on the average mean scores on the Shirom–Melamed burnout questionnaire, respondents were categorized into three groups: healthy referents with scores below 2.75; intermediate (2.75 to less than or equal to 4.75), and burnout with scores greater than 4.75 on a discrete scale ranging from a low of 1 (almost never, for example, tired, to a high of 7, almost always). Figure 16.4 depicts the results for this validation.

Both of the above methods suggest that the cut-off value for healthy controls on the fatigue scale should be around 35%. Fatigued groups score around 55%. Severely fatigued or "burnout" subjects score 60% or higher.

16.9
Fatigue Development Over Time – Risk Factors and Protective Factors

Using longitudinal data in the HealthIT study, running over a 1-year period, we were interested in identifying risk factors as well as protective (salutogenetic)

Mean Fatigue Scores

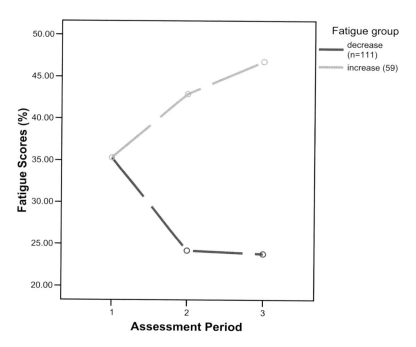

Fig. 16.5. Development of fatigue over a one year period. Assessments were done at baseline (1), at 6 months (2) and at 12 months (3). Results are covaried for initial fatigue scores.

factors for the development of fatigue. The sample was divided into participants whose scorings on the fatigue scale increased continuously during the 1-year prospective study, and those that continuously decreased their fatigue scores. In Fig. 16.5, results are depicted for these two groups of participants. The mean starting fatigue score was 35%, which was suggested by our prior validation studies to be the upper limit for normal fatigue scores.

There was a significant time–fatigue group interaction over the 1-year study period ($p < 0.001$). Furthermore, fatigue scores at baseline were a codeterminant of the development of fatigue over time ($p < 0.0001$). Thus, higher initial scorings on the fatigue scale might actually function as an early warning sign for future development of severe fatigue.

In the final step, we were interested in identifying possible psychosocial and biological predictors of changes in fatigue scores over time. Changes in stress, ratings of future prospects and serum testosterone between the first and the second assessments, 6 months apart, were used to predict changes in fatigue scale scorings during the same period.

As shown in Table 16.2, changes in fatigue scorings were predicted in model 1

Tab. 16.2. Results from the linear regression analysis, using changes in fatigue scores as the dependent variable.

Model		Unstandardized Coefficients		Standardized Coefficients	t	Sig.
		Beta	Std. Error	Beta		
1	(Constant)	−3.452	0.807		−4.280	0.000
	DSTRESS 21	0.171	0.041	0.270	4.163	0.000
2	(Constant)	−3.086	0.800		−3.858	0.000
	DSTRESS 21	0.167	0.040	0.265	4.167	0.000
	DFUTURE 21	−0.146	0.047	−0.198	−3.118	0.002

by changes in self-rated stress during the same 6-month period (DSTRESS 21). That is, increased stress ratings predicted increased fatigue. The model explained 7% of the variance in changes in self-rated fatigue.

In model 2, changes in self-rated beliefs about future prospects (DFUTURE 21) predicted changes in fatigue scorings during the same period. That is, in addition to increased stress, decreased belief about future prospects related to increased fatigue. This model explained 11% of the variance in changes in fatigue scorings.

We also looked at biological predictors. None of the biological predictors, such as changes in brain natriuretic hormone, a peptide (BNP), serum prolactin, chromogranin A, or serum cortisol, predicted changes in fatigue scorings during the same 6-month period. However, changes in serum testosterone predicted changes in fatigue scorings. As expected the association was inverse (standardized Beta −0.21. $R^2 = 0.46$).

This study indicates that chronic stress is a predictor of fatigue development, while a positive view of future prospects appears to be acting as a salutogenetic or protective factor. Serum levels of testosterone, a recognized anti-stress hormone, is counteracting the development of fatigue. Testosterone has been shown in numerous studies to be sensitive to various stressors and is often a more sensitive biological stress indicator than many other stress markers. Testosterone levels decrease in serum during long-term stressor exposure.

In summary, the current chapter discusses the concept of fatigue and attempts to separate it from various disorders characterized by fatigue along with a range of other symptoms. A five-item scale presented is suggested to be of interest in measuring fatigue. The scale has been validated using various other scales but has also established tentative cut-off values for nonfatigue states versus severe fatigue. It is suggested that future research into fatigue more clearly separates fatigue and fatigue states from other disorders, such as depression and dysthymia.

It is also of interest to identify in further detail the molecular mechanisms behind fatigue-related states and also to attempt to separate this form of fatigue from other fatiguing illnesses' conditions.

Medically nonexplained fatigue syndromes, such as CFS, most probably represent a heterogeneous group of disorders with a multifactorial pathophysiology including disturbances to the neuro–endocrine–immune (NEI) systems. One recent suggestion has considered CFS as a neuro–endocrine–immune dysfunction syndrome. Because the hypothalamic–pituitary–adrenocortical (HPA) axis plays an important role in the NEI interaction it has been suggested as a pathway linking factors such as sleep disturbances, inactivity and immunological dysfunctions to fatigue disorders. From the actual literature, however, we conclude that there is no specific change to the HPA axis in CFS. Although the association to the HPA axis is established, a direct causal link has not yet been demonstrated. Evidence to date support the notion that in later stages of CFS and related disorders, there can be HPA axis changes, which in turn can lead to progression and preservation of fatigue and other symptoms.

References

ARNETZ B. Staff perception of the impact of health care transformation on quality of care. Int J Qual Health Care 1999 11:345–351.

BAROFSKY I, LEGRO MW. Definition and measurement of fatigue. Rev Infect Dis 1991;13[suppl 1]:S94–S97.

BULTMAN U, KANT I, KASL S, et al. Fatigue and psychological distress in the working population: psychometrics, prevalence, and correlates. J Psychosom Res 2002;52:445–452.

CHALDER T, BERELOWITZ G, PAWLIOKOWSKA T, et al. Development of a fatigue scale. J Psychosom Res 1993;37:147–153.

DAVID A, PELOSI A, MCDONALD E, et al. Tired, weak, or in need of rest: fatigue among the general practice attenders. Br Med J 1990;301:1199–1202.

DITTNER AJ, WESSELY SC, BROWN RG. The assessment of fatigue. A practical guide for clinicians and researchers. J Psychosom Res 2004;56:157–170.

FUKUDA K, STRAUS SE, HICKIE I, SHARPE MC, DOBBINS JG, KOMAROFF A. The chronic fatigue syndrome. A comprehensive approach to its definition and study. Ann Intern Med 1994;121:953–959.

HEIM C, BIERL C, NISENBAUM R, WAGNER D, REEVES WC. Regional prevalence of fatiguing illnesses in the United States before and after the terrorist attacks of September 11, 2001. Psychosom Med 2004;66:672–678.

LEWIS G, WESSELY S. The epidemiology of fatigue: more questions than answers. J Epidemiol Community Health 1992;46:92–97.

LOGE JH, EKEBERG O, KAASA S. Fatigue in the general Norwegian population: normative data and associations. J Psychosom Res 1998;45:53–65.

MELAMED S, UGARTEN U, SHIROM A, KAHANA L, LERMA Y, FROOM P. Chronic burnout, somatic arousal and elevated salivary cortisol levels. J Psychosom Res 1999;46:591–598.

SHAPIRO CM. Editorial. Chronic fatigue – chronically confusing but growing information. J Psychosom Res 2004;56:153–155.

SKAPINAKIS P, LEWIS G, MAVREAS V. Temporal relations between unexplained fatigue and depression: Longitudinal data from an international study in primary care. Psychosom Med 2004;66:330–335.

SLUITER JK, VAN DER BEEK AJ, FRINGS DRESEN MH. The influence of work characteristics on the need for recovery and experienced health: a study on coach drivers. Ergonomics 1999;42:573–583.

TAYLOR RR, JASON LA, TORRES A. Fatigue rating scales: an emperical comparison. Psychol Med 2000;30:849–856.

VERCOULEN JH, SWANINK CM, FENNIS JF, et al. Dimensional assesment of chronic fatigue syndrome. J Psychosom Res 1994;38:383–392.

17

The Role of Stress in the Etiology
of Medically Unexplained Syndromes

James Rubin and Simon Wessely

17.1
Medically Unexplained Syndromes

Physical symptoms are a normal part of our everyday life. In any given month about 80% of us will experience at least one somatic symptom, although only a minority will seek medical advice from their general practitioner as a result. For those who do, thorough investigation typically reveals no organic cause in about a third of cases. Such "medically unexplained" complaints are also common outside of primary care, with no fewer than 54% of consultations by frequent attenders at specialist gastroenterology clinics being the result of medically unexplained symptoms [1]. The corresponding figures for neurology (50%), cardiology (34%), rheumatology (33%) and orthopedics (30%) are similarly high.

Although many patients experience only one or two discrete medically unexplained symptoms, such as headaches, fatigue or nausea, others present with more complex symptom clusters for which no pathophysiological cause can be found. These clusters are often given labels such as chronic fatigue syndrome (CFS), electromagnetic sensitivity (ES), fibromyalgia or irritable bowel syndrome (see Table 17.1).

Whilst these illnesses can often be difficult and frustrating to treat, that they require treatment is not in question. CFS, for example, is linked to greater levels of disability than congestive heart failure, type II diabetes, multiple sclerosis or recent acute myocardial infarction [2], is strongly associated with emotional distress and disorder, and has a poor prognosis if left untreated.

Although it is sometimes assumed that each of these illnesses is a discrete entity with its own risk factors, correlates and appropriate management strategies, in many respects the similarities between them are more striking than the differences. For example, almost all of these syndromes are more commonly reported by women than by men, emotional disorders tend to be unusually prevalent in each, and each is characterized by difficulties in forming a therapeutic relationship between doctor and patient [3]. Similarities also exist between the symptoms that must be used to diagnose the illnesses in the absence of any accepted physiological abnormalities, with many patients who initially present with one medically unex-

Stress in Health and Disease. Edited by Bengt B. Arnetz and Rolf Ekman
Copyright © 2006 WILEY-VCH Verlag GmbH & Co. KGaA, Weinheim
ISBN: 3-527-31221-8

Tab. 17.1. Labels given to the medically unexplained syndromes encountered in different specialties.

Specialty	Syndrome labels
Allergy	Multiple chemical sensitivity, total allergy syndrome
Cardiology	Atypical chest pain, effort syndrome
Dentistry	Burning mouth syndrome, intolerance to dental amalgam, atypical facial pain
Ear, nose and throat	Globus syndrome
Gastroenterology	Irritable bowel syndrome, food intolerance
Gynecology	Premenstrual syndrome, chronic pelvic pain
Infectious diseases	Chronic fatigue syndrome/myalgic encephalomyelitis
Military health	Gulf War syndrome
Occupational health	Electromagnetic sensitivity, sick building syndrome
Rheumatology	Fibromyalgia

plained syndrome also meeting the diagnostic criteria for several others. This phenomenon may partly be explained by another similarity between the syndromes: their heterogeneity. Even within diagnostic categories there is often a wide disparity in terms of the symptoms experienced by patients. For example, within ES, no coherent syndrome of symptoms has yet been detected [4], with the same being true of other medically unexplained illnesses. It is perhaps unsurprising, then, that a considerable degree of overlap exists between these illnesses, with many patients reporting two or more at the same time or changing their self-diagnosis from one label to another as time goes by.

Research into treatments for medically unexplained illnesses also shows a degree of convergence. In most cases, reducing exposure to a putative toxic agent, be it dental amalgam, electromagnetic fields or exercise, is not effective in reducing symptoms. Instead, many of the syndromes have been shown to respond well to psychological treatments and in particular to cognitive behavioral therapy (CBT) [5]. Although there is also some evidence for the efficacy of other, illness-specific, treatments, such as hydrocortisone for CFS or smooth muscle relaxants for irritable bowel syndrome, this generalized efficacy of CBT suggests that common psychological or behavioral factors probably contribute to the chronic symptoms that characterize each illness.

Such similarities have led some authors to suggest that the individual medically unexplained syndromes are best seen as different labels for the same underlying processes [3], with the diagnosis given to any particular patient having more to do with which medical speciality he or she happens to be referred to first and which new disease is currently prominent in the mass media than to any objective features of their condition. What these common underlying processes are is still uncertain, but some have suggested that stress may play an important etiological role. In this chapter, we review the evidence linking psychosocial stress to medically unexplained syndromes and discuss some of the possible mechanisms which may explain this association. Two syndromes in particular are used to illustrate these links: CFS and ES. The first of these, CFS, is conventionally defined as severe and debilitating fatigue which has been present for at least 6 months, is inexplicable in terms of any recognized organic or psychiatric pathology, and which co-occurs with four or more other symptoms such as impaired memory or concentration, sore throat, muscle pain, headaches, or tender lymph nodes. ES is less well-defined but includes any patients who report medically unexplained symptoms which they believe to be caused or exacerbated by exposure to weak electromagnetic fields such as those emitted by computers, domestic appliances, mobile phones, or overhead power lines.

17.2
Evidence for an Association with Psychosocial Stress

17.2.1
Life Events as Risk Factors for Illness Onset

When patients with CFS are asked to list any factors which they think contributed to the onset of their illness, stressful life events tend to figure relatively highly. For example, in one study by Salit [6], 134 consecutive patients with CFS who had been referred to his clinic for assessment were asked to recall whether any stressful events had occurred in the year prior to the onset of their illness. As a control, 35 healthy participants were asked the same question regarding any stressful events experienced in the past 12 months. Of the CFS patients, 85% recalled one or more life events prior to their illness onset, compared to just 6% of controls who reported life events in the past year. In a similar fashion, Ray et al. [7] interviewed 60 CFS patients about any factors which they thought may have contributed to their illness onset. "Stressful circumstances" such as strained or broken relationships, bereavement or moving house were mentioned by 77% of the sample, while 82% mentioned "doing too much," being overworked, for example, having a large number of family responsibilities or "burning the candle at both ends."

Other studies using more formalized life event questionnaires such as the Holmes and Rahe Social Readjustment Rating Scale have tended to confirm these findings. For instance, in a study 46 CSF patients were asked to complete an abbreviated version of this scale with reference to the year prior to their illness onset, while a control group of 46 healthy participants were asked to complete it with reference to the 12 months prior to a "very difficult period" in their lives [8]. Negative events were nearly twice as prevalent in the immediate period prior to CFS as compared to prior to the control group's difficult periods. Several other studies, each using slightly different controls and questionnaires, have since replicated these results. Not all researchers have found this association, however. For example, Lewis et al. [9] compared 47 CFS patients, 47 irritable bowel syndrome patients and 30 healthy controls in terms of the number and severity of life events experienced in the 2 years prior to their illness onset or, for the controls, prior to interview. Although CFS patients were more likely to report having bought or moved house before their illness, no overall differences were found between the three groups in terms of the incidence or severity of life events.

In general then, although most case control studies suggest that life events may help to trigger CFS, it seems that experiencing a stressful upheaval is not a necessary precondition for developing the illness. It may be best to treat the findings of these studies with a degree of caution, however, as there are still several areas of uncertainty surrounding their methodology. In particular, each study relies heavily on the accuracy of patients' recall for stressful events that may have occurred several years previously, as well as on their ability to discriminate events that preceded their illness from those which followed it. This is particularly problematic in the context of CFS, as many patients with this illness experience a gradual onset of their symptoms. As a result, it may sometimes be difficult for patients to remember whether stressful events such as strained relationships or depression were a possible cause of their illness or were actually the result of their slowly deteriorating health. Case control studies may also produce artificially inflated estimates of the number of life events experienced prior to illness onset as a result of recall bias, with the mere act of receiving a diagnosis prompting individuals to try to remember possible triggering events that fit with their mental models of what might cause their particular illness.

Part of the solution to these problems is to use prospective cohort studies to examine the effects of life events on patients known to be at risk of developing CFS. One such at-risk group consists of patients who are newly diagnosed with infectious mononucleosis (IM), a fatigue-related illness which is reported as a triggering factor by many CFS patients [6]. So, for example, Bruce-Jones et al. [10] followed up a group of 155 IM patients for 6 months following their diagnosis, of whom 14 eventually developed medically unexplained chronic fatigue. At 6 months post-IM diagnosis, patients were asked to report any severe life events or difficulties that they had experienced in the 6 months before and after contracting IM: patients with chronic fatigue were no more likely than those without to have experienced stressful life events or difficulties, although the low statistical power of this study may have prevented a small but important association from being detected. In a separate study using a similar design, Buchwald et al. [11] followed up 142 IM patients for 6 months. In this sample experiencing a "threatening event" more than 6 months prior to IM onset was associated with the development of chronic fatigue. Thus, although it is possible to question how valid chronic fatigue following acute IM is as a model for full-blown CFS, the results of these studies do seem to imply that the association between stressful life events and CFS onset found by many case control studies is not merely the result of recall bias.

17.2.2
Occupational Stress and "Technostress" as Risk Factors for Illness Onset

Although the onset of CFS seems to be associated with stressful life events, research into the etiology of other medically unexplained syndromes has focused on different forms of stress. In particular, the seemingly close relationship between many of these syndromes and the working environment has led some to examine the role of occupational stress in their etiology. For example, chronic lower back pain, repetitive strain injuries, sick building syndrome and ES all frequently develop within the workplace and can be exacerbated by the working environment. In ES patients who are still able to attend work, for instance, more symptoms tend to be reported following days spent at work than during leisure days. Although it might be argued that this relationship is caused by the presence of greater electromagnetic fields in the office, this seems an unlikely explanation as blind and double-blind provocation studies have repeatedly shown that patients who report ES do not tend to react to the presence of increased electromagnetic fields with increased symptoms [12]. Instead, several studies point to occupational stress as being a key mediating factor in the relationship, with ES patients typically reporting more perceived psychosocial stress than healthy controls, a finding that is particularly true when the stress assessments are made at work.

As might be expected in a syndrome that often manifests itself as an apparent intolerance to items of modern office equipment, stress relating specifically to an individual's interaction with modern technologies may be of particular relevance in the development of ES. Interest in this area has focused on whether technostress might play a role in the etiology of the condition. Technostress is the term used for the mental and physiological arousal experienced when a worker attempts to satisfy the increased demands for productivity that modern technologies appear to allow, yet without feeling that he or she has all the necessary skills to master that technology. These problems in human–computer interaction can be especially frustrating where the employee is interested and motivated in his or her work and hence actively tries to cope with their perceived increase in workload. Unfortunately, evidence relating to the notion of technostress as one of the causes of ES is still limited, but some authors have found that ES sufferers who report a particular intolerance to their computers are more likely than their healthy colleagues to be unsatisfied with the information they have about their computer systems, to be sceptical about their computers, to feel unable to substitute other work for computer work and to be unable to control or assess the amount and type of work that they are expected to do. On the other hand, others have suggested that having too much control over computer work may be associated with ES in users of modern technologies, while still others have been unable to find any significant correlation either way.

Thus although more research is required to tease out the exact relationship between occupational stress and ES, it does seem that individuals who report this illness are also more likely to experience stress in their workplace and stress associated with their interactions with the apparently "toxic" technology. These effects are not limited to ES and similar findings have been also reported for repetitive strain injury, back pain and sick building syndrome.

17.2.3
Stress as an Exacerbating Factor in Medically Unexplained Illnesses

A common complaint amongst patients with CFS is that their symptoms are made worse by physical and mental stress. An interesting example of this can be found in a unique study of CFS sufferers from South Florida who experienced the full impact of Hurricane Andrew in 1992. Those sufferers who lived in areas that were severely affected by the disaster were significantly more likely to experience a relapse and to report large increases in CFS-related symptoms than those who lived in unaffected areas of the state [13]. While the physical upheaval involved in the evacuation and subsequent reconstruction effort undoubtedly contributed to this effect, the main predictor of relapse in these patients was the individual's own subjective distress response.

Although it is impossible to recreate this type of severe and chronic stressor in the laboratory, experimental studies have shown that similar effects can be elicited to lesser extent by relatively mild stressors. For example, tasks such as solving difficult anagrams have been shown to provoke an increase in symptoms in CFS patients that is greater than that experienced by patients with either muscular dystrophy or a psychiatric diagnosis.

This association between acute stress and increased symptoms is not found in all medically unexplained illnesses, however. For example, work days that are characterized by high levels of occupational stress do not seem to cause any increase in symptom severity in ES sufferers when compared to low-stress work days. Similar results have also been found under laboratory conditions, for example, in one experimental provocation study which required ES patients to complete a task which mimicked stressful computer work. Although the participants in this study did find the task subjectively stressful, it did not elicit any increase in their symptom severity.

Although psychosocial stress may be relevant as a potential risk factor for the initial development of medically unexplained syndromes and may also serve to exacerbate symptoms in some conditions, it would therefore appear that high levels of stress are not necessary for the subsequent maintenance of these ill-

---

Key Points from Section 17.1 and 17.2
- Medically unexplained syndromes can be chronic and debilitating.
- There are striking similarities between the different syndromes.
- There is evidence that stressful life events and occupational stress are risk factors for the onset of CFS and ES respectively.
- Stress may also exacerbate symptoms following illness onset.

nesses. Furthermore, it is worth noting that although stress may exacerbate symptoms in some conditions, the persistent avoidance of stressors by patients does not necessarily lead to an improved quality of life. In CFS, for example, the use of avoidance strategies to cope with stressful situations in day to day life is actually associated with increased, rather than decreased, levels of fatigue and disability.

17.3
Possible Mechanisms

Although many studies have shown an association between psychosocial stress and medically unexplained syndromes, why this association exists is still a matter for debate. Several mechanisms have been proposed which might explain the relationship but a lack of good quality data means that most remain somewhat speculative. Five possible mechanisms are outlined below.

17.3.1
Negative Mood as a Mediating Variable

Most of the medically unexplained syndromes show a strong association with emotional distress [3]. As many patients with these syndromes also respond to antidepressants, some authors have suggested that these illnesses should be seen as a form of "affective spectrum disorder" [14]. If correct, one potential mechanism through which stress might trigger or exacerbate medically unexplained syndromes is by increasing the risk or severity of emotional disorder in patients who are already at risk of somatizing their negative mood and interpreting it in terms of a physical illness. In support of this, it is certainly the case that life events or chronic stressors can cause emotional distress and are, for example, a significant predictor of emotional disorder in patients newly diagnosed with IM [10]. At present, however, the theory that medically unexplained illnesses are simply a form of affective disorder remains speculative. In particular it is worth noting that, although common, not all patients with medically unexplained syndromes do experience significant emotional distress.

17.3.2
Symptom Amplification

An alternative psychological mechanism is that suggested by Barsky and Borus [15]. These researchers have proposed that medically unexplained syndromes are best understood as a process of symptom amplification, whereby various psychosocial factors encourage a patient to focus their attention on a set of symptoms that might otherwise have proved transient and benign. The four factors they propose as central to this process include the belief that one is sick, holding expectations that certain exposures will result in certain symptoms, the reinforcing effect of adopting the sick role, and experiencing stress and distress. With respect to this final factor, it has long been recognized that psychosocial stress can have a major impact on symptom amplification by increasing a person's sensitivity to innocuous bodily sensations, increasing the likelihood that a sensation, when detected, will be labeled as an adverse symptom, increasing the likelihood that clusters of symptoms will be interpreted as implying the presence of a disease, and making it more probable that medical care will be sought as a result [16]. Of course, stress can also be the direct cause of bodily sensations such as fatigue or racing heart that may themselves be liable to such amplification. Furthermore, given that suffering from an apparently inexplicable ailment can itself be a potent source of stress, in some syndromes the potential exits for a vicious circle of stress, symptom amplification and sickness to develop and contribute to the perpetuation of the illness.

A large amount of experimental evidence exists to support the role of psychosocial stress in symptom amplification in healthy volunteers and patients with organic pathologies [15, 16]. As such it would be surprising if this mechanism was not also involved in the development or exacerbation of medically unexplained syndromes. Exactly how much of a role it plays and whether it is the sole mechanism responsible for the relationship between these syndromes and stress has yet to be established.

17.3.3
Classical Conditioning

Certain medically unexplained syndromes such as ES and multiple chemical sensitivity are characterized by an association between symptom occurrence and specific triggering stimuli, such as computers or particular odors. Given that double-blind exposures to these stimuli typically fail to elicit greater symptom severity than exposure to a suitable sham substance [12], some have proposed that these associations may be the result of classical, or Pavlovian, conditioning. According to this idea, repeated pairing of an initially neutral stimulus (the conditioned stimulus, for example a computer or odor) with a symptom-eliciting event (the unconditioned stimulus) may eventually result in presentation of the conditioned stimulus alone being sufficient to elicit the symptoms. This effect has been demonstrated in several studies by Van den Bergh and colleagues, who have shown that the somatic complaints and respiratory responses that result from inhalation of carbon-dioxide-enriched air can, after relatively few pairings with a foul-smelling odor, subsequently be elicited by presentation of the odor alone [17]. This effect has even been found for pairings between carbon-dioxide-induced symptoms and being asked to imagine a negative scenario such as being trapped in an elevator, suggesting that simply believing oneself to be in a hazardous environment, regardless of the presence of any physical cues, may be sufficient to result in symptom onset once the conditioning has taken hold.

As many of the stimuli that trigger symptoms in medically unexplained illnesses are also sources of psychosocial stress, it may be that in some cases the stress response itself serves as the original unconditioned stimulus in this process of conditioning. For example, stressful work with a computer may result in physiological changes such as increased dermal blood flow and higher levels of thyroxin and estradiol, which can in turn contribute towards symptoms such as burning and itching sensations. After experiencing these symptoms several times as a result of stressful computer work, the patient may come to associate the computer or the working environment with their symptoms, until simply being near to the computer in the case of ES, or entering the office in the case of sick building syndrome, is enough to elicit the same reaction. Whether the mechanisms underlying these conditioned responses are physiological, psychological or both is still uncertain, although experimental studies in which ES sufferers are exposed to real and sham electromagnetic fields have so far found no compelling evidence of any neuroendocrine or dermal correlates to the skin symptoms that are elicited by both types of exposure. It may therefore be that psychological processes such as expectations and symptom amplification are the key factors in driving this conditioning (see Section 17.3.2).

17.3.4
Chronic Neuroendocrine Dysfunction

Numerous studies have examined the role of chronic neuroendocrine dysfunction in the etiology of medically unexplained syndromes in general and CFS in particular. Many of these, though by no means all, have found CFS to be linked to low basal cortisol levels [18]. That these low levels may be etiologically important in the condition is suggested by two double blind placebo-controlled trials of hydrocortisone replacement therapy for CFS, both of which reported modest improvements in health as a result of the pharmacological treatment. Although it is not yet clear when it is during the pathogenesis of CFS that low cortisol develops, one suggestion is that the neuroendocrine abnormality may be a preexisting trait which predisposes some people to develop chronic fatigue after they experience a physiological or psychosocial stressor. Furthermore, as some evidence exists to suggest that critical or traumatic life events can cause dysregulation of the neuroendocrine system, it has also been suggested that this low cortisol may be the key mediating variable which explains the relationship between life events and the onset of CFS.

Although this is an intriguing hypothesis, the results of several studies have failed to provide support for it. In particular, two prospective cohort studies of groups at risk of developing chronic fatigue have not found any association between preexisting low cortisol and subsequent fatigue status [18]. Meanwhile it has also been demonstrated that when CBT is used to normalize the daily routines of patients with CFS their cortisol levels also tend to return to normal. It therefore appears that the low cortisol levels found in some CFS patients are more likely to be the result of the behavioral changes that are typical of the illness rather than being its primary cause. The mechanism to explain the relationship between life events and CFS onset may therefore need to be sought elsewhere.

17.3.5
Cardiovascular and Neuroendocrine Responses to Acute Stressors

The fact that psychosocial stress can exacerbate symptoms in some medically unexplained illnesses has led to several studies which have attempted to identify possible physiological mechanisms underlying this phenomenon. In particular, several studies have focused on putative abnormalities in the autonomic and cardiovascular responses to stress. For example, LaManca et al. [19] examined the cardiovascular responses to stressful cognitive tasks in 19 CFS patients. In comparison to the responses of a healthy control group, the CFS patients showed significantly reduced heart rate and systolic and diastolic blood pressure changes when asked to perform the tasks. Moreover, those patients who were most severely affected by CFS showed the greatest blunting of their cardiovascular responsiveness. Similar effects have also been observed in other studies of CFS and idiopathic chronic fatigue, leading some to suggest that patients with CFS may have abnormalities in the central mechanisms responsible for regulating their blood pressure response to stressors, and that this in turn can result in cerebral hypoperfusion and a worsening of symptoms [19]. On the other hand, findings of increased cardiovascular responsiveness to stressors have also been reported by some, while others have suggested that any blunting of the cardiovascular response that does exist may be restricted to a subgroup of patients who suffer from a less severe form of the illness. Furthermore, as it is also possible for abnormal autonomic and cardiovascular responses to be the result of cardiovascular deconditioning, it may be that CFS and the low activity levels that go with it are the cause rather than the consequence of these phenomena. However, given that blunted cardiovascular responses have been observed even where CFS patients are compared to non-exercising sedentary controls, this particular explanation for these findings seems unlikely.

It is unclear whether these findings extend to other medically unexplained syndromes. For example, studies which have examined the response of ES participants to cognitive stressors have tended to observe heightened, rather than reduced cardiovascular responsiveness, while studies of ES patients subjected to external stimuli such as audiotones or flickering light also suggest a degree of hyperresponsiveness.

Abnormal neuroendocrine responses to stressors have also been examined as a feature of medically unexplained illness, and one study has recently reported a lower cortisol response to the naturalistic stress of awakening in CFS patients [20]. A separate study using the same paradigm did not observe any such effect, however, while another observed no effect of social stress on cortisol response in CFS, although a reduced adrenocorticotropic hormone (ACTH) response was found.

Thus, although a range of abnormal physiological responses to stress have been reported in medically unexplained illnesses, no consensus has yet been reached as to precisely what variables are affected, which patient groups are involved, whether hyper- or hyporesponsiveness best characterizes the abnormality, and what role the abnormalities play in the etiology of the syndromes. Clearly, more work is needed in this area.

Key Points from Section 17.3
- Psychological theories may partly explain the association between stress and medically unexplained syndromes, but at the moment they remain speculative.
- Chronic neuroendocrine dysfunction seems unlikely as a complete explanation for the associations.
- Intriguing findings regarding cardiovascular and autonomic hyper- and hyporesponsiveness to stressors have been reported, but these require replication and extension.

17.4
Implications for Diagnosis

The presence of high levels of psychosocial stress is not a necessary requirement for the diagnosis of any of the medically unexplained syndromes. Nevertheless, identifying the presence and source of stress may assist in the treatment of the disorder. Furthermore, regardless of its role in the etiology of a patient's complaints, high levels of stress and negative mood are themselves quality-of-life issues and may therefore be deserving of treatment in their own right. For these reasons, patients presenting with persistent medically unexplained symptoms and syndromes should be assessed for mood disorder using standard interviews or self-report questionnaires.

17.5
Implications for Treatment

The association between stress and medically unexplained syndromes has various implications for treatment. Several studies, for example, have examined the efficacy of using antidepressants in illnesses such as fibromyalgia, irritable bowel syndrome and CFS. While such treatments have often proved effective, it appears that their efficacy in treating the symptoms of medically unexplained illnesses may be independent of their effects on emotional distress. The exact mechanism underlying their modest efficacy in these syndromes therefore remains unclear.

Numerous other studies have demonstrated the efficacy of an alternative treatment for medically unexplained syndromes, namely CBT [5, 21], the underlying theory of which is that the way an individual perceives and thinks about their illness strongly influences how they act and feel. Accordingly, the reason why medically unexplained syndromes can be so disabling and persistent may be that, regardless of the initial causes, the long-term maintenance of the illness is due to a self-perpetuating cycle of cognitions, behaviors and symptoms. As shown in

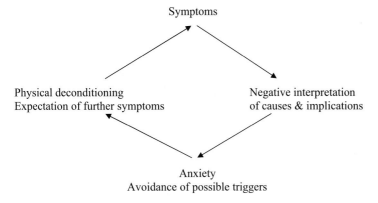

Fig. 17.1. Cognitive–behavioral model of medically unexplained syndromes.

Fig. 17.1, it is believed that when a patient with a medically unexplained syndrome experiences a symptom, they form certain negative assumptions about the causes and implications of it. These assumptions then produce high levels of anxiety and also promote avoidance of the assumed trigger, the fear-avoidance model. The knock-on effects of this can then include physical deconditioning, particularly if the assumed trigger for the symptom involves exercise, and an increased expectation of symptoms the next time the assumed trigger is encountered. Unfortunately, both of these factors will tend to make symptoms more likely to return in future. The fear and depression that result from this apparently intractable vicious circle only serve to make the patient's condition worse.

CBT aims to provide a route out of this cycle by providing patients with the skills needed to alter their patterns of thinking and behavior. The specific goals of the treatment are usually identified through negotiation with the patient and help to provide concrete milestones which can be used to judge progress. These goals are often very pragmatic. For example, the patient's main aim may be to resume a particular hobby, to be able to go shopping again or to be able to visit relatives despite the presence of feared stimuli in their homes. To help the patient achieve these goals, the therapist must identify any maladaptive beliefs that the patient holds about their illness and help them to find ways of testing or reframing these beliefs. In this regard, it is often important to help patients overcome the idea that the presence of symptoms implies that long-term damage has been done to their health ("catastrophizing"). This can be done by suggesting alternative interpretations for symptoms; they might be due to anxiety, for example, or they may be a transient consequence of having undertaken unaccustomed or excessive exercise. Where necessary it can also sometimes be helpful to teach patients relaxation techniques if anxiety is a major problem for them. While these strategies can be taught by a therapist, it is only outside the therapy room that they can be effectively practiced. Another key feature of CBT is therefore the use of homework, in which patients are encouraged to keep diaries of their symptoms, record the automatic assumptions they make about their causes or meaning, and also record and evaluate possible alternative explanations for them.

CBT is a broad treatment package which incorporates several therapeutic elements. As such it is not certain whether there is any one "active ingredient" in it that is responsible for its efficacy. However, as many CBT treatments include some element of "stress inoculation", it is possible that this is one of its key components. Although a recent review of the efficacy of CBT across a range of medically unexplained syndromes concluded that its impact on physical symptoms did not correlate with its impact on standard measures of psychological distress [21], it is still possible that more subtle stress-related effects may be important factors in its success, by reducing distressing thoughts about symptoms, for example, or increasing a patient's perceived control over their illness.

Key Points from Sections 17.4 and 17.5
- Patients with medically unexplained illnesses should be assessed for emotional distress, which may require treatment in its own right.
- Cognitive behavioral therapy has been found to improve the quality of life of patients with many forms of medically unexplained illness.
- The "key ingredients" of cognitive behavioral therapy are unknown, but it is very unlikely that stress reduction is the sole mechanism underlying its efficacy.

Others have suggested that different features of CBT may be more important. In particular the fact that it promotes increased physical activity and improved cardiovascular fitness has been suggested as the most important factor by some, particularly when used for CFS. In support of this, several studies have shown that graded exercise therapy can also be effective as a treatment for CFS [5], although interestingly, objectively assessed improvements in physical fitness do not predict which patients will benefit from graded exercise. It may therefore be that a key component of graded exercise therapy is not the exercise *per se*, but more the improved sense of control over the illness that being able to exercise gives to the patient.

Other studies have suggested that, although reducing overall levels of stress may not be necessary for symptomatic improvements to be seen in medically unexplained syndromes, improvements in certain key stress-related variables may be helpful. For example, one trial of standard acupuncture versus sham acupuncture for ES patients noted improvements in symptoms in both conditions, and also found that both interventions had been effective in improving the ability to relax following a day at work [22]. It is therefore possible that temporary decrements in technostress helped to mediate the success of this intervention. Even the simple reassurance that treatment is available may be effective in reducing symptoms in some medically unexplained syndromes, with 50% of ES patients in one trial reporting improved health after having spent 6 months on a waiting list for CBT. Again, such an effect may have been the result of reductions in stress associated with the perception that one's illness is untreatable.

Where psychosocial stress is present in patients with a medically unexplained illness, attempts to treat the illness should therefore also include attempts to treat the distress. Whether such an approach by itself can lead to a complete cure in these conditions remains doubtful, however.

Questions Yet to be Answered

- Do the same psychophysiological processes underlie all medically unexplained syndromes or do important differences exist in terms of their etiology and appropriate management?
- Why do certain stressors act as risk factors for the onset of medically unexplained syndromes? Are there physiological or psychological mechanisms that can explain this association? Are these associations specific for certain syndromes, or general for all syndromes?
- Why does CBT work for medically unexplained syndromes? Does it encourages greater physical activity, for example, or give patients a better sense of control over their illness?
- Is CBT effective for all patients with medically unexplained syndromes? Are there certain subgroups for whom it is less effective?

References

1 S. Reid, S. Wessely, T. Crayford, M. Hotopf. 2001. Medically unexplained symptoms in frequent attenders of secondary heath care: retrospective cohort study. *Br Med J* 322:1–4.

2 A. Komaroff, L. Fagioli, T.H. Doolittle, B. Gandek, M.A. Gleit, R.T. Guerriero, R.J. Kornish, N.C. Ware, J.E. Ware, D.W. Bates. 1996. Health status in patients with chronic fatigue syndrome and in general population and disease comparison groups. *Am J Med* 101:281–290.

3 S. Wessely, C. Nimnuan, M. Sharpe. 1999. Functional somatic syndrome: one or many? *Lancet* 354:936–939.

4 M. Roosli, M. Moser, Y. Baldinini, M. Meier, C. Braun-Fahrlander. 2004. Symptoms of ill health ascribed to electromagnetic field exposure – a questionnaire survey. *Int J Hyg Environ Health* 207:141–150.

5 P. Whiting, A.-M. Bagnall, A.J. Sowden, J.E. Cornell, C.D. Mulrow, G. Ramirez. 2001. Interventions for the treatment and management of chronic fatigue syndrome: a systematic review. *J Am Med Assoc* 286:1360–1368.

6 I.E. Salit. 1997. Precipitating factors for the chronic fatigue syndrome. *J Psychiatr Res* 31:59–65.

7 C. Ray, S. Jefferies, W. Weir, K. Hayes, S. Simon, F. Akingbade, P. Marriott. 1998. Making sense of chronic fatigue syndrome: patients' accounts of onset. *Psychol Health* 13:99–109.

8 T. Theorell, V. Blomkvists, G. Lindh, B. Evengard. 1999. Critical life events, infections, symptoms during the year preceding chronic fatigue syndrome (CFS): an examination of CFS patients and subjects with a non-specific life crisis. *Psychosom Med* 61:304–310.

9 S. Lewis, C.L. Cooper, D. Benne. 1994. Psychosocial factors and chronic fatigue syndrome. *Psychol Med* 24:661–671.

10 W.D.A. Bruce-Jones, P.D. White, J.M. Thomas, A.W. Clare. 1994. The

effect of social adversity on the fatigue syndrome, psychiatric disorders and physical recovery, following glandular fever. *Psychol Med* 24:651–659.

11 D. BUCHWALD, T.D. REA, W.J. KATON, J.E. RUSSO, R.L. ASHLEY. 2000. Acute infectious mononucleosis: characteristics of patients who report failure to recover. *Am J Med* 109:531–537.

12 G.J. RUBIN, J. DAS MUNSHI, S. WESSELY. 2005. Electromagnetic hypersensitivity: a systematic review of provocation studies. *Psychosom Med* 67:224–252.

13 S.K. LUTGENDORF, M. ANTONI, G. IRONSON, M.A. FLETCHER, F. PENEDO, A. BAUM, N. SCHNEIDERMAN, N. KLIMAS. 2004. Physical symptoms of chronic fatigue syndrome are exacerbated by the stress of Hurricane Andrew. *Psychosom Med* 57:310–323.

14 A.J. GRUBER, J.I. HUDSON, H.G.J. POPE. 1996. The management of treatment-resistant depression in disorders on the interface of psychiatry and medicine. Fibromyalgia, chronic fatigue syndrome, migraine, irritable bowel syndrome, atypical facial pain, premenstrual dysphoric disorder. *Psychiatr Clin North Am* 19:51–69.

15 A.J. BARSKY, J.F. BORUS. 1999. Functional somatic syndromes. *Ann Intern Med* 130:910–921.

16 J.W. PENNEBAKER. 1982. The psychology of physical symptoms. Springer Verlag, New York.

17 O. VAN DEN BERGH, W. WINTERS, I. VAN DIEST. 2002. Learning subjective health complaints. *Scand J Psychol* 43:147–152.

18 A.J. CLEARE. 2003. The neuroendocrinology of chronic fatigue syndrome. *Endocr Rev* 24:236–252.

19 J. LaMANCA, A. PECKERMAN, S.A. SISTO, J. DeLUCA, S. COOK, B.H. NATELSON. 2001. Cardiovascular response of women with chronic fatigue syndrome to stressful cognitive testing before and after strenuous exercise. *Psychosom Med* 63:756–764.

20 A.D.L. ROBERTS, S. WESSELY, T. CHALDER, A. PAPADOPOULOS, A.J. CLEARE. 2004. Salivary cortisol response to awakening in chronic fatigue syndrome. *Br J Psychiatry* 184:136–141.

21 K. KROENKE, R. SWINDLE. 2000. Cognitive–behavioral therapy for somatization and symptom syndromes: A critical review of controlled clinical trials. *Psychother Psychosom* 69:205–215.

22 B.B. ARNETZ, M. BERG, I. ANDERZEN, T. LUNDEBERG, E. HAKER. 1995. A nonconventional approach to the treatment of "environmental illness". *J Occup Environ Med* 37:838–844.

18
Oxidative Inflammatory Stress in Obesity and Diabetes

Paresh Dandona, Ahmad Aljada, Ajay Chaudhuri, and Husam Ghanim

18.1
Introduction

This chapter, dedicated to oxidative and inflammatory stress in obesity and diabetes, attempts to (a) define oxidative and inflammatory stress, (b) describe these mechanisms as relevant to obesity and diabetes, (c) describe the role of glucose in the pathogenesis of oxidative and inflammatory stress, (d) describe the antioxidant and antiinflammatory effect of insulin, (e) relate these processes to how it may affect the brain, and (f) define some exciting new directions in which future investigations are likely to proceed. Oxidative and inflammatory stresses are related to our day-to-day activities, including eating, drinking, and exercise as well as disease states. Recent observations have elucidated not only an understanding of what constitutes oxidative and inflammatory stress, but also how they are induced. These observations have linked those stresses to daily activities and lifestyles in addition to linking them to disease entities.

18.2
Oxidative Stress

Oxidative stress is defined as a condition characterized by an excess of reactive oxygen species (ROS) which results in oxidative damage of lipids, proteins, amino acids and nucleic acids. ROS are either free radicals (FRs), reactive anions containing oxygen atoms, or molecules containing oxygen atoms that can either produce FRs or are chemically activated by them. A compound becomes a FR by gaining an electron, or by losing an electron. The term ROS is a collective term that includes not only oxygen-centered radicals such as: superoxide (O_2^-) and hydroxyl (OH), but also some nonradical derivatives of oxygen such as hydrogen peroxide (H_2O_2), singlet oxygen and hypochlorous acid (HOCl). This extra electron provides the FR with an extremely high reactivity in terms of affinity, rates of reaction and the diversity of molecular types [1]. ROS including O_2^- are generated through the metabolic activities mediated by the electron transport chain and by the enzyme

Stress in Health and Disease. Edited by Bengt B. Arnetz and Rolf Ekman
Copyright © 2006 WILEY-VCH Verlag GmbH & Co. KGaA, Weinheim
ISBN: 3-527-31221-8

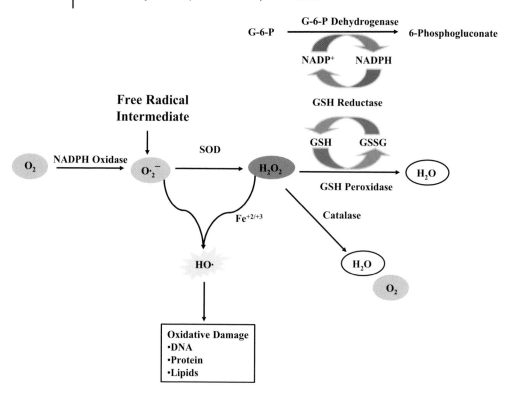

Fig. 18.1. Cell damage is induced by reactive oxygen species (ROS). Under normal conditions, ROS are cleared from the cell by the action of superoxide dismutase (*SOD*), catalase, or glutathione (*GSH*) peroxidase. The main damage to cells results from the ROS-induced alteration of macromolecules such as polyunsaturated fatty acids in membrane lipids, essential proteins, and DNA. GSH = reduced glutathione, GSSG = oxidized glutathione, NADPH = nicotine adenine dinucleotide phosphate.

NADPH oxidase, which is located in cell membranes, especially the polymorphonuclear leucocyte and the monocyte [2]. The O_2^- radical is converted either spontaneously or through superoxide dismutase in combination with water (H_2O) to form H_2O_2. The latter forms hydroxyl radical (OH) following a reaction with Fe^{2+}. O_2^- and OH are highly reactive and are able to react with and disrupt lipids, amino acids proteins and nucleic acids including DNA (Fig. 18.1). Thus, they can damage all biological molecules.

The function of O_2^- generated by the membrane NADPH oxidase is to mediate the destruction of bacteria during and following phagocytosis. The destruction of the bacteria is mediated by peroxidation of membrane lipids as well as oxidative damage of the membrane and intranuclear proteins. Oxidative damage of proteins may lead to the disruption of enzyme systems and that of DNA to abnormalities in genetic material [1]. These comments are relevant not only to the mechanisms involved in bacterial killing but also in damage to one's own body when an excess of ROS are generated in the absence of infection, as in diabetes and obesity.

In addition to causing damage to biological molecules, O_2^- also mediates biological signaling: O_2^- activates a nuclear translocated protein, nuclear factor κB (NFκB), and an activation protein-1, key proinflammatory transcription factors [3]. Both of the proteins are redox sensitive. Thus, O_2^- leads to the induction of inflammation. Therefore, oxidative stress and inflammatory stress are closely linked.

18.3
Inflammatory Stress

Inflammation is classically related to infection, injury and autoimmunity resulting in several disease entities. However, the last decade has seen (a) the definition of inflammation in molecular terms; (b) the emerging evidence that obesity and type 2 diabetes are chronic, low grade inflammatory states; (c) macronutrient intake induces proinflammatory and oxidative stress; and (d) insulin exerts ROS-suppressive and antiinflammatory effect.

The definition of inflammation in molecular terms is the translocation of the key proinflammatory transcription factor, NFκB, from the cytoplasm into the nucleus. In the nucleus, it binds to the promoters of over 200 genes which transcribe mRNA for a variety of proinflammatory proteins including cytokines, adhesion molecules and chemokines [3]. This major trigger for NFκB translocation of the nucleus is the O_2^- radical as mentioned above.

It is of interest that macronutrient intake stimulates processes similar to those triggered by endotoxin and other agents. Thus, glucose and a fast food meal increase intranuclear NFκB binding, thus increasing the gene transcription of proinflammatory cytokines (molecules) like tumor necrosis factor (TNFα) in peripheral blood mononuclear cells (MNC) [4–7]. The oxidative and inflammatory stress induced by glucose and a fast food (900 kcal) meal lasts for at least 2–3 h. It is also relevant that the intake of glucose, fat and a fast food meal result in an increase in ROS, in particular O_2^- radical generation [5, 8]. Thus, O_2^- may contribute to the activation of the inflammatory cascade and the translocation of NFκB to the nucleus. All of these stimuli lead to an increase in O_2^- generation by approximately 100% over the basal. Oxidative stress lasts for at least 2 h after glucose challenge, while that after a fast food meal lasts for more than 3 h.

In this context, it is important to mention that a meal equicaloric to the fast food meal mentioned above but rich in fruit and fiber does not cause either oxidative or inflammatory stress. Thus, it is possible to make rational choices in terms of food selection to avoid oxidative and inflammatory stress. Isocaloric amounts of alcohol and orange juice also do not cause oxidative or inflammatory stress [6].

18.4
Oxidative Stress in Obesity and Diabetes

Increased oxidative stress has been associated with type 2 diabetes for a long time. Elevated ROS generation by MNC in diabetes was described in early 1980s, especially in patients with hypertriglyceridemia. Evidence of increased lipid peroxidation and increased oxidizability of low density lipoproteins (LDLs) has also been shown to occur in diabetes. In addition, there is evidence that increased protein carbonylation occurs in this condition. Finally, it has been shown that DNA in the nuclei of circulating MNC in diabetics is markedly damaged due to oxidative stress [9].

The initial description of obesity-related oxidative stress is more recent, but conceptually it is an extension of the fact that macronutrient intake induces oxidative stress since the obese consume an excess of macronutrients. The obese show evidence of increased lipid peroxidation as reflected in increased plasma concentration of thiobarbituric acid reacting substances (TBARS) and other products of lipid peroxidation. These patients also have increased concentrations of chemically modified proteins and oxidatively damaged amino acids. Caloric restriction and weight loss in the obese have been shown to lead to a fall in these indices within 4 weeks [10]. In addition, there is a marked fall in ROS generation following dietary restriction. Clearly, oxidative stress, elevated in the obese, is dependent upon macronutrient intake and it decreases markedly with dietary restriction. It is relevant that a fast in normal subjects also results in a 35–50% reduction in ROS generation by MNC respectively at 24 and 48 h [11]. We can conclude, therefore, that macronutrient intake is the major determinant of ROS generation and oxidative stress. Since the administration of vitamin E and C prior to glucose intake prevents an increase in ROS and O_2^- generation and also prevents NFκB activations, it can also be suggested that glucose-induced NFκB-based inflammatory stress is induced through O_2^- generation. Thus, a mere lifestyle change with a reduction in macronutrient intake may reduce both oxidative and inflammatory stress.

Thus, the occurrence of oxidative and inflammatory stress is partly due to the act of living itself. Daily metabolic activities, especially high caloric intake, generate oxidative stress through the electron transport chain and NADPH oxidase activation [5]. An increase in these metabolic activities will generate greater oxidative stress and a reduction in these activities will reduce oxidative stress. An increase in macronutrient intake, carbohydrates and fats in particular, would increase oxidative stress and inflammatory stress. Obesity, a result of chronic excessive macronutrient intake, would therefore, be associated with chronic oxidative stress and inflammatory stress.

The reduction in oxidative and inflammatory stress with a restriction in macronutrient intake suggests that one way to prevent oxidative and inflammatory damage leading to atherosclerosis and related complications would be through a change in lifestyle. In this light, the effect of exercise is not understood fully. However, it is known that exercise causes oxidative stress acutely, while when exercise is taken regularly there is a diminution in inflammatory stress. Fully trained athletes and marathon runners have plasma concentrations of complement reacting protein (CRP), an inflammatory mediator, that are significantly lower than those in controls [12].

The evidence that chronic low grade inflammation is a part of obesity was demonstrated in animals associated with an increase in the constitutive expression of TNFα, a cytokine in adipose tissue [13]. This observation initiated the concept of adipocytokines (adipokines) and brought the participation of inflammatory mechanisms into the pathogenesis of metabolic disease. Since TNFα interferes with insulin signaling, it follows that inflammatory mechanisms may be related to the pathogenesis of insulin resistance in obesity and diabetes. Further investigation in this area may reveal the sites/mechanisms involved in the pathogenesis of insulin resistance in obesity and type 2 diabetes. A preliminary study with an aspirin derivative in humans shows promising results in terms of glucose and triglyceride lowering [14]. It is of interest that aspirin was used in the treatment of diabetes prior to the discovery of insulin in 1921. More recently, certain other small proteins which are induced by proinflammatory stimuli like TNFα have been shown to interfere with insulin signal transduction. Elucidation of their mode of action, generation and suppression should lead to a better understanding of the pathogenesis and the treatment of insulin resistance.

Recent work has also shown that the MNC in the obese has an increase in intranuclear NFκB binding. In addition, these cells express increased levels of several inflammatory mediators [15]. The inflammatory status of these cells is associated with a decrease in insulin signaling as reflected in insulin receptor phosphorylation and an increase in the level of the small inflammation-associated molecules which interfere with insulin signaling. Thus, MNC may (a) contribute to the increased plasma concentrations of inflammatory mediators; (b) contribute to arterial atherosclerosis, which is a chronic inflammation; and (c) reflect the insulin-resistant and proinflammatory state of the obese.

Recent work shows that the macrophages in the stromal tissue occupying the interstitial spaces of adipose tissue are the major source of inflammatory cytokines from the adipose tissue. These macrophages also stimulate preadipocytes and adipocytes into secreting cytokines. Furthermore, it has been shown that monocytes migrate from the circulation transendothelially into the adipose tissue, based on the increased expression of chemokines. Monocytes from the circulation become macrophages in adipose tissue. This is similar to their classical role in atherogenesis: monocytes move across the arterial endothelium to form inflammatory foci in the arterial wall. Monocytes in these foci take up oxidized LDL to form lipid-laden foam cells which become fatty streaks, the initial lesion of atherosclerosis. Thus, the circulating MNC in an inflammatory milieu will set up atherogenesis in the arterial wall and inflammation in adipose tissue. This explains why obesity, atherosclerosis and inflammation and diabetes coexist. It also explains why atherogenesis occurs in the obese even before diabetes appears.

As far as diabetes is concerned, hyperglycemia and its proinflammatory effects get added to those related to obesity and insulin resistance. Thus, the overall inflammatory state is enhanced, as is atherogenesis (Fig. 18.2). This is reflected in enhanced risk of acute myocardial infarction (AMI) and stroke in diabetes, the magnitude of which is greater than that observed in obesity. The evidence that inflammatory mechanisms feature in type 2 diabetes came soon afterwards with the demonstration that diabetics have an elevated concentration of sialic acid in plasma [16]. Type 2 diabetics have been shown to have elevated plasma concentrations of CRP, TNFα and other proteins involved in inflammation.

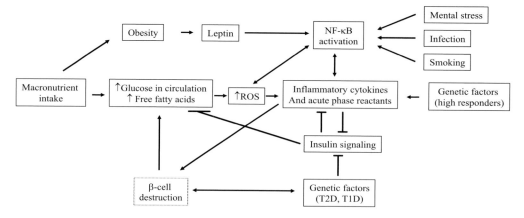

Fig. 18.2. Reactive oxygen species (*ROS*) generation and inflammation by macronutrient intake. *NF-κB* Nuclear factor κB. Adapted from Dandona et al. [7].

18.5
Antioxidant and Antiinflammatory Effect of Insulin

Recent work has shown that insulin suppresses the expression of inflammatory proteins and NFκB binding, *in vitro*, in human aortic endothelial cells. It also suppresses ROS generation by MNC in these cells. Insulin also causes the suppression of NFκB binding and other proinflammatory transcription factors. Consistent with these effects, insulin suppresses the genes regulated by these three transcription factors. The antioxidant and antiinflammatory effects of insulin were also confirmed in patients with acute myocardial infarction observed with insulin therapy [17]. Recent studies in experimental animals also confirm the antiinflammatory effects of insulin. Endotoxin-induced inflammation was prevented by insulin in rats and pigs. Burn- and trauma-induced inflammation was also suppressed by insulin.

The recent data on the action of insulin in acute myocardial infarction also suggests that it may have a cardioprotective effect in humans. Indeed, in experimental acute myocardial infarction, treatment with insulin led to a reduction in the size of the infarct through a cell protective effect [18].

Relevant to the above data on the antiinflammatory effect of insulin is a recent study showing that the restoration of normoglycemia by an infusion of insulin in a large series of patients in a surgical intensive care unit (ICU) led to a 50% reduction in mortality in addition to a marked reduction in other complications like renal failure the need for blood transfusions, ICU neuropathy and the incidence of bacteremia [19]. The restoration of normoglycemia in these patients was associated with a fall in CRP concentrations, consistent with a proinflammatory effect of glucose and an antiinflammatory effect of insulin. In a recent study, the same group demonstrated mitochondrial changes in association with hyperglycemia in the same series of patients. The mitochondrial changes were prevented in patients infused with insulin. The authors suggested that these changes were due to oxidative stress. The reversal of the mitochondrial changes with insulin is consistent with the findings that glucose induces oxidative stress and that insulin suppresses it.

The antiinflammatory effect of insulin may be related to the anticatabolic (or anabolic) effect of insulin in inflammatory states. This area needs further investigation. Since insulin-resistant states of obesity and type 2 diabetes are associated with several cancers, it is possible that resistance to insulin predisposes to neoplasia. This too needs further investigation.

18.6
Mental Stress and Inflammation

The relationship of psychological stress to oxidative and inflammatory stress still requires exploration. However, there are beginnings of such data. It has been shown that persons who look after patients with chronic serious stresses like cancer and Alzheimer's disease have elevated interleukin-6 (IL-6) concentrations in their plasma when compared with controls and that these elevated levels do not return to normal after the demise of the patients [20]. Whether such an elevation of a proinflammatory cytokine affect other organ systems and contributes to insulin resistance needs to be demonstrated. In addition, there is a paradox when considering the relationship between mental stress and proinflammatory changes. Stress normally leads to the activation of the hypothalamic–pituitary–adrenocortical (HPA) axis and an increase in the secretion of corticosteroids. Corticosteroids are known to suppress O_2^- generation and NFκB binding [21]. These actions suppress inflammatory processes. Corticosteroids also suppress the other major proinflammatory transcription factor, activator protein-1 and the genes regulated by them, matrix metalloproteinases. These actions of glucocorticoids explain why stressed individuals do not have adequate immune responses to vaccination and have a greater vulnerability to infection. However, glucocorticoids also induce hyperglycemia through enhanced gluconeogenesis through the induction of S6 kinase which interferes with insulin action. Glucocorticoids also induce hyperlipidemia and hypertension which may promote atherogenesis. Glucocorticoid-induced hyperglycemia and diabetes may also add to this atherogenic action. In addition, glucocorticoids may interfere with insulin-induced nitric oxide (NO) release and nitric oxide synthase (NOS) expression endothelium, and thus impair the vasodilatory responses to endothelium-mediated stimuli. NO is a potent vasodilator and a major modulator of tissue perfusion. The paradox of the antiinflammatory drugs, corticosteroids, causing atherogenesis and deaths due to cardiovascular events is best reconciled by the facts mentioned above: interruption with insulin signaling, hyperlipidemia and the suppression of NO.

18.7
Atherogenesis and Insulin

Since O_2^- radical generated following macronutrient intake activates NFκB and AP-1, two major proinflammatory transcription factors that are redox sensitive, oxidative stress is closely associated with inflammatory stress. The oxidative and inflammatory stress in obesity involves the circulating MNC and the endothelial cells as well as the adipocytes. Since the MNC and the endothelial cells directly participate in atherogenesis, obesity is atherogenic in the long term.

The effect of insulin is suppressive of O_2^- and ROS generation and inflammatory responses. These effects are observed in the MNC and endothelial cells. Thus, the effect of insulin is potentially antiatherogenic in the long term. Any insulin-resistant state is therefore, likely to be proinflammatory and proatherogenic as in obesity. It is of interest that two recent studies in experimental animals support an antiatherogenesis role for insulin.

18.8
The New Paradigm

These observations also take us into a new paradigm regarding the relationship between macronutrient intake and insulin generation/action. For 80 years since the discovery of insulin, we have lived with a metabolic paradigm. The recent observations take us into an inflammatory paradigm. Thus, while macronutrient intake provides an ongoing proinflammatory, oxidative stress signal, insulin provides a tonic antioxidant and antiinflammatory effect. It would therefore be of interest to examine whether the deliberate removal of insulin signaling by a knock out of the insulin receptor or other elements in insulin signal transduction would result in a proinflammatory state.

18.9
Future Horizons

The fact that glucose is proinflammatory and that insulin has opposite effects has implications in the pathogenesis of several systemic phenomena. In particular, they relate to the process of aging and Alzheimer's disease. Diabetes and obesity are known to induce atherosclerosis prematurely, probably through oxidative stress and atherosclerosis. Atherosclerosis is a condition related to aging. In addition, it is now known that in Alzheimer's disease, atherosclerotic changes in the cranial and cerebral arteries coexist with intracerebral plaques of Alzheimer's disease. The pathogenesis of the plaques is related to inflammatory processes.

It is also of note that neurons and glial cells possess the insulin receptor. However, little is known about the specific actions of insulin on the brain. In neuronal cultures, insulin promotes dendrite formation. Insulin is also known to act on the hypothalamic neurons to suppress appetite. Intracerebroventricular infusion of insulin leads to the suppression of food intake. The specific deletion of the insulin receptor in neurons in mice leads to obesity and hypogonadotrophic hypogonadism. In this respect, it is of great interest that a recent report shows that type 2 diabetes is associated with hypogonadotrophic hypogonadism in as many as 33% of patients suffering from this condition [22].

There are recent data to show a loss of cognitive function, the rapidity of information processing and in mental flexibility in diabetics. Since diabetes is atherogenic and proinflammatory, it is possible that diabetes is a risk factor for Alzheimer's disease. In addition, loss or lack of control of diabetes leads to depression, anxiety and psychosocial distress. Whether these changes lead to specific oxidative and inflammatory stress beyond what is related to hyperglycemia needs to be critically analyzed. Clearly, this area of investigation is in its infancy and needs further investigation and development.

References

1 DJORDJEVIC VB. Free radicals in cell biology. *Int Rev Cytol.* 2004;237:57–89.
2 BABIOR BM, LAMBETH JD, NAUSEEF W. The neutrophil NADPH oxidase. *Arch Biochem Biophys.* 2002;397:342–344.
3 BARNES PJ, KARIN M. Nuclear factor-kappaB: a pivotal transcription factor in chronic inflammatory diseases. *N Engl J Med.* 1997;336:1066–1071.
4 ALJADA A, MOHANTY P, GHANIM H, ABDO T, TRIPATHY D, CHAUDHURI A, DANDONA P. Increase in intranuclear nuclear factor kappaB and decrease in inhibitor kappaB in mononuclear cells after a mixed meal: evidence for a proinflammatory effect. *Am J Clin Nutr.* 2004;79:682–690.
5 MOHANTY P, HAMOUDA W, GARG R, ALJADA A, GHANIM H, DANDONA P. Glucose challenge stimulates reactive oxygen species (ROS) generation by leucocytes. *J Clin Endocrinol Metab.* 2000;85:2970–2973.
6 DHINDSA S, TRIPATHY D, MOHANTY P, GHANIM H, SYED T, ALJADA A, DANDONA P. Differential effects of glucose and alcohol on reactive oxygen species generation and intranuclear nuclear factor-kappaB in mononuclear cells. *Metabolism.* 2004;53:330–334.

7 DANDONA P, ALJADA A, BANDYOPADHYAY A. Inflammation: the link between insulin resistance, obesity and diabetes. *Trends Immunol.* 2004;25:4–7.
8 MOHANTY P, GHANIM H, HAMOUDA W, ALJADA A, GARG R, DANDONA P. Both lipid and protein intakes stimulate increased generation of reactive oxygen species by polymorphonuclear leukocytes and mononuclear cells. *Am J Clin Nutr.* 2002;75:767–772.
9 DANDONA P, THUSU K, COOK S, SNYDER B, MAKOWSKI J, ARMSTRONG D, NICOTERA T. Oxidative damage to DNA in diabetes mellitus. *Lancet.* 1996;347:444–445.
10 DANDONA P, MOHANTY P, GHANIM H, ALJADA A, BROWNE R, HAMOUDA W, PRABHALA A, AFZAL A, GARG R. The suppressive effect of dietary restriction and weight loss in the obese on the generation of reactive oxygen species by leukocytes, lipid peroxidation, and protein carbonylation. *J Clin Endocrinol Metab.* 2001;86:355–362.
11 DANDONA P, MOHANTY P, HAMOUDA W, GHANIM H, ALJADA A, GARG R, KUMAR V. Inhibitory effect of a two day fast on reactive oxygen species

(ROS) generation by leucocytes and plasma *ortho*-tyrosine and *meta*-tyrosine concentrations. *J Clin Endocrinol Metab.* 2001;86:2899–2902.

12 MATTUSCH F, DUFAUX B, HEINE O, MERTENS I, ROST R. Reduction of the plasma concentration of C-reactive protein following nine months of endurance training. *Int J Sports Med.* 2000;21:21–24.

13 HOTAMISLIGIL GS, SHARGILL NS, SPIEGELMAN BM. Adipose expression of tumor necrosis factor-alpha: direct role in obesity-linked insulin resistance. *Science.* 1993;259:87–91.

14 YUAN M, KONSTANTOPOULOS N, LEE J, HANSEN L, LI ZW, KARIN M, SHOELSON SE. Reversal of obesity- and diet-induced insulin resistance with salicylates or targeted disruption of Ikkbeta. *Science.* 2001;293:1673–1677.

15 GHANIM H, ALJADA A, HOFMEYER D, SYED T, MOHANTY P, DANDONA P. Circulating mononuclear cells in the obese are in a proinflammatory state. *Circulation.* 2004;110:1564–1571.

16 PICKUP JC, MATTOCK MB, CHUSNEY GD, BURT D. NIDDM as a disease of the innate immune system: association of acute-phase reactants and interleukin-6 with metabolic syndrome X. *Diabetologia.* 1997;40:1286–1292.

17 CHAUDHURI A, JANICKE D, WILSON MF, TRIPATHY D, GARG R, BANDYOPADHYAY A, CALIERI J, HOFFMEYER D, SYED T, GHANIM H, ALJADA A, DANDONA P. Anti-inflammatory and profibrinolytic effect of insulin in acute ST-segment-elevation myocardial infarction. *Circulation.* 2004;109:849–854.

18 JONASSEN AK, SACK MN, MJOS OD, YELLON DM. Myocardial protection by insulin at reperfusion requires early administration and is mediated via Akt and p70s6 kinase cell-survival signaling. *Circ Res.* 2001;89:1191–1198.

19 VAN DEN BERGHE G, WOUTERS P, WEEKERS F, VERWAEST C, BRUYNINCKX F, SCHETZ M, VLASSELAERS D, FERDINANDE P, LAUWERS P, BOUILLON R. Intensive insulin therapy in the critically ill patients. *N Engl J Med.* 2001;345:1359–1367.

20 KIECOLT-GLASER JK, PREACHER KJ, MACCALLUM RC, ATKINSON C, MALARKEY WB, GLASER R. Chronic stress and age-related increases in the proinflammatory cytokine IL-6. *Proc Natl Acad Sci U S A.* 2003;100:9090–9095.

21 ALJADA A, GHANIM H, ASSIAN E, MOHANTY P, HAMOUDA W, GARG R, DANDONA P. Increased IkappaB expression and diminished nuclear NF-kappaB in human mononuclear cells following hydrocortisone injection. *J Clin Endocrinol Metab.* 1999;84:3386–3389.

22 DHINDSA S, PRABHAKAR S, SETHI M, BANDYOPADHYAY A, CHAUDHURI A, DANDONA P. Frequent occurrence of hypogonadotropic hypogonadism in type 2 diabetes. *J Clin Endocrinol Metab.* 2004;89:5462–5468.

19
The Metabolic Syndrome

Christian Berne and Per Björntorp [†]

Christian Berne has revised Per Björntorp's chapter. Per Björntorp passed away in 2004.

19.1
Introduction

The metabolic syndrome, also called insulin resistance syndrome, denotes a group of risk factors for cardiovascular disease, among which insulin resistance is a key factor. The combination of abdominal obesity, with primarily intraabdominal (visceral) fat, and type 2 diabetes, impaired glucose tolerance or impaired fasting glucose, dyslipidemia characterized by high triglyceride levels and low high-density lipoprotein (HDL) cholesterol ("good cholesterol") and high blood pressure entails a significantly increased risk of developing or ultimately dying of cardiovascular disease. The metabolic syndrome implies a high probability of developing diabetes, which in turn significantly increases the risk of cardiovascular disease and microvascular diabetic complications in the eyes, kidneys and nervous system.

19.2
History

Since the beginning of the 20th century, physicians have noted that certain diseases often occur in the same individuals. Patients with myocardial infarction commonly suffer from diabetes, and *vice versa*. The origin of the metabolic syndrome can be traced back to observations that certain symptoms, clinical findings or pathological changes were found to precede the development of atherosclerosis, myocardial infarction and type 2 diabetes. As early as the 1920s, Swedish physician E. Kylin published a series of articles where he described his observation that diabetes and hypertension often appear together. Along with German researchers, he coined the term "das Hypertonie-Hyperglykämie-Hyperurikämie Syndrom" (hypertonic–hyperglycemic–hyperuricemic syndrome). The association between atherosclerosis and myocardial infarction was established early in obese patients, prediabetics with hypertension, by Spanish physician Maranon. As far back as 100 years

Stress in Health and Disease. Edited by Bengt B. Arnetz and Rolf Ekman
Copyright © 2006 WILEY-VCH Verlag GmbH & Co. KGaA, Weinheim
ISBN: 3-527-31221-8

ago, a connection to increased activity in the sympathetic nervous system was also suggested.

In the late 1940s, French researcher J. Vague divided obesity into different groups. He differentiated between abdominal obesity, common in men, and the predominantly female distribution of fat to the hips. He referred to the two forms of fat distribution as android and gynoid respectively, popularly known as "apple" and "pear" shapes. However, it wasn't until the end of the 1980s that Swedish research presented the increased risk abdominal fat implies for ischaemic heart disease, diabetes and stroke.

Risk factors for ischaemic heart disease, stroke and type 2 diabetes may be present in various combinations in different individuals, who subsequently develop one or several of these conditions. In the 1980s, G. Reaven described "syndrome X," connecting the aforementioned risk factors to these common diseases. Hence, the idea of the metabolic syndrome was born.

We can imagine a tip-of-the-iceberg phenomenon. The part of the iceberg that peeks above the clinical horizon may vary, and under the surface are the factors that give rise to the clinical manifestations.

19.3
Metabolic Syndrome

19.3.1
Definition

There is as yet no widely accepted definition of the metabolic syndrome; however, the main components have been agreed upon. The previous WHO definition de-

Tab. 19.1. Definition of the metabolic syndrome.

New IDF worldwide definition for use in clinical practice

Abdominal circumference ≥ 94 cm (Europid men) or ≥ 80 cm (Europid women). For other populations cf. below.

+ two of the following four criteria

Raised triglycerides: ≥ 1.7 mmol/l*

Reduced HDL-cholesterol: <1.03 mmol/l (men) or <1.29 mmol/l (women)*

Raised blood pressure: systolic BP ≥ 130 or diastolic BP ≥ 85 mm Hg*

Raised fasting plasma glucose (FPG ≥ 5.6 mmol/l) or previously diagnosed type 2 diabetes

• South Asians and Chinese ≥ 90 cm (M), ≥ 80 cm (F) Japanese ≥ 85 cm (M), ≥ 90 cm (F).

• Ethnic South and Central Americans, use South Asians values.

• Sub-Saharan Africans, Eastern Mediterranean and Middle East (Arab) populations, use European data.

* or treatment for the specific dyslipidemia, or for hypertension, respectively.

(www.idf.org)

manded measuring the patient's insulin resistance and was not of any use in clinical practice. Table 19.1 shows the most recent definition of metabolic syndrome, which provides a good indication of what a tenable definition should include.

There is as a disease can be good reason that the designation of the metabolic syndrome questioned. The sum of the components undoubtedly constitutes a strong risk factor for cardiovascular disease. However, the metabolic syndrome is appearing at an increasing rate in countries where it was previously a virtually unknown concept, as modern Western lifestyle is adopted with its negative features of physical inactivity and excessive intake of energy and stress. To denounce this as a pathological state could in the long run lead to the problem being medicalized, and it could therefore be questioned.

19.3.2
Prevalence and Causes

The background to metabolic syndrome is multifactorial, with lifestyle, external stressors, metabolism and genetic factors contributing to varying degrees. The absence of a generally accepted definition makes the prevalence difficult to determine precisely. Figures between 5 and 25% of the adult population of the Western world have been suggested. The prevalence increases somewhat with age and a general increase is underway worldwide. Considerable variation between ethnic groups indicates a significant genetic component. Insulin resistance is 50% due to heredity and 50% due to lifestyle factors such as physical inactivity, increased energy intake and stress. Low birthweight with intrauterine growth inhibition has been linked to insulin resistance, high blood pressure and increased mortality in cardiovascular disease (the Barker hypothesis, described below).

A possible cause of the metabolic syndrome's increase in so many countries, not least in Asia, may be that natural selection has favored insulin resistance over time. In times of starvation a lower degree glucose metabolism is favored in the muscles, and when food is bountiful, storage of the energy in the fat tissue is favored. Such a metabolism would have increased man's chance of survival during our hunter–gatherer era (the "thrifty gene" hypothesis). In the metabolic syndrome, energy is predominantly stored in the visceral fat, from which it can most easily be mobilized in case of starvation. If a long period of selective pressure is at the root of today's metabolic syndrome, it is most likely that it is polygenetically inherited, i.e., it is impossible to pinpoint single genes as the main cause of the syndrome. Phenotypic variations in various populations, such as lower body mass index (BMI) and abdominal circumference in Asia than in Western Europe, and variations in the risk for cardiovascular disease support this view.

Stress, anxiety/depression and lack of sleep have, together with smoking and overconsumption of alcohol, been associated with the development of the metabolic syndrome. Important links between these factors and the development of the syndrome may be increased central activity of the sympathetic nervous system and increased activity in the hypothalamic–pituitary–adrenal (HPA) axis (described below).

19.3.3
Insulin Resistance

The condition of insulin resistance implies that an abnormally large amount of insulin is required to achieve an adequate response, e.g., to lower the blood glucose. It results in a compensatory increase in insulin secretion and high insulin levels in the blood (hyperinsulinemia).

Insulin resistance is expressed as a decreased insulin-dependent glucose uptake into the skeletal muscles and poorer inhibition of the liver's glucose production. As the liver produces too much glucose and less is taken up peripherally, the blood glucose begins to rise. In the adipocytes, lipolysis increases leading to a greater release of free fatty acids from the adipose tissues. In metabolic syndrome, the majority of these fatty acids are released from the visceral fat surrounding the intestines, which depending on the degree of abdominal obesity, makes up 6–20% of the body's total fat. According to many researchers, abdominal obesity is central in the pathogenesis of the metabolic syndrome.

19.3.4
The Role of Abdominal Obesity

An alternative explanation centers on abdominal obesity as the primary factor underlying the array of abnormalities in metabolism and circulatory regulation. The abdominal fat has a sensitive system for releasing free fatty acids, which are then transported directly via the portal vein to the liver, which in turn uses them to synthesize very low density lipoproteins (VLDL), predominantly consisting of triglycerides. Insulin resistance in the liver cells causes the hepatic glucose production to increase, as do the high blood levels of free fatty acids, which contribute to high blood glucose. The blood insulin levels increase further as the liver's ability to break the hormone down decrease. Insulin's ability to stimulate lipoprotein lipase diminishes. Lipoprotein lipase is an enzyme that breaks down triglycerides, and its decreased activity partially explains the lower levels of HDL cholesterol. These changes result in dyslipidemia, hyperglycemia and hyperinsulinemia, i.e., the components of the metabolic syndrome (Fig. 19.1) with the exception hypertension, which could possibly be linked to the hyperinsulinemia. The link between abdominal fat and blood pressure is weaker than that to the other components of the syndrome. It is important to note that the level of cholesterol in the blood, another important risk factor for cardiovascular disease lacks a clear connection to insulin resistance and the metabolic syndrome.

19.3.5
Adipose Tissue as an Endocrine Organ and Site of Synthesis for Inflammatory Markers

Today, the notion that the adipose tissue is a mere center for energy storage has been abandoned. Fat is considered a hormonally active tissue that produces the

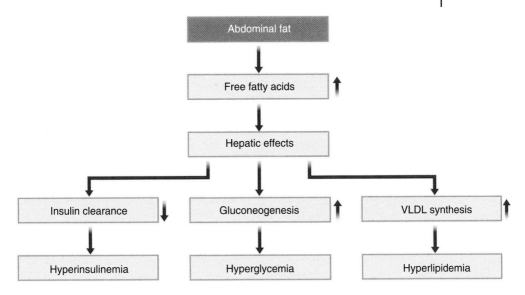

Fig. 19.1. The central role of abdominal fat in metabolic syndrome.

appetite-regulating hormone leptin and adiponectin, which affects insulin sensitivity. Low levels of adiponectin have been linked with cardiovascular disease. The adipose tissue is the site of synthesis of angiotensin II, an important hormone in blood pressure regulation. It also contains enzyme systems important for the metabolism of glucocorticoids and estrogen. Cytokines such as interleukin-6 (IL-6) and TNF-α (Tumor Necrosis Factor α) may in various ways be involved in the genesis of obesity and insulin resistance. The levels of these factors appear to be partially regulated by the level of stress, and are affected by cortisol, estrogen and testosterone.

19.4
Hormones in Metabolic Syndrome

19.4.1
Cortisol

It has been known for some time that overproduction of cortisol leads to insulin resistance and a state resembling the metabolic syndrome, as can be observed in patients with Cushing's syndrome. Glucocorticoids are involved in a multitude of metabolic processes, including glucose and fat metabolism, insulin sensitivity, growth and differentiation of adipose tissue. Cortisol induces abdominal obesity by increasing the activity of lipoprotein lipase, an enzyme necessary for the uptake of fatty acids into adipose tissue. Fat mobilization is further inhibited upon binding to the glucocorticoid receptor, a nuclear transcription factor, which implies that it controls the expression of various genes that affect the body's stress response. The glucocorticoid receptor concentration is high in visceral fat, making cortisol's fat-accumulating effect particularly prominent in this region. The same effect arises in patients who are subjected to longer periods of exogenous glucocorticoid administration to alleviate, e.g., asthma or rheumatoid arthritis. When the medication is discontinued, cortisol's effects gradually diminish. If the adrenals are removed from mice in some of the most common hereditary mouse models for obesity (obob), their weight is normalized.

Cortisol also inhibits the production of insulin in insulin-secreting pancreatic beta-cells, a possible contribution to the disturbed glucose metabolism in the metabolic syndrome. The effects of glucocorticoids are not only determined by the levels circulating in the blood and the expression of glucocorticoid receptors, but also by tissue-specific intracellular metabolism by the enzyme 11β-hydroxysteroid dehydrogenase (11βHSD), which exists in two forms. 11βHSD-1 converts inactive cortisone to the active form cortisol and is primarily expressed in the liver, adipose tissue and central nervous system. 11βHSD-2 contributes to the kidney's elimination of cortisol, where it protects the renal mineralocorticoid receptors from cortisol's effects. The mineralocorticoids are vital for regulating electrolyte balance and blood pressure.

Increased 11βHSD-1 activity is a possible explanation for the increased effect of stress hormones in the metabolic syndrome. 11βHSD-1 has been given increased attention in recent years as drugs have been developed to decrease insulin resistance by targeting the enzyme.

19.4.2
Sex Hormones and Growth Hormone

Sex hormones and growth hormone (GH) often function in synergy, and have effects opposite to those of the glucocorticoids. The balance between these hormones and cortisol may be of essence in the development of the metabolic syndrome.

The components of the metabolic syndrome can be observed in male patients lacking testosterone, female patients lacking estrogen and patients of either sex lacking GH. When the missing hormone is substituted so that normal hormone levels for the patient's age are achieved, the risk factors for cardiovascular disease that constitute the metabolic syndrome diminish or disappear entirely.

The underlying mechanisms are the following. Testosterone works with GH to inhibit uptake of fatty acids into the adipose tissue via lipoprotein lipase, and has strongly stimulating effects on the mobilization of fatty acids. Testosterone binds to specific androgen receptors, which are high in concentration in the abdominal fat. High levels of testosterone stimulate upregulation of such receptors. The insulin sensitivity in skeletal muscles decreases when testosterone levels are low, and can be restored when extra testosterone is administered.

Estrogen has similar effects in women. It is known that postmenopausal women accumulate abdominal fat, but the mechanisms for this development are incompletely understood. At this stage of life, women's risk of cardiovascular disease begins to approach that of men. Estrogen replacement therapy partially normalizes the components of the metabolic syndrome.

Concentrations of androgens, male sex hormones, are generally low in women and their effects are completely different than in men. Slight increases in free testosterone levels in women have been strongly linked to the metabolic syndrome.

Androgen production in women with the metabolic syndrome is seated primarily in the adrenals, with possible contribution from the ovaries. Decreased levels of sex-hormone-binding globulin (SHBG) contribute to the high levels of free testosterone. If women are given testosterone they develop abdominal fat; the exact mechanisms for this are, however, unclear.

It is most likely that there is an optimal testosterone concentration for both sexes, being ten times higher in men than in women. Exceeding the limit leads to the metabolic syndrome in both men and women. Androgens are a stronger contributor to metabolic syndrome than cortisol in women, while the opposite is true for men.

A decrease in sex hormones and/or GH may contribute to the development of the metabolic syndrome and enhance the risk of its development via the stress hormone cortisol, by shifting the balance between these groups of hormones to cortisol's advantage.

There is an important connection between the secretion of cortisol, sex steroids and GH. Cortisol secretion is stimulated by the HPA axis. If this axis is hyperactive

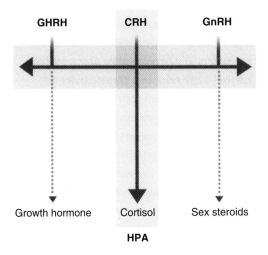

Fig. 19.2. Inhibition of the gonad axis and the growth hormone axis through increased activity in the hypothalamus–pituitary–adrenal (*HPA*) axis (CRH–cortisol). *GHRH* Growth hormone releasing hormone, *CRH* corticotropin releasing hormone, *GnRH* gonadotropin releasing hormone.

for a sufficient period of time, central gonad and GH axes are inhibited. The dysfunction of a combined increase in cortisol secretion and decrease in sex hormone and GH secretion can therefore stem from a primary overactivity in the HPA axis due to an increase in stimulation or sensitivity (Fig. 19.2). Such changes in hormone balance are possible contributors to the development of metabolic syndrome.

19.4.3
Measuring Cortisol

Many studies on obesity have analyzed cortisol levels, and produced varying results. One cause of this discrepancy may be that few of the studies have considered the distribution of the fat when selecting subjects.

The methods used have often been too insensitive or unspecific to measure functional increases in cortisol secretion, e.g., during stress. New techniques must therefore be utilized that are unaffected by the stress that the test itself implies for subjects not accustomed to the hospital or laboratory environments where such tests are conducted. Concentration measurements in saliva are an excellent alternative, since saliva can easily be delivered at any time during a normal day and also reflects the free, active fraction of circulating cortisol.

The regulation of the HPA axis is exceptionally sensitive to environmental factors and mental influences. Experiencing stress just prior to measuring salival cortisol, the memory of previous stress or expectation of future stress, or simply being in a good or bad mood affects the test results. Therefore, it is necessary to perform such tests under everyday conditions to avoid artifacts or deviation from the natural pattern of cortisol secretion. Owing to large circadian variations in HPA axis activity, single values are of little use. A picture of the regulation over the course of a full day, preferably over 24 h, is needed. Daily curves of salival cortisol show large variation within populations and three separate groups with different secretion patterns have been identified (Fig. 19.3).

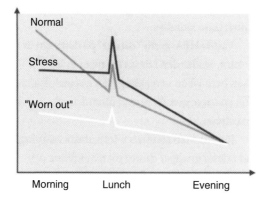

Fig. 19.3. Salival cortisol in middle-aged men, tested over the course of an average workday.

19.4.4
Circadian Variation in Cortisol Secretion

Normally, cortisol levels are high upon awakening, and then decrease rapidly over the course of the morning. After a standardized lunch, which may be used as a physiological stimulator of the HPA axis, the values increase, to subsequently decrease over the afternoon and evening. This pattern may be observed in about one-third of middle-aged Swedish men and women.

In about 25% a slightly different daily curve is observed. These subjects report they experienced stress at the time of the test. Their morning values are lower and do not decrease prior to lunch. Eating a midday meal triggers a greater cortisol secretion than usual. After lunch the values fall to a normal level. Such a pattern implies a larger total secretion over the course of a day. The test subjects that portray such curves have probably experienced stress for some time prior to examination.

Finally, a small portion of the population – less than 10% – show low morning values and little variation over the course of the day, including after stimulation of the axis by means of food intake. Such regulation of the HPA axis has earlier been observed in patients with long-term neuroendocrine dysfunction, e.g., posttraumatic stress syndrome but also in clinical conditions such as fibromyalgia and other chronic pain.

The differences between these three types of curve (Fig. 19.3) may be due to a deviance from the norm to a gradually aggravated state due to stress. The cause of this "wearing out" of the HPA axis is unknown.

If results from other studies of these groups are analyzed, one finds abdominal fat and other components of metabolic syndrome in the group that displays an increased, stress-related cortisol secretion. It is probable that this increased cortisol secretion contributes to the development of metabolic syndrome.

However, there is also a connection to the metabolic syndrome in the small group of subjects with low cortisol secretion. This group is also characterized by low testosterone levels in the men, low GH secretion, hypertension and higher heart rate. It is unlikely that cortisol is the cause of the metabolic changes in this group, but it is possible that the decreased levels of the other hormones may be responsible, via the mechanisms of dysregulated balance described previously. Hypertension and a high pulse indicate activation of the sympathetic nervous system, which in turn may lead to increased mobilization of free fatty acids, which increases insulin resistance.

19.5
Hypertension

Increased blood pressure is a component of the metabolic syndrome. Some connect the high pressure to hyperinsulinemia, since this stimulates the central sympathetic nervous system and may cause fluid retention, which in turn increases the

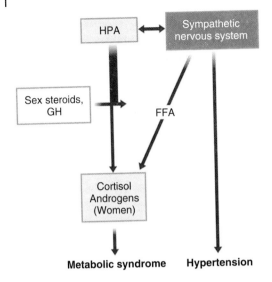

Fig. 19.4. Interaction between stress axes and hormonal and metabolic consequences. *HPA* Hypothalamus–pituitary–adrenal axis, *GH* growth hormone, *FFA* free fatty acids.

blood pressure. The results are ambiguous, however. Upon acute administration, insulin causes vasodilation, an effect which, however, may shift to vasoconstriction in certain groups, primarily overweight subjects.

The elevated blood pressure in metabolic syndrome may also be connected with the activation of the HPA axis, which is often stimulated simultaneously with the sympathetic nervous system. These functions are strongly connected on several levels, and in reality it is difficult to activate one axis independently of the other. It is likely that insulin potentiates the activation of the sympathetic nervous system. The parallelism between blood pressure and insulin may in reality be due to concerted activation of both stress axes (Fig. 19.4).

Glucocorticoids also inhibit the normal vasodilation caused by nitrous oxide, contribute to increased production of vasoconstricting angiotensin II and potentiate catecholamines' vessel constricting effects. All of these mechanisms may contribute to increased blood pressure upon activation of the HPA axis. Increased stimulation of renal mineralocorticoid receptors could, by causing fluid retention, also add to a volume-dependent hypertension.

Another hormone that stimulates the central sympathetic nervous system is leptin, an appetite-regulating hormone produced in adipose tissue. Leptin production increases with increased fat stores. Activation of the leptin receptors in the hypothalamus may contribute to the increase in blood pressure seen in metabolic syndrome.

19.6
Stress Axes

The classic stress axes consist of the HPA axis and the central sympathetic axis. Stress is a term encompassing a great number of factors, including subjectively experienced mental stress, threats registered by our sensory organs, toxins, infections, trauma, pain and fever, as described in more detail in other chapters. As stress factors are so multifaceted and difficult to define, with different effects on the individual, some researchers simply define stress as situations in which the stress axes are affected. People with metabolic syndrome show statistical connections with several of these stress factors.

As described above, people with increased daily cortisol secretion often report that they experienced stress on the day of the test, and have curves characterized by a condition of stress for a long period before the testing date. People with irregular cortisol secretion often report psychosocial and socioeconomic difficulties. Some examples of such include living alone or being divorced, having a weak economy, problems in professional life due to dissatisfaction in leadership or colleagues, etc. One can naturally assume that such situations involve frequent strain of various forms, which lead to stress reactions that are causing more or less constant activation of the stress axes, which in turn may lead to development of the metabolic syndrome.

The Whitehall Study, an extensive examination of English employees, illustrates this exceptionally well. It found that a socioeconomic gradient is inversely proportional to visceral abesity associated with the metabolic syndrome. Other studies have shown connections between experienced stress and pathologic regulation of the HPA axis, and that long periods of low socioeconomic status exacerbate the symptoms. This may be the explanation for the socially unequal distribution of conditions such as myocardial infarction and type 2 diabetes. High alcohol consumption and smoking are common in people with the metabolic syndrome. Alcohol's quantitative effect is difficult to evaluate due to the known problem that a large proportion of alcohol abuse goes unreported, but is probably a significant factor.

There are also clear connections between depression and various anxiety disorders and the metabolic syndrome. These conditions are not necessarily manifested as psychiatric illness, but also have a subclinical form. Use of antidepressants or anxiety-suppressing medication is common, as are various forms of sleeping difficulties. Lack of sleep has been shown to produce a strong stress activation, with subsequent insulin resistance, particularly tangible in sleep apnea, where there are strong links with abdominal obesity, diabetes and hypertension. Both clinically manifest anxiety and panic anxiety display an excessive activation of the HPA axis and sympathetic nervous system, and it is likely that the same applies in subclinical cases.

A connection has been suggested between chronic activation of the HPA axis and inflammatory markers and chronic infections that may cause, e.g., tooth loss and increase the risk of myocardial infarction. The increased HPA activity could

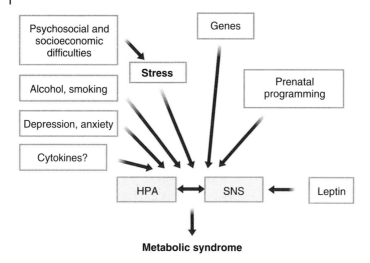

Fig. 19.5. Summary of known factors that activate stress
centers and show connections to the metabolic syndrome. *HPA*
Hypothalamus–pituitary–adrenal axis, *SNS* sympathetic
nervous system.

increase the sensitivity to infection by depressing the immune system; alternately, infections might activate the HPA axis via cytokines.

Studies have shown that mental stress stimulates the production of proinflammatory cytokines such as interluekin-6 and TNF-α, which are formed in the adipose tissue and in turn increase the production of components in the inflammatory response, which has increasingly been linked to the metabolic syndrome and atherosclerotic disease.

The above indicates that our present hectic and competition-focused lifestyle is an important cause of HPA axis activation, with possible secondary development of the metabolic syndrome. In some cases, this lifestyle may lead to "burnout", dominated by psychological symptoms, but whose physical consequences, e.g., the metabolic syndrome, have yet to be determined. Physical inactivity is likely to be involved in the problem. Physical activity counteracts many of the stress factors mentioned above, and also has strong therapeutic effects on both abdominal obesity and insulin resistance. A summary is presented in Fig. 19.5.

19.6.1
Genetic Factors

There is most likely a polygenetic genetic predisposition underlying the metabolic syndrome. The HPA axis is strongly influenced by genes that steer the central regulation of the HPA axis and sympathetic nervous system may be of great importance. The connection between cortisol secretion and the metabolic syndrome has also been shown to be stronger in Asian populations that in West European ones.

Monozygotic twins display daily cortisol secretion curves that are virtually identical, even in smaller details such as the time and magnitude of individual secretion peaks.

Individuals with increased stress-induced cortisol secretion sometimes show signs of decreased function in the glucocorticoid receptors in their central nervous system, whose function is vital for feedback regulation of the HPA axis. This may be due to downregulation of the number of receptors, long term exposure to high levels of cortisol, or genetic mutations causing disturbed receptor function. There is a genetic change in individuals with poorly regulated cortisol secretion that has also been strongly linked to the metabolic syndrome.

19.7
Other Conditions

19.7.1
Depression

Melancholic depression implies a significantly increased risk of developing cardio-vascular disease and type 2 diabetes. Reviews of epidemiological literature indicate a connection of varying strength between depression, overweight, abdominal fat and metabolic syndrome. Even if the connections are statistically established, the mechanisms remain unclear, partially because established risk factors are rarely measured.

Depression increases the activity in the sympathetic nervous system as well as the HPA axis. Individuals who present symptoms of depression but who fail to meet the criteria for the diagnosis of melancholic depression, show abnormal regulation of the HPA axis and often display components of the metabolic syndrome. In melancholy depression there is a clearly increased prevalence of abdominal obesity. The increased risk of myocardial infarction and diabetes may be mediated by the presence of the metabolic syndrome, partially evoked by the neuroendocrine and autonomic disorders described in depression.

A small study of selective serotonin reuptake inhibitors (SSRIs), the most common form of antidepressant used today, showed that disturbances of the HPA axis and sympathetic nervous system were normalized at the same time as various components of the metabolic syndrome were improved in a group of men with the metabolic syndrome and subclinical symptoms of depression, prior to any effects on the symptoms of depression.

19.7.2
The "Small Baby Syndrome"

Barker and associates has shown that children with lower birthweight than expected for the duration of the pregnancy develop the metabolic syndrome as adults, a finding confirmed by a long line of subsequent studies. Recently, an increased cortisol secretion indicating increased HPA axis sensitivity to ACTH has been shown. This higher sensitivity appears to be programmed already *in utero*.

Research on animal models have shown that immune stress and exposure to glucocorticoids in rat fetuses results in increased HPA axis sensitivity in adulthood. The effect is especially strong on the feedback control of the HPA axis, possibly due to effects on the establishment of glucocorticoid receptors in the hippocampus. The adult rats show signs identical to the metabolic syndrome, with low testosterone levels in males and high levels in females.

The small baby syndrome is therefore likely to be one of numerous paths to the development of metabolic syndrome through hypersensitivity in the HPA axis. It is as yet impossible to determine the importance of fetal influence compared with stress in the surroundings. The sensitivity of the HPA axis and central nervous system probably vary depending on prenatal programming and genetic factors, which entail varying responses to environmental stress in adult years (Fig. 19.5).

19.7.3
Stress and Obesity

Whereas mental stress in healthy test subjects increases insulin sensitivity despite an acute reaction from both the sympathetic nervous system and the HPA axis, the opposite has been found in overweight subjects, whose blood pressure increases. In obesity the administration of dexamethasone, a cortisol analogue, gives a decreased suppression of cortisol production, an indication that the feedback regulation of the HPA axis is not functioning optimally.

It is well-known that patients with Cushing's syndrome and those treated with glucocorticoids alike often develop an increased appetite and subsequently typical abdominal obesity. The question that arises is whether stress-induced cortisol secretion can instigate the development of obesity. Controlled tests showing that exposure to glucocorticoids are followed by increased food intake, even after stress, support this theory.

One could thereby expect that the phenomenon of "stress eating" in fact exists, since stress is followed by increased cortisol production. To this, one may add that eating under stress is frequently haphazard and rushed, often while on the go. The feeling of being full and intake control are weakened, all of which may contribute to weight gain. The global obesity epidemic has surfaced and been exacerbated in recent decades as processes are automated and computerized, and we find ourselves in a constantly hurried state. Physical inactivity surely plays an important role as a causative factor, but an increased energy intake secondary to increased stress may very well contribute to the development of obesity and thereby be connected with metabolic syndrome.

19.8
Prevention and Therapy

One might summarize the metabolic syndrome as a multiple endocrine disorder based on environmental factors, which are especially prominent in a competitive, high-tech society which generates stress reactions. Prevention of such reactions demands either personal training in stress management or extensive societal reformation.

From a global perspective, the connection does not only apply to modern Western society's high-tech development. The greatest increases in diabetes and metabolic syndrome today are seen in e.g., Asia and South America, where urbanization with crowded living conditions, social deprivation, unemployment and physical inactivity may be important underlying causes.

Some concrete examples of measures against this development follow below. In the past decades, substantial improvements have been made in the physical work environment. Noise and air pollution have been reduced and better injury prevention introduced. However, little has been done to improve the psychological work environment, which still features monotonous work at a fast pace and out of the individual's control, overtime etc. Instead, much indicates a decline in such aspects of quality in work environment. The time has come for further improvements in this area.

One of the most efficient methods to prevent or treat stress and the metabolic syndrome is physical activity. Exercise counteracts experiences of stress, probably by stimulating endorphin production. Moreover, exercise is probably the most efficient way to increase insulin sensitivity in the skeletal muscles' glucose transporters. Both dyslipidemia and hypertension are positively affected by physical activity. It is efficient in preventing and treating obesity. It is thereby a causal treatment of the metabolic syndrome, and at present the one truly effective treatment that attacks the full spectrum of psychological and physical factors in the metabolic syndrome and stress. Lifestyle changes in the population are the only realistic and cost efficient cures for metabolic syndrome, which otherwise threatens to become an area for unprecedented medicalization, to alleviate the consequences of the unbeneficial development of man's psychosocial environment.

19.9
Summary

The metabolic syndrome is a group of symptoms that constitute risk factors for cardiovascular disease, type 2 diabetes and stroke. The syndrome encompasses insulin resistance, abdominal obesity, dyslipidemia and hypertension. It is a scientific challenge to find a common denominator for these symptoms and thereby for the metabolic syndrome. Insulin resistance and accumulation of abdominal fat have been held forth as primary pathogenetic factors, but are insufficient to explain the entire genesis of the syndrome.

A concerted stimulation of the HPA axis and the central nervous system commonly occurs during stress. The resulting endocrine dysfunction, increased cortisol and in women increased secretion of adrenal androgens, with simultaneous secondary inhibition of growth and sex hormones, leads to abdominal fat accumulation. Insulin resistance follows and leads to hyperinsulinemia and dyslipidemia.

Patients with metabolic syndrome have now been shown to have abnormal endocrine regulation and sympathetic nervous systems. There is also a connection between subjectively experienced stress and supposedly stress-induced factors, e.g., psychosocial handicap, socioeconomic difficulties, use of stimulants and symptoms of depression and anxiety. Other conditions with similar neuroendocrine disorders, such as Cushing's disease and melancholy depression, also lead to development of the metabolic syndrome.

Prevention and therapy ought primarily to focus on lifestyle factors, including stress. Physical activity has positive effects on both central and peripheral abnormalities in metabolic syndrome and is at present the best-known alternative for prevention and treatment. Therapy for the endocrine disorders has been attempted with significant success, but has not yet been sufficiently tested for public use.

References

Björntorp P. Visceral obesity: a "civilization syndrome". Obesity Res 1993;1:206–222.

Björntorp P. Neuroendocrine perturbations as a cause of insulin resistance. Diabetes Metab Res Rev 1999;15:1–15.

Reaven G.M. Role of insulin resistance in human disease. Diabetes 1988;37:1595–1607.

Seematter G, Binnert C, Martin JL, Tappy L. Relationship between stress, inflammation and metabolism. Curr Opin Clin Nutr Metab Care 2004;7:169–173.

Tomlinson J.W., Walker E.A., Bujalska I.J., Draper N., Lavery G.G., Cooper M.S., Hewison M., Stewart P.M. 11β-Hydroxysteroid dehydrogenase type 1: a tissue-specific regulator of glucocorticoid response. Endocr Rev 2004;25:831–866.

Walker B.R. Steroid metabolism in metabolic syndrome X. Best Practice Res Clin Endocrinol Metab 2001;15:111–122.

Wang M. The role of glucocorticoid action in the pathophysiology of the metabolic syndrome. Nutr Metab 2005;2(3):1–14.

20
Chronic Pain: the Diathesis–Stress Model

Yuan Bo Peng, Perry N. Fuchs, and Robert J. Gatchel

20.1
Introduction

Nowhere do psychiatric and medical pathologies interface more prominently than in pain disorders. The most promising work conducted thus far has embraced a biopsychosocial interdisciplinary approach in which the mental health needs of the patient require careful evaluation and treatment, along with the concurrent physical pain problem. Patients with chronic pain are at increased risk for depression, suicide (which is identified by the Surgeon General as one of the top public health concerns in the USA), and sleep disorders. As pain becomes more chronic, emotional factors play an increasingly dominant role in the maintenance of dysfunction and suffering [1]. Affective disorders, anxiety disorders and substance abuse disorders are the three major psychiatric concomitants of chronic pain [1]. The importance of psychopathology in pain comorbidity is further evidenced by the potentially common pathogenetic mechanisms involved in psychiatric disorders, such as depression and pain. Both nociceptive and affective pathways coincide anatomically. Furthermore, norepinephrine and serotonin, the two neurotransmitters most implicated in the psychopathology of mood disorders, are also involved in the gate-control mechanisms of pain. Finally, antidepressants have been found to have a mitigating effect on chronic pain, even at doses considered subtherapeutic for depression. Table 20.1 summarizes the major concomitants of chronic pain.

There is a strong comorbidity of chronic pain and psychopathology.

20.2
A Conceptual Model of the Transition from Acute to Chronic Pain and Emotional Distress

Our past research is based upon a broad conceptual model which proposes three stages that may be involved in the transition of acute low back pain (ALBP) into chronic low back pain (CLBP) disability and accompanying psychosocial distress

Stress in Health and Disease. Edited by Bengt B. Arnetz and Rolf Ekman
Copyright © 2006 WILEY-VCH Verlag GmbH & Co. KGaA, Weinheim
ISBN: 3-527-31221-8

Tab. 20.1. Comorbid conditions/symptoms associated with chronic pain.

- Axis I clinical disorders, especially affective disorders, anxiety disorders and substance abuse disorders

- Axis II personality disorders

- Sleep disorders

- Overall increase in emotional distress

- Pain behaviors, such as bracing, guarded movements, and decreased activities of daily living

- Fear and avoidance of physical activity

---

[2] (Fig. 20.1). To summarize, it is proposed that *Stage 1* is associated with emotional reactions such as fear, anxiety, etc., as a consequence of the perception of pain during the acute phase. Pain or hurt is usually associated with harm, and so there is a natural emotional reaction to the potential for physical harm. If the pain persists past a reasonable acute period of time (2–4 months), this leads to the progression into *Stage 2*, which is associated with a wider array of psychological reactions and problems, such as learned helplessness–depression, distress–anger, somatization, etc., that are the result of suffering with the now more chronic nature of pain. The form these problems take will depend upon the *premorbid* or preexisting psychosocial characteristics of the individual, as well as current socioeconomic conditions. Thus, for a person with a premorbid problem with depression who is seriously affected economically by loss of a job due to pain, depressive symptomatology may be exacerbated during this stage. Similarly, for someone

STAGE 3: CHRONIC PAIN (acceptance of the "sick role" and demonstration of abnormal illness behaviors)

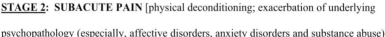

STAGE 2: SUBACUTE PAIN [physical deconditioning; exacerbation of underlying psychopathology (especially, affective disorders, anxiety disorders and substance abuse)]

STAGE 1: ACUTE PAIN (initial anxiety and concern about the pain)

Fig. 20.1. The transition from acute to chronic pain stages.

who has some significant personality disorder, such a disorder may begin to severely hamper the ability to effectively cope with the stress of chronic pain. This model does *not* propose that there is one primary preexisting "pain personality." It is assumed that there is a general nonspecificity in terms of the relationship between personality–psychosocial problems and pain. This is in keeping with the research that has not found any such consistent personality syndrome. Moreover, even though there is a relationship usually found between pain and certain psychiatric problems such as depression, the nature of the relationship between the two variables remains inconclusive. Some, but not all, patients develop depression secondary to chronic pain. Others show depression as the primary syndrome, of which pain is a symptom. Moreover, factors that mediate the relationship between depression and pain remain largely unknown [1]. Thus, it is assumed that patients "bring with them" certain predisposing psychosocial characteristics that differ from one patient to the next, and that may be exacerbated by the stress of attempting to cope with pain. Indeed, the relationship between stress and exacerbation of mental health problems has been documented [2]. Other researchers have also recently proposed a similar diathesis–stress model of pain and psychopathology. That work will be discussed later in this chapter.

This conceptual model proposes that as the "layer" of behavioral/psychological problems persists, it leads to the progression into *Stage 3* which can be viewed as the acceptance or adoption of a "sick role" during which patients are excused from their normal responsibilities and social obligations. This may become a potent reinforcer for not becoming "healthy." The medical and psychological "disabilities" or "abnormal illness behaviors" are consolidated during this phase. There has been research consistently demonstrating the important psychological changes that occur as a pain patient progresses from the acute to more chronic phases, such as the changes. Kinney et al. [3] Minnesota Multiphasic Personality Inventory (MMPI) have also documented differences in the prevalence of psychopathology in ALBP and CLBP patients. More specifically, 68% of the chronic patients had a current axis I disorder, compared to 23% of the acute patients. The chronic patients had more major depression (46%) and anxiety disorders (25%) than the acute patients (8% and 10%, respectively). This conceptual model also proposes that superimposed on these stages is what is known as the physical "deconditioning syndrome." This refers to a significant decrease in physical capacity (strength, flexibility and endurance) due to disuse and the resultant atrophy of the injured area. There is usually a two-way pathway between the physical deconditioning and the above stages.

There is clear transition from acute pain (associated with little psychopathology) to more chronic stages (associated with greater comorbidity of psychopathology).

20.2.1
Data Supporting the Conceptual Model

As Dersh and colleagues [1] have reviewed, a great deal of research data supportive of this conceptual model have been accumulated over the last decade. Various investigations have documented high rates of psychopathology and various types of chronic pain, as well as higher rates of psychopathology in chronic versus acute pain patients, and decreased rates after successful treatment of chronic pain. For example, besides the earlier reviewed study by Kinney and colleagues [3], other investigations also revealed elevated prevalences of depressive disorders, anxiety disorders, substance use disorders, "somatization," and personality disorders in CLBP patients e.g., [4] Indeed, rates of major depressive disorder range from 34% to 57% in these studies, compared to rates of 5–26% in the general population. More recent studies have also documented elevated rates of psychopathology in other types of chronic pain conditions, including headaches, temporomandibular disorders, pelvic pain, and fibromyalgia syndrome.

Support for this model can also be found from studies demonstrating that psychosocial variables are potent predictors of pain and disability chronicity. In fact, attempts to predict which individuals with ALBP will go on to develop chronic disabilities, including a poor response to rehabilitation treatment, have demonstrated that psychosocial factors are better predictors than physical factors in failure to return to work after a spinal injury (see [5]). For example, Gatchel, Polatin and Mayer [6] evaluated whether a comprehensive assessment of psychosocial characteristics is useful in characterizing those ALBP patients who subsequently develop chronic pain disability problems (as measured by job work status at 1 year postevaluation). In this study, all patients were administered a standard battery of psychological assessment tests within 6 weeks of acute lumbar spine pain onset. A structured telephone interview was conducted 1 year after the psychological assessment in order to evaluate return-to-work status. Logistic regression analyses, conducted to differentiate between those patients who were back at work at 1 year versus those who were not, revealed the importance of only psychosocial factors in correctly identifying 90.7% of the cases. There were no differences between the two groups for the physician-rated severity of the initial back injury or the physical demands of the job to which patients had to return. These results clearly demonstrated the presence of a robust "psychosocial disability factor" that is associated with those injured workers who are likely to develop CLBP disability problems. Such results again highlight the fact that chronic pain disability reflects more than just the presence of some physical symptomatology or a single psychosocial characteristic; it is a complex psychosocioeconomic phenomenon. In fact, many investigators have argued that only a small amount of the total disability phenomenon in someone complaining of chronic back pain can be attributed to physical impairment [7].

20.2.2
Base Rates of Psychopathology

When one views earlier results from the National Institute of Mental Health (NIMH) epidemiologic study on 1-month prevalence of various mental disorders in the general population [8], it is not surprising that there are often psychiatric problems associated with chronic pain patients because the base rates for such problems in the general population are quite high. For example, these statistics indicated that the prevalences for anxiety disorders, affective disorders, and substance abuse are 7.3, 5.1 and 3.8% of the population, respectively. Symptoms of schizophrenia are 1.7%. Therefore, 15.4% of the noninstitutionalized population has some significant mental health disorder. In an earlier study of *lifetime* prevalences of these above disorders assessed across three sites, there were even higher rates. More recently, Narrow and colleagues [9] have presented revised prevalence estimates of mental disorders in the USA that were somewhat lower. However, they used a clinical significance criterion (e.g., unable to work or engage in usual activities due to symptoms) which lowered these rates. Nevertheless, one can easily argue that these disorders will become greatly exacerbated under the stress of chronic pain disability. These NIMH prevalence statistics also do not take into account the equally prevalent personality disorders such as antisocial, borderline, and paranoid personalities, estimated to be between about 10–18% in the general population.

20.3
The Diathesis–Stress Model

Subsequent to Gatchel's introduction of a diathesis–stress model of chronic pain [2], other investigators have amplified the importance of such a model. For example, Weisberg and Keefe [10] presented a diathesis–stress model of personality disorders in chronic pain to explain the discrepancy between the rates of those disorders in the general population and in the chronic pain population. According to the 4th edition of the *Diagnostic and Statistical Manual of Mental Disorders* (DSM-IV), "Personality traits are enduring patterns of perceiving, relating to, and thinking about the environment and one's self that are exhibited in a wide range of social and personal contacts. Only when personality traits are inflexible and maladaptive and cause significant functional impairment or subjective distress do they constitute personality disorders" ([11], p. 630). Personality disorders are thought to develop during childhood and adolescence and must be evident by late adolescence or early adulthood. Work by Weisberg and Keefe [10] posits that personality disorders develop as an interaction between an underlying personality predisposition (i.e., a diathesis) and the extreme stress of pain and its physical, psychological, and social consequences (thus, a diathesis–stress model). Again, in this model disorder is a consequence of acute and subacute pain, and it also can perpetuate chronic, disabling pain. Indeed, it is well-established that personality disorders are highly prevalent in patients with chronic pain. Comparisons with other psychiatric and medical populations support the observation that chronic pain patients demonstrate high levels of personality psychopathology [12]. The rate in the general population ranges from 0.5% to 3%, according to the DSM-IV [11]. Moreover, in outpatient psychiatric clinical populations, the prevalences vary greatly. One study of more than 18 000 individuals reported a prevalence rate of 12.9% [13]. The reader is referred to Weisberg and Keefe [10] for a further review of these data.

There has been much written concerning the history of the diathesis–stress model. Biological predispositions have been assigned a primary role in the etiology of physical illness as far back as the time of Hippocrates. Hippocrates believed that pain arose when one humor was in excess or depleted. Plato believed that pain occurred not only from peripheral stimulation but also from emotions in the soul and the heart. More modern studies of diatheses have focused on genetic vulnerabilities that predispose individuals to disease. For example, discoveries of genetic markers for some types of breast cancer, Parkinson's disease, and for Huntington's disease and neurofibromatosis reflect this trend. Of course, the presence of a genetic marker does not necessarily imply that there is an underlying biological predisposition, but it is one of the closest measurements available for assessing genetic predisposition, other than specific gene typing. Genetic markers have also been identified in psychiatric disorders, such as schizophrenia and depression. In addition, psychological or social diatheses have been proposed as the medical model has evolved into a more biopsychosocial approach [14]. Moreover, the gene that appears to control the analgesic properties of morphine has been recently isolated [15]. This suggests that there might be a genetic predisposition for the degree to which people experience pain and respond to analgesic compounds. Thus, there are a number of biopsychosocial diatheses that need to be considered in any comprehensive diathesis–stress model.

Of course, the stress component of this model is just as important to consider. The recognition of the influence of stress on health is a relatively recent advance in our conceptualization of health and illness [16]. The forerunner of recent research on stress was Hans Selye's general adaptation syndrome [17] which initially highlighted the importance of environmental factors on disease. Subsequently, Lazarus and Folkman [18] provided a general conceptualization of stress as the physiological, psychological or mental influences that exert pressure on the organism, taxing or exceeding its capacity to respond. The emerging field of psychoneuroimmunology has also increased our understanding of the complex connection between stress and illness. This area of research has demonstrated that, during times of stress, immune functioning weakens e.g., [19] leaving one more susceptible to minor illnesses such as the common cold or flu. Psychosocial stressors that tax the immune system include negative life events such as marital discord and bereavement, as well as work stressors.

As Weisberg and Keefe [10] have noted, the importance of both underlying diatheses and of stress have been recognized in illness models for years. However, these two concepts were never unified into one model until the early 1960s, when the diathesis–stress model of schizophrenia was developed. This model viewed schizophrenia as developing as an interaction between a biological or genetic substrate (a diathesis) and the expression of that substrate under stressful conditions (the stress). It is the interaction of these two components that produce the onset of schizophrenia. This conceptualization of the diathesis–stress model continued to develop with the introduction of the biopsychosocial model of illness. The biopsychosocial model extends the previously overly simplistic and reductionistic view of medical illness to one that includes biological, psychological, and social influences. Several aspects of an individual's environment, and how they interact with biological factors, must be understood in order to better understand illness. This diathesis–stress model of pain has been further expanded by recent work by Melzack and associates to be discussed next.

20.3.1
Melzack's Neuromatrix Theory of Pain and Emotional Distress

In the past, many researchers have reported a relationship between stress-induced musculoskeletal activity and pain symptoms [20]. However, surprisingly, a formal model concerning the relationship between pain and stress was not proposed until quite recently. Melzack [21] proposed the neuromatrix theory of pain, which conceptualizes chronic pain not as solely caused by neuromechanisms of sensory transmission but, rather, as also involving genetic contributions and the neural–hormonal mechanisms of stress. Pain is not a purely perceptual phenomenon, but the injury that has caused the pain also disrupts the body's homeostatic regulation systems which, in turn, produce stress and the initiation of complex programs to restore homeostasis. Melzack argues that recognizing the role of the stress system in pain processes significantly broadens the conceptualization of chronic pain and our ability to understand it. Indeed, chronic pain is a stressor that will "tax" the stress system. Prolonged activation of the stress regulation systems will ultimately generate breakdowns of muscle, bone and neural tissue that, in turn, will cause more pain and produce a vicious cycle of pain–stress reactivity. Turk and Monarch [22] have recently provided a more comprehensive review of the heuristic features of this model.

One particular stress-related measure that Melzack suggests to be important in the above pain–stress cycle is cortisol. As Melzack points out, along with the activation of the sympathetic nervous system, "cortisol sets the stage for the stress response." He goes on to state that

"... cortisol plays a central role because it is responsible for producing and maintaining high levels of glucose for the response. At the same time, cortisol is potentially a highly destructive substance because, to ensure a high level of glucose, it breaks down the protein in muscle and inhibits the ongoing replacement of calcium in bone."

Indeed, cortisol is the main hormonal product of the hypothalamic–pituitary–adrenal axis in humans. Although increased cortisol secretion is considered an adaptive response mechanism of the organism when stressed (for purposes of energy mobilization), prolonged secretion can lead to negative effects such as muscle atrophy, impairment of growth and tissue repair, immune system suppression, etc. Melzack suggests that cortisol will serve as a good marker of the degree of stress that should closely parallel the development of chronic pain. Melzack's neuromatrix theory of pain and stress provides an ideal theory-driven methodology to use in diathesis–stress research for evaluating the overall biopsychosocial efficacy of our early intervention approach. Fortunately, reliable measures of cortisol can be easily obtained in a noninvasive manner in human subjects. For example, results have shown that cortisol level after morning awakening, assessed by sampling saliva, is a reliable biological marker for adrenocortical activity. Extensive other research has shown that salivary cortisol provides an accurate index of free plasma cortisol. Studies with human subjects have also demonstrated a close relationship between stress and salivary cortisol levels.

There is growing empirical support for the diathesis–stress model of chronic pain.

20.4
Summary and Conclusions

As pain becomes more chronic in nature, psychosocial factors begin to play an increasingly dominant role in the maintenance of pain behavior and suffering. This has resulted in the need for a more comprehensive biopsychosocial model of pain. A conceptual model of the transition from acute to chronic pain was presented in which it is assumed that the type of psychosocial distress displayed by patients who become subacute or chronic depends on the premorbid or preexisting personality/psychological characteristics of that individual. One of the major psychosocial concomitants or sources of distress that health care professionals must be prepared to deal with when treating chronic pain patients in psychopathology. Elevated rates of depressive, somatoform, anxiety, substance abuse and personality disorders have been identified as the most common diagnostic categories. Although these aspects are unique to the relationship between chronic pain and each specific type of psychopathology, a diathesis–stress model is emerging as the most dominant overarching theoretical perspective. In this model, diatheses are conceptualized as preexisting semidormant characteristics of the person prior to the onset of chronic pain, which are then activated by the stress of this chronic condition, eventually resulting in diagnosable psychopathology. There is now a growing amount of research addressing the pain–stress relationship in the context of the diathesis–stress model of chronic pain.

Acknowledgements

The writing of this chapter was supported in part by grants No. 2R01 DE10713, 2R01 MH46452 and 1K05 MH071892 from the National Institutes of Health and grant No. DAMD17-03-1-0055 from the Department of Defense.

References

1 DERSH J, POLATIN P, GATCHEL R. Chronic pain and psychopathology: research findings and theoretical considerations. *Psychosom Med.* 2002;64:773–786.

2 GATCHEL RJ. Psychological disorders

and chronic pain: cause and effect relationships. In: GATCHEL RJ, TURK DC (eds.) *Psychological Approaches to Pain Management: A Practitioner's Handbook.* Guilford, New York. 1996, pp 33–52.

3 KINNEY RK, GATCHEL RJ, POLATIN PB, FOGARTY WJ, MAYER TG. Prevalence of psychopathology in acute and chronic low back pain patients. *J Occup Rehab.* 1993;1993:95–103.

4 FISHBAIN DA, GOLDBERG M, MEAGHER BR, STEELE R, ROSOMOFF H. Male and female chronic pain patients categorized by DSM-III psychiatric diagnostic criteria. *Pain.* 1986;26:181–197.

5 GATCHEL RJ, GARDEA MA. Psychosocial issues: their importance in predicting disability, response to treatment, and search for compensation. *Neurol Clin.* 1999;17(1):149–166.

6 GATCHEL RJ, POLATIN PB, MAYER TG. The dominant role of psychosocial risk factors in the development of chronic low back pain disability. *Spine.* 1995;20(24):2702–2709.

7 WADDELL G, MAIN CJ, MORRIS EW. Chronic low back pain, psychologic distress, and illness behavior. *Spine.* 1984;5:117–125.

8 REGIER DA, BOYD JH, BURKE JD, et al. One-month prevalence of mental disorders in the United States. *Arch Gen Psychiatry.* 1988;45:977–986.

9 NARROW WE, RAE DS, ROBINS LN, REGIER DA. Revised prevalence estimates of mental disorders in the United States: using a clinical significance criterion to reconcile 2 surveys' estimates. *Arch Gen Psychiatry.* 2002;59:115–130.

10 WEISBERG JN, KEEFE FJ. Personality disorders in the chronic pain population: basic concepts, empirical findings, and clinical implications. *Pain Forum.* 1997;6(1):1–9.

11 American Psychiatric Association. *Diagnostic and Statistical Manual of Mental Disorders, 4th Edn.* APA, Washington. 1994.

12 GATCHEL RJ, POLATIN PB, MAYER TG,

GARCY PD. Psychopathology and the rehabilitation of patients with chronic low back pain disability. *Arch Phys Med Rehab.* 1994;75:666–670.

13 FABREGA H, ULRICH R, PILKONIS A, MEZZICH J. Personality disorders diagnosed at intake at a public psychiatric facility. *Hosp Community Psychiatry.* 1993;44(2):159–162.

14 GATCHEL RJ. Comorbidity of chronic mental and physical health disorders: the biopsychosocial perspective. *Am Psychologist.* In Press.

15 FUCHS PN, ROZA C, SORA I, UHL G, RAJA SN. Characterization of mechanical withdrawal responses and effects of mu, kappa and delta opioid agonists in normal and mu opioid receptor knockout mice. *Brain Res.* 1999;821:480–486.

16 BAUM A, GATCHEL RJ, KRANTZ DS (eds.) *An Introduction to Health Psychology, 3rd edn.* McGraw-Hill, New York. 1997.

17 SELYE H. The general adaptation syndrome and the diseases of adaptation. *J Clin Endocrinol.* 1946;6:117.

18 LAZARUS R and FOLKMAN J. *Stress, Appraisal, and Coping.* Springer, New York. 1984.

19 ADER R, FELTON D, and COHEN N (eds.) *Psychoneuroimmunology.* Academic, San Diego. 1990.

20 KEEFE FJ, DOLAN EA. Correlation of behavior and muscle activity in patients with myofacial pain dysfunction syndrome: facial pain. *J Craniomandibular Disord.* 1988;2: 181–184.

21 MELZACK R. Pain and stress: a new perspective. In: GATCHEL RJ, TURK DC (eds.) *Psychosocial Factors in Pain: Critical Perspectives.* Guilford, New York. 1999.

22 TURK DC, MONARCH ES. Biopsychosocial perspective on chronic pain. In: TURK DC, GATCHEL RJ (eds.) *Psychological Approaches to Pain Management: A Practitioner's Handbook, 2nd edn.* Guilford, New York. 2002.

21
Emotional Stress, Positive Emotions, and Psychophysiological Coherence

Rollin McCraty and Dana Tomasino

21.1
Introduction

Chris, a 45-year-old business executive with a family history of heart disease, was feeling extremely stressed, fatigued, and generally in poor emotional health. A 24-hour heart rate variability analysis[i] revealed abnormally depressed activity in both branches of his autonomic nervous system, suggesting autonomic exhaustion ensuing from mal-adaptation to high stress levels. His heart rate variability was far lower then would be expected for his age and was below the clinical cut-off level for significantly increased risk of sudden cardiac death. In addition, Chris's average heart rate was abnormally high at 102 beats per minute, and his heart rate did not drop at night as it should.

Upon reviewing these results, his physician concluded that it was imperative that Chris take measures to reduce his stress. He recommended that Chris begin practicing a set of emotional restructuring techniques that had been developed by the Institute of HeartMath. These positive emotion-focused techniques help individuals learn to self-generate and sustain a beneficial functional mode known as psychophysiological coherence, characterized by increased emotional stability and by increased synchronization and harmony in the functioning of physiological systems.

Concerned about his deteriorating health, Chris complied with his physician's recommendation. Each morning during his daily train commute to work, he practiced the Heart Lock-In technique, and he would use the Freeze-Frame technique in situations when he felt his stress levels rise.[ii]

---

i) The analysis of heart rate variability (HRV), a measure of the naturally occurring beat-to-beat changes in heart rate, provides an indicator of neurocardiac fitness and autonomic nervous system function. Abnormally low 24-h HRV is predictive of increased risk of heart disease and premature mortality. HRV is also highly reflective of stress and emotions.

ii) The Heart Lock-In tool is an emotional restructuring technique, generally practiced for 5–15 min, that helps build the capacity to sustain the psychophysiological coherence mode for extended periods of time. The Freeze-Frame technique is a 1-min positive emotion refocusing exercise used in the moment that stress is experienced to change perception and modify the psychophysiological stress response. The steps of these techniques are presented later in this chapter.

At first Chris was not aware of the transformation that was occurring. His wife was the first to notice the change and to remark about how differently he was behaving and how much better he looked. Then his coworkers, staff, and other friends began to comment on how much less stressed he appeared in responding to situations at work and how much more poise and emotional balance he had. A second autonomic nervous system assessment, performed six weeks after the initial one, showed that Chris's average heart rate had decreased to 85 beats per minute and it now lowered at night, as it should. Significant increases were also apparent in his heart rate variability, which had more than doubled! These results surprised Chris' physician, as 24-hour heart rate variability is typically very stable from week to week, and it is generally quite difficult to recover from autonomic nervous system depletion, usually requiring much longer than six weeks.

In reflecting on his experience, Chris started to see how profoundly his health and his life had been transformed. He was getting along with his family, colleagues, and staff better than he could remember ever having enjoyed before, and he felt much more clearheaded and in command of his life. His life seemed more harmonious, and the difficulties that came up at work and in his personal relationships no longer created the same level of distress; he now found himself able approach them more smoothly and proactively, and often with a broadened perspective.

The true story of Chris' transformation is not an isolated example, but rather is only one of many similar case histories illustrating the profound transformations that have taken place when people have learned to self-manage their stress using these heart-based, positive emotion-focused tools. In this chapter, we describe two core tools of the HeartMath system, the Freeze-Frame and Heart Lock-In techniques, and then explore the scientific basis of their effectiveness. This discussion is built upon a conceptual framework that emphasizes the emotional component of the experience of stress and the proposition that truly transforming stress requires intervention at the emotional level. To understand how stress is generated and processed in the brain and body, we present a model of emotion, based on Pribram's theory, in which the brain functions as a complex pattern-matching system. From this perspective, it is shown that the heart is a key component of the emotional system, with the patterns of its extensive inputs to the brain making an important contribution to emotional experience. We also provide an overview of the Institute of HeartMath's research on the physiological correlates of positive emotions, which has led to the characterization of a distinctive mode of psychophysiological functioning known as *psychophysiological coherence*. Through the use of tools and technologies that foster positive emotions and psychophysiological coherence, individuals can effectively initiate a "repatterning" process, whereby habitual emotional patterns underlying stress are replaced with new, healthier patterns that establish increased emotional stability, mental acuity, and physiological efficiency as a new familiar baseline or norm.

21.2
The Emotional Basis of Stress

The term "stress" has become one of the most widely exercised words in everyday vernacular. People describe themselves as "stressed" when stuck in traffic and also when experiencing the dissolution of a long-term relationship. Preparing for an examination, having difficulty communicating with a coworker, dealing with serious illness in the family, and adjusting to new living or working conditions can all be "stressful". But what is the common thread that unites these diverse experiences, making them worthy of a common descriptor? What defines the essence of the experience of "stress"?

A widely accepted model of stress involves the perception and appraisal of a stimulus as threatening, and the consequent activation of set of physiological reactions characterized as the "stress response". Thus, stress research has traditionally been oriented towards studies examining the cognitive processes that influence the perception of stress (a cognitive perspective) or the body's response to stress (a physiological perspective). Surprisingly, however, comparatively little attention has been given to the role of the emotional system in the stress process. From a psychophysiological perspective, emotions are central to the experience of stress; indeed, it is the *emotions* activated in response to perceiving a stimulus as threatening – feelings such as anxiety, irritation, frustration, helplessness, or hopelessness – that are truly what we are experiencing when we describe ourselves as "stressed". All of the above examples of "stressors" – whether minor inconveniences or a major life changes – are experienced as stressful to the extent that they trigger emotions such as these.

While mental processes clearly play a role in stress, it is most often unmanaged emotions that provide fuel for their sustenance. It is well-recognized that thoughts carrying an emotional charge are those that tend to be perpetuated in our conscious awareness. It is also emotions – more than thoughts alone – that activate the physiological changes comprising the stress response. Our own research has clearly shown that a purely mental activity, such as cognitively recalling a past situation that provoked anger, does not produce nearly as profound an impact on physiological processes as actually engaging the emotion associated with that memory: actually reexperiencing the *feeling* of anger. It is the emotion that activates the autonomic nervous system (ANS) and hypothalamic–pituitary–adrenal axis, leading to changes in the activity and function of the body's systems and organs. Thus, many of the deleterious effects of stress on the brain and body are in fact physiological repercussions of negative emotions.

In essence, stress is conceptualized here as *emotional unease* – the experience of which ranges from low-grade feelings of emotional unrest to intense emotional turmoil. It is further contended that stress arises not only in direct response to external situations or events, but also, to a large extent, involves the ongoing internal emotional processes and attitudes individuals perpetuate even in the absence of any identifiable extrinsic stimulus. Recurring feelings of agitation, worry, and anxiety; anger, judgmentalness, and resentment; discontentment and unhappiness;

insecurity and self-doubt often consume a large part of our emotional energy and disrupt our feeling world even as we are engaged in the flow of everyday life and not necessarily confronted with a specific, current "stressor". Indeed, many people do not realize the extent to which these internalized habitual emotional patterns dominate their internal landscape, diluting and limiting positive emotional experience, and eventually becoming so familiar that "stress" essentially becomes a defining part of their sense of self-identity [1, 2].

21.3
Breaking the Stress Cycle: The Power of Positive Emotions

Although most stress has an emotional source, it is interesting to observe that most of the widely used stress management interventions do not directly focus on emotions. For example, relaxation has long been seen as the ultimate remedy for stress; many individuals believe that if they could just learn to relax then they would be healthier and happier. Relaxation is a helpful and beneficial process in that it temporarily draws attention away from distressing feelings and reduces physiological arousal, thereby promoting regeneration of the body. However, relaxation techniques generally do not address the unmanaged emotions that are the root cause of stress; nor do they seek to transform the deeper, recurring emotional patterns that give rise to stress-producing feelings. Without these more fundamental changes at the emotional level, any relief from stress that is experienced is likely to be short-lived.

Other techniques commonly used to manage stress are derived from cognitive–behavioral psychotherapy. The cognitive–behavioral model operates from the theory that maladaptive thoughts drive unhealthy behaviors and that these thoughts should therefore be the focus of therapeutic intervention. Cognitive-behavioral therapy by definition excludes emotions as a primary focus for attention, and although emotions may be explored, they are seen as a consequence of maladaptive thoughts. According to the cognitive model, all emotions follow a cognitive assessment of sensory input, which then leads to a behavioral response. The basic theoretical framework on which cognitive-behavioral methods are based, thus, is that if emotions always follow thought, then by changing one's thoughts, one can gain control over one's emotions.

In the last decade, however, research in the neurosciences has made it quite clear that emotional processes operate at a much higher speed than thoughts, frequently bypassing the mind's linear reasoning process entirely [3]. Further, although emotions can be induced by thoughts, they may also arise from unconscious associations triggered by external or internal events. In other words, not all emotions follow thoughts; emotions often occur independently of the cognitive system and, moreover, can significantly bias or color the cognitive process and its output or decision [3, 4]. For this reason, a therapeutic focus on thought processes alone may often fail to identify the fundamental cause of an emotional disturbance and thus fail to resolve it. In some cases, try as one might to rectify one's thinking, one can fall short of achieving emotional relief simply because the underlying maladaptive emotional pattern may be driven largely by unconscious triggers that operate independently of the intellect.

Further insight is gained from current research in neuroscience, which is confirming that emotion and cognition can best be thought of as separate but interacting functions and systems, which communicate via bidirectional neural connections between the neocortex and emotional centers such as the amygdala. These connections allow emotion-related input to modulate cortical activity and cognitive input from the cortex to modulate emotional processing. However, research indicates that within the brain, neural connections from the emotional system to the cognitive system are stronger and more numerous than those flowing from the cognitive to the emotional system [3] (Fig. 21.1). This provides a physiological basis for the common experience that emotional arousal can readily dominate the mental landscape, yet it is usually far more difficult to willfully turn off strong emotions through thought alone. Likewise, it is generally one's emotional experience, rather than solely cognitive activity, that is the strongest motivator of attitudes, decisions, and behavior.

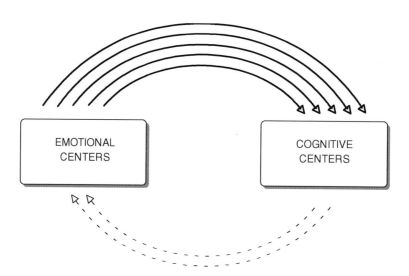

Fig. 21.1. Simplified representation illustrating the asymmetry in the neural connections between the emotional and cognitive systems in the brain. The neural connections that transmit information from the emotional centers to the cognitive centers in the brain are stronger and more numerous than those that convey information from the cognitive to the emotional centers. This accounts for the powerful influence of input from the emotional system on virtually all stages of cognitive processing involved in functions such as attention, perception, and memory, as well as on higher-order thought processes. Conversely, the comparatively limited influence of input from the cognitive system on emotional processing helps to explain why it is so difficult to modulate our emotions through thought alone.

This is why strategies that encourage "positive thinking" – *without also engaging positive feelings* – may frequently provide only temporary, if any, relief from emotional distress. While the individual may make a conceptual shift (which is important), the fundamental source of stress and driver of unhealthy behavior – the underlying maladaptive emotional pattern – remains largely intact. This understanding of how the cognitive and emotional systems interact has significant implications for emotion regulation interventions: it suggests that *intervening at the level of the emotional system itself* is a more direct, efficient, and powerful way to override and transform the maladaptive patterns underlying unhealthy psychological, behavioral, and physiological stress responses.

More specifically, it is proposed that the *activation of positive emotions* plays a critical role in breaking the stress cycle by effectively transforming stress at its source. The transformative power of positive emotions is far from being a new concept, having been noted for centuries by religious scholars, artists, scientists, medical practitioners, and lay authors alike. However, scientific exploration of these experiences has been for the most part lacking. Overshadowed by the prevailing pathology-oriented paradigm of modern psychology, positive emotions have only recently been reexamined in a scientific light [5]. Hardly surprisingly, a growing body of such research is now beginning to provide objective evidence of the centrality of positive emotions to optimal functioning in nearly all spheres of human experience. Positive emotions have been demonstrated to improve health and increase longevity [6, 7]. They have also been shown to affect the way we think and address challenges, increasing cognitive flexibility, creativity, receptivity, and innovative problem solving. Positive emotions further shape our behavior, promoting helpfulness, generosity, and effective cooperation. In short, it is suggested that positive emotions are critical to our effective adaptation to life's challenges, and to our growth and development as human beings [1, 8, 9].

Intriguingly, research is now beginning to reveal some of the underlying physiological processes that may help explain *how* positive emotions improve health, enhance cognitive function, and promote constructive behavior. As described in detail below, we have found that positive emotions are associated with a specific physiological state characterized by increased system-wide coherence, which in turn is associated with improved physiological functioning, emotional stability, and cognitive performance.

21.4
Positive Emotion-Focused Tools and Techniques

The recent Positive Psychology movement has emphasized the importance of encouraging not only the reduction of negative emotions, but also the cultivation of positive emotions in daily life. Yet, psychology has seen a notable scarcity of interventions that focus directly and systematically on increasing positive emotional experiences. Recognizing this need many years ago, D. Childre, founder of the Institute of HeartMath, undertook the development of practical, heart-based positive emotion-focused tools and techniques, which are designed to facilitate the self-regulation of emotions [2, 10]. Collectively known as the HeartMath system, these tools are intentionally designed as simple, easy-to-use interventions that can be adapted to virtually any culture, setting, or age group. They are free of religious or cultural bias, and most people feel a positive emotional shift and experience a broadened perception the first time they use them.

Briefly, these interventions combine a shift in the focus of attention to the area around the heart (where many people subjectively feel positive emotions) with the intentional self-induction of a sincere positive emotional state, such as appreciation. We have found that appreciation is one of the most concrete and easiest of the positive emotions for individuals to self-induce and sustain for longer periods.

Here we describe two of the core HeartMath tools, the Freeze-Frame and Heart Lock-In techniques, which are the tools that were used in Chris' case history that opened this chapter.

21.4.1
Freeze-Frame: A Positive Emotion Refocusing Technique

Freeze-Frame is a positive emotion refocusing exercise that enables individuals to intervene *in the moment* to greatly reduce or prevent the stress created from inappropriate or unproductive emotional triggers and reactions. The technique's name is derived from the concept that conscious perception works in a way that is analogous to watching a movie, in that each moment is perceived as an individual perceptual frame. When a scene becomes stressful, it is possible and helpful to freeze that perceptual frame and isolate it in time so that it can be observed from a more detached and objective viewpoint – similar to putting a VCR on pause for the moment. We have found that the process of intentionally deenergizing and temporarily disengaging from distressing thoughts and emotions can be greatly facilitated by shifting one's attention to the physical area around the heart (center of the chest) and self-generating a sincere positive feeling, such as appreciation. This process prevents or interrupts the body's normal stress response and also facilitates higher cognitive faculties that are normally compromised during stress and negative emotional states. This sharpens one's discernment abilties, increases resourcefulness, and often facilitates a perceptual shift, which allows the original stressor to then be assessed and addressed from a broader, more emotionally balanced perpective.

The Freeze-Frame technique consists of five simple steps, which can be effectively applied in real time in the midst of a stressful situation or day-to-day activities (e.g., while driving, sitting in a meeting, interacting with others, etc.). The tool can be used effectively in less than 1 min.

21.4.1.1   The Steps of Freeze-Frame

1. Take a time-out so that you can temporarily disengage from your thoughts and feelings, especially stressful ones.

2. Shift your focus of attention to the area around your heart. Now feel your breath coming in through your heart and going out through your solar plexus.
Practice breathing this way a few times to ease into the technique.

3. Make a sincere effort to activate a positive feeling.
Allow yourself to feel genuine appreciation or care for some person, some place, or something in your life.

4. Ask yourself what would be an efficient, effective attitude or action that would balance and destress your system.
Your ability to think more clearly and objectively is enhanced based on the increased coherence you've created in steps 2 and 3. You can view the issue now from a broader, more balanced perspective. Ask yourself what you can do to help minimize future stress.

5. Quietly sense any change in perception or feeling, and sustain it as long as you can.
Heart perceptions are often subtle. They gently suggest effective solutions that would be best for you and all concerned.

The key elements of the technique are: *shift* (to the area of the heart), *activate* (a positive feeling), and *sense* (what is the best perspective or attitude for this situation). In most training contexts, individuals are first led through several exercises designed to aid them in identifying their deepest core values and the people, places, or events they truly appreciate and care about. This helps them with step 3, where they are asked to self-generate a feeling of appreciation or other positive emotion, which is an important aspect of the technique's effectiveness.

An important way in which Freeze-Frame is distinguished from various other stress management interventions is that it is designed to enable individuals to intercede in the moment that stress is being experienced, rather than try to recuperate after the fact. The benefits of this cannot be overstated. Using Freeze-Frame in the heat of the moment saves tremendous amounts of energy that otherwise would have been drained and often prevents hours of emotionally induced wear and tear on the body and psyche. It can also reduce the time and energy spent dealing with the consequences of impulsive decisions or emotionally charged reactions, such as regret, embarrassment, guilt, accidents, and damaged relationships.

One of the long-term benefits to be gained from the practice of emotion refocusing techniques such as Freeze-Frame is increased emotional awareness, a fundamental step in the process of improving emotional well-being. In addition to helping people modify their responses to stressful events in the external environment, such techniques also help individuals identify and modify more subtle internal stressors (i.e., persistent self-defeating and energy-depleting thought patterns and feelings, such as anxiety, fear, hurt, resentment, judgmentalism, perfectionism, and projections about the future). As individuals practice "freezing the frame" when feeling inner emotional unrest, they gain increased awareness of the habitual mental and emotional processes that underlie their stress, and become more able to catch the onset of these feelings and patterns, thus diminishing their influence.

21.4.2
Heart Lock-In: An Emotional Restructuring Technique

Heart Lock-In is an emotional restructuring technique that is generally taught as a companion tool to Freeze-Frame. The Heart Lock-In technique focuses on building the capacity to sustain heartfelt positive emotions and their associated benefits for longer periods. This technique is generally practiced for a few minutes at a time, although longer sessions may be used as well. If desired, practice of this technique may also be facilitated by music specifically created to promote emotional balance and augment the favorable psychological and physiological effects of positive affective states [11].

21.4.2.1 **The Steps of Heart Lock-In**

1. Gently shift your attention to the area around your heart.
2. Shift your breathing so that you are breathing in through the heart and out through the solar plexus.
3. Activate a genuine feeling of appreciation or care for someone or something in your life.
4. Make a sincere effort to sustain feelings of appreciation or care while directing them to yourself and others.
5. When you catch your mind wandering, gently focus your breathing back through the heart and solar plexus and reconnect with feelings of care or appreciation.

After you're finished, sincerely sustain your feelings of care and appreciation as long as you can. This will act as a cushion against recurring stress or anxiety.

The key elements of the technique are: *focus* (in the area of the heart), *appreciate*, and *sustain* (positive feelings). In the midst of life's perpetual activity, the Heart Lock-In offers a simple way to cultivate and amplify heartfelt positive feelings and their nourishing effects on the body and psyche. This process is typically accompanied by feelings of deep peacefulness, harmony, and a sense of inner warmth, and is often an effective means to diffuse accumulated stress and negative feelings. Also, in quieting the normal stream of mental dialogue through this process, many report the spontaneous emergence of increased intuitive clarity and insight relative to problems or troublesome issues.

Studies conducted across diverse populations in laboratory, organizational, educational, and clinical settings have demonstrated that HeartMath positive emotion-focused techniques are effective in producing both immediate and sustained reductions in stress, together with improvements in many dimensions of psychosocial well-being. Moreover, these interventions have also been shown to give rise to significant improvements in key health and performance-related measures. For a review of outcome studies, see [1, 11]. Collectively, results indicate that such techniques are easily learned and used, produce rapid improvements, have a high rate of compliance, and are readily adaptable to a wide range of demographic groups.

21.5
The Scientific Basis of the HeartMath Techniques

We now turn to examining, from a psychophysiological perspective, the scientific basis of the positive emotion-focused tools described here. This discussion will lead us through a systems model of how emotions are generated and processed, explain the important role of the heart in the emotional system, and describe the psychophysiological changes associated with the induction of positive emotional states.

21.5.1
The Generation of Emotions: A Pattern-Matching Process

Recent years have seen the emergence of a new understanding of how the brain functions, as well as of the brain–body dynamics involved in emotional processing. Rather than assembling thoughts and feelings from bits of data like a digital computer, the brain is an analog processor that relates whole concepts or patterns to one another and looks for similarities, differences, and relationships between them. This new way of understanding brain processes has also challenged long-held views of how emotions are generated. Psychologists once maintained that emotions were purely mental expressions generated by the brain alone. We now know, instead, that emotions have as much to do with the body as they do with the brain: thus, the emergence of emotional experience results from the ongoing interaction between the brain, the body, and the external environment.

Our research finings support a systems model of emotion that includes the heart, brain, and the nervous and hormonal systems as fundamental components of a dynamic, interactive network that underlies the emergence of emotional experience [12]. This model is based on the theory of emotion first proposed by Pribram [13], in which the brain functions as a complex pattern-identification and -matching system. In this model, past experience builds within us a set of familiar patterns, which are instantiated in the neural architecture. Inputs to the brain from both the external and internal environments contribute to the maintenance of these patterns via a feedback process. Within the body, the patterns of activity of many processes provide constant rhythmic inputs with which the brain becomes familiar. These include the heart's rhythmic activity; digestive, respiratory, and hormonal rhythms; and activation patterns of muscular tension, particularly facial expressions. These inputs are continuously monitored by the brain and help organize sensory perception, cognition, feelings, and behavior.

Recurring input patterns from prior experience form a stable backdrop, or *reference pattern*, against which the input patterns from present experience are compared. According to this model, current patterns that match the reference pattern are processed and experienced as "familiar," and therefore do not produce a change in emotional arousal or experience. However, when an input pattern in the present is sufficiently different from the reference pattern, a discontinuity or *mismatch* occurs. This mismatch, or *departure from the familiar pattern*, is what underlies the generation of feelings and emotions.

Once a reference pattern is established, in order to maintain stability, the neural systems attempt to maintain a match between the reference pattern, current inputs, and future behaviors. When the input to the brain does not match the existing reference pattern, an adjustment must be made to achieve control and return the system to stability. One way to reestablish stability is by executing an outward action. We are motivated to eat if we feel hungry, to run away or fight if threatened, to do something to draw attention to ourselves if feeling ignored, etc. Alternatively, we can gain control and reestablish stability by making an internal adjustment (without any overt action). For example, a confrontation at work may lead to feelings of anger, which can prompt inappropriate behavior (e.g., outward actions such as shouting, fighting, etc.). However, through intentional internal adjustments, we can self-manage our feelings in order to inhibit these responses, reestablish stability, and maintain our job. Ultimately, when we achieve stability through our efforts, the results are feelings of satisfaction and gratification. By contrast, when there is a failure to assert control to reestablish psychophysiological stability, feelings such as anxiety, panic, annoyance, apprehension, hopelessness, or depression result.

In short, since our psychophysiological systems are designed to maintain stability, returning to the familiar reference pattern gives us a sense and feeling of security, while remaining in unfamiliar territory causes unrest. Importantly, this is true even if the established reference pattern is one of chaos and confusion: *if the reference pattern becomes maladapted, the system will still strive to maintain a match to that pattern, even though it may be dysfunctional.*

In addition to processes that monitor the inputs and controls for maintaining stability (pattern-matching) in the here-and-now, there are also matching processes that appraise the degree of congruity or incongruity between the past and the now and between the now and the projected future. Inputs to the neural systems are appraised and compared to memories of past outcomes associated with similar inputs or situations. These prospective appraisals can be either optimistic or pessimistic. If the historical outcomes of similar situations are positive (resulting in the ability to maintain control and reestablish stability), an optimistic affect (e.g., interest, confidence, or hope) will result.

On the other hand, if the appraisal does not result in a projected ability to return to stability, the current inputs are accompanied by pessimistic feelings about the future (e.g., annoyance, apprehension, hopelessness, or depression). A pessimistic appraisal can be due to the expectation of failure to achieve stability based on outcomes of past experiences of similar situations, or to a lack of experience in the projected future situation. However, as we encounter novel situations, experience new inputs, and learn new strategies to reestablish and maintain stability, we expand our repertoire of successful outcomes. The more repertoires available, the more likely a novel input will be appraised optimistically, with a high probability of success in maintaining stability. Once we learn how to handle new challenges effectively and maintain stability, the strategy (complex pattern) for dealing with the challenge also becomes familiar and part of our repertoire. It is through this process that we mature, increasing our internal self-control and management of emotions as well as our ability to respond effectively to external situations.

This model provides a psychophysiological basis for understanding why chronic stress can be so difficult to change. Through repeated experiences of stress, the brain learns to recognize the patterns of psychophysiological activity associated with "stress" as familiar, and therefore "comfortable". To the extent that these patterns of activity become part of our baseline reference, the system then automatically strives to maintain a match with these habitual psychophysiological patterns, through a feedback process, despite their detrimental impact on health, emotional well-being, and behavior. Without effective intervention, stress can thus become self-perpetuating and self-reinforcing.

However, as the system is in a dynamic relationship with its environment, this model also incorporates the means for change and development. Through a *feedforward* process, like resetting a thermostat, as new input patterns are consistently experienced and thus reinforced in the neural architecture, they become familiar to the system, and the reference pattern is thus modified and fed forward to a new stability. Once the new reference pattern is stabilized, the system then strives to maintain a match with inputs that characterize this new baseline.

Usually this process occurs automatically and unconsciously. *However, such a feedforward, repatterning process can also be intentionally initiated.* This occurs as a pattern-matching operation in which the individual deliberately holds and projects a new emotional or behavioral pattern into the future as a target of achievement, in Pribram's terms [14]. Holding the new pattern as a target in this way causes the psychophysiological systems to feed forward as new patterns of input are experienced and processed. Essentially, the system makes continual adjustments in its patterns of activity until a match is achieved between the target and the current pattern of system activity. Eventually, if this process is sustained, a new baseline is created in which the new pattern is instantiated in the system as the reference pattern. It is on this principle that the HeartMath technology is based. To further understand the processes by which these techniques work, it is necessary to examine the key role of the heart in this model.

21.5.2
More Than a Pump: The Heart's Key Role

The model of emotion described here highlights the critical function of afferent (ascending) input from the bodily organs to the brain in contributing to the input patterns that ultimately determine emotional experience [12, 13]. Although complex patterns of activity originating from many different bodily organs and systems are involved in this process, it has become clear that the heart plays a particularly important role. The heart is the primary and most consistent source of dynamic rhythmic patterns in the body. Furthermore, the afferent networks connecting the heart and cardiovascular system with the brain are far more extensive than the afferent systems associated with other major organs. To add to this, it is now established that the heart is a sophisticated information encoding and processing center, with an intrinsic nervous system sufficiently sophisticated to qualify as a "little brain" in its own right. Its circuitry enables it to learn, remember, and make functional decisions independent of the cranial brain, and its rhythmic input to the brain reflects these processes [15].

The heart also functions as a sensory organ, and is particularly sensitive and responsive to changes in a number of other psychophysiological systems. For example, heart rhythm patterns are continually and rapidly modulated by changes in the activity of either branch of the ANS, and the heart's extensive intrinsic network of sensory neurons also enables it to detect and respond to variations in hormonal rhythms and patterns [15]. Finally, the heart is itself an endocrine gland that manufactures and secretes multiple hormones and neurotransmitters [16].

Thus, with each beat, the heart not only pumps blood, but also continually transmits dynamic patterns of neurological, hormonal, pressure, and electromagnetic information to the brain and throughout the body [16]. An extensive body of research has shown, moreover, that cardiac afferent input not only exerts homeostatic effects on cardiovascular regulatory centers in the brain, but also influences the activity and function of higher brain centers involved in perceptual, cognitive, and emotional processing, see [16] for a review. The multiple and continuous inputs from the heart and cardiovascular system to the brain, are, therefore, a major contributor in establishing the familiar reference pattern against which the current input of the "now" is compared. It follows, also, from this model that *changes* in the heart's patterns of activity can have an immediate and profound impact on emotional perception and experience.

Given this connection between heart rhythm patterns and emotion, it would be predicted that interventions that enable individuals to *intentionally* change the pattern of the heart's rhythmic activity should modify one's emotional state. In fact, people commonly use just such an intervention when feeling stress: simply altering their breathing rhythm by taking several slow, deep breaths. Most people do not realize, however, that an important reason breathing techniques are effective in helping to shift one's emotional state is because changing one's breathing rhythm modulates the heart's rhythmic activity. The modulation of the heart's rhythm by respiratory activity is referred to as respiratory sinus arrhythmia.

While it can provide short-term relief from stress, cognitively directed, paced breathing is difficult for most people to maintain longer than a few minutes. On the other hand, we have found that characteristic, sustained shifts in the heart's rhythmic activity can be generated through the intentional self-induction of positive emotions. As we discuss next, this process has system-wide repercussions.

21.5.3
The Physiology of Positive Emotions

In the early stages of our research examining how psychophysiological patterns change during stress and different emotional states, we sought to determine which physiological variables were most sensitive and responsive to changes in emotion. In analyzing many different physiological measures, we discovered that the rhythmic beating patterns of the heart were consistently the most reflective of changes in emotional states, in that they covaried with emotions in real time.

Specifically, we examined the natural fluctuations in heart rate, known as heart rate variability (HRV) or *heart rhythms*, which are a product of the dynamic interplay of many of the body's systems. Short-term (beat-to-beat) changes in heart rate are largely generated and amplified by the interaction between the heart and brain via the flow of neural signals flowing through the efferent and afferent pathways of the sympathetic and parasympathetic branches of the ANS. HRV is thus considered a measure of neurocardiac function that reflects heart–brain interactions and ANS dynamics.

Utilizing HRV analysis, we have demonstrated that distinct heart rhythm patterns characterize different emotional states [16, 17]. In general, emotional stress – including emotions such as anger, frustration, and anxiety – leads to heart rhythm patterns that appear *incoherent*: erratic, disordered, and jagged (Fig. 21.2). Overall, compared to a neutral baseline state, this indicates less synchronization in the reciprocal action of the parasympathetic and sympathetic branches of the ANS. This desynchronization in the ANS, if sustained, taxes the nervous system and bodily organs, impeding the efficient synchronization and flow of information throughout the psychophysiological systems. Furthermore, as studies have shown that prefrontal cortex activity is reflected in HRV via modulation of the parasympathetic branch of the ANS, this increased disorder in heart rhythm patterns is also likely indicative of disorder in higher brain systems.

In contrast, sustained positive emotions, such as appreciation, care, compassion, and love, generate a smooth, ordered, sine-wave-like pattern in the heart's rhythms. Relative to a neutral baseline, this reflects increased synchronization between the two branches of the ANS and a general shift in autonomic balance towards increased parasympathetic activity. As is visually evident (Fig. 21.2) and also demonstrable by quantitative methods [16, 17], heart rhythms associated with positive emotions such as appreciation are clearly more *coherent* than those generated during a negative emotional experience such as frustration.

We observed that these associations appeared to hold true in studies conducted in both laboratory and natural settings, and for both spontaneous emotions and intentionally generated feelings. An important point to emphasize is that although heart *rate* or the *amount* of HRV can also covary with emotional changes, our findings showed that it is the larger scale *pattern* of the heart's rhythmic activity that is most directly related to emotional dynamics.

Taking this research further, we also observed that when positive emotional states are intentionally maintained, coherent heart rhythm patterns can be sus-

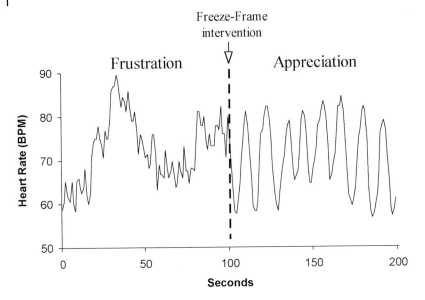

Fig. 21.2. Emotions are reflected in heart rhythm patterns. The real-time heart rate variability (heart rhythm) pattern is shown for an individual making an intentional shift from a self-induced state of frustration to a genuine feeling of appreciation by using the Freeze-Frame positive emotion refocusing technique (at the dotted line). It is of note that when the recording is analyzed statistically, the *amount* of heart rate variability is found to remain virtually the same during the two different emotional states; however, the *pattern* of the heart rhythm changes distinctly. Note the immediate shift from an erratic, disordered (incoherent) heart rhythm pattern associated with frustration to a smooth, harmonious, sine-wave-like (coherent) pattern as the individual uses the positive emotion refocusing technique and self-generates a heartfelt feeling of appreciation.

tained for longer periods, which also leads to increased synchronization and entrainment between the heart's rhythm and the activity of multiple bodily systems. Based on the distinctive set of physiological and psychological correlates that are consistently observed in such states across diverse subject populations, we have introduced the term *psychophysiological coherence* to describe this particular mode of functioning [16].

21.5.4
Psychophysiological Coherence

At the physiological level, the psychophysiological coherence mode is characterized by increased order, efficiency, and harmony in the activity and interactions of the body's systems, encompassing phenomena such as autocoherence, entrainment, synchronization, and resonance [1, 16]. As described above, this mode is associated with increased coherence in the heart's rhythmic activity (autocoherence), which manifests as a sine-wave-like heart rhythm pattern oscillating at a frequency of approximately 0.1 Hz. Thus, in this mode the HRV power spectrum is dominated by a narrow-band, high-amplitude peak near the center of the low frequency range (Fig. 21.3).

Further, during the psychophysiological coherence mode, there is increased cross-coherence or entrainment among the rhythmic patterns of activity generated by different physiological oscillatory systems. Because the heart is the body's most powerful rhythmic oscillator, generating the strongest rhythmic wave pattern, as the heart's rhythm becomes more coherent it can drive other oscillatory systems into entrainment with it. Typically, entrainment is observed between heart rhythms, respiratory rhythms, and blood pressure oscillations; however, other biological oscillators, including very low frequency brain rhythms, craniosacral rhythms, and electrical potentials measured across the skin, can also become entrained [16].

Finally, psychophysiological coherence is characterized by increased synchronization between the activity of the heart and brain. Specifically, we have found that the brain's alpha rhythms exhibit increased synchronization with the cardiac cycle during this mode [1, 16].

In terms of physiological functioning, the coherence mode confers a number of benefits to the system. These include: (a) resetting of baroreceptor sensitivity, which is related to improved short-term blood pressure control and increased respiratory efficiency; (b) increased vagal afferent traffic, which is involved in the inhibition of pain signals and sympathetic outflow; (c) increased cardiac output in conjunction with increased efficiency in fluid exchange, filtration, and absorption between the capillaries and tissues; (d) increased ability of the cardiovascular system to adapt to circulatory requirements; and (e) increased temporal synchronization of cells throughout the body. This results in increased system-wide energy efficiency and conservation of metabolic energy [16]. These observations support a link between positive emotions and increased physiological efficiency, which may partially explain the growing number of documented correlations between positive emotions, improved health, and increased longevity. We have also shown that practicing techniques that increase physiological coherence is associated with both short-term and long-term improvement in several objective health-related measures, including enhanced humoral immunity [18] and an increased dehydroepiandrosterone (DHEA)/cortisol ratio [19].

Psychophysiological coherence is similarly associated with beneficial psychological correlates, including reduced perception of stress, sustained positive affect, and a high degree of mental clarity and emotional stability. We have also found that the coherence mode is associated with significant improvement in cognitive performance [1, 16].

It is important to note that the psychophysiological coherence mode is both physiologically (as shown in Fig. 21.3) and psychologically distinct from a state of relaxation. At the physiological level, relaxation is characterized by an overall reduction in ANS outflow and a shift in ANS balance towards increased parasympathetic activity. The coherence mode is also associated with an increase in parasympathetic

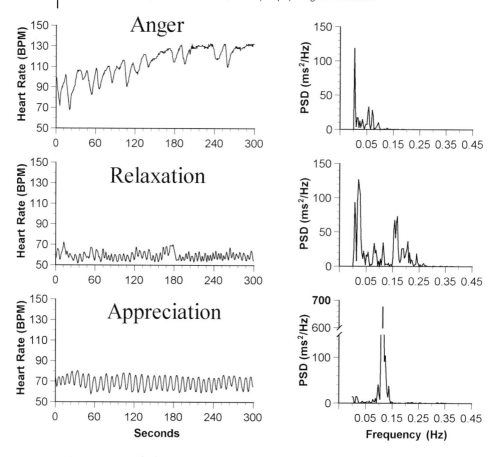

Fig. 21.3. Heart rhythm patterns during different psychophysiological states. The graphs to the *left* are heart rate tachograms, which show beat-to-beat changes in heart rate. To the *right* are shown the heart rate variability power spectral density (*PSD*) plots of the tachograms at *left*. Anger is characterized by a lower frequency, disordered heart rhythm pattern and increasing heart rate. As can be seen in the corresponding power spectrum to the *right*, the rhythm during anger is primarily in the very low frequency band, which is associated with sympathetic nervous system activity. Relaxation produces a higher frequency, lower amplitude heart rhythm, indicating reduced autonomic outflow. In this case, increased power in the high frequency band of the power spectrum is observed, reflecting increased parasympathetic activity (the relaxation response). In contrast, sustained positive emotions such as appreciation are associated with a highly ordered, smooth, sine-wave-like heart rhythm pattern, indicative of the psychophysiological coherence mode. As can be seen in the corresponding power spectrum, the coherence mode is associated with an unusually high-amplitude peak (note the scale difference) in the low frequency band, centered around 0.1 Hz. This indicates system-wide resonance, increased synchronization between the sympathetic and parasympathetic branches of the nervous system, and entrainment between the heart rhythm pattern, respiration, and blood pressure rhythms. The psychophysiological coherence mode is also associated with increased parasympathetic activity, thus encompassing a key element of the relaxation response, yet it is physiologically distinct from relaxation because the system is oscillating at its natural resonant frequency (~0.1 Hz) and there is increased harmony and synchronization in nervous system and heart–brain dynamics. In addition, the coherence mode does not necessarily involve a lowering of heart rate *per se*, or a change in the amount of variability, but rather a change in heart rhythm pattern.

activity, thus encompassing a key element of the relaxation response, but is physiologically distinct from relaxation because the system is oscillating at its natural resonant frequency and there is increased harmony and synchronization in nervous system and heart–brain dynamics [16]. Further, unlike relaxation, the coherence mode does not necessarily involve a lowering of heart *rate per se*, or a change in the *amount* of HRV, but rather a change in heart rhythm *pattern*.

Not only are there fundamental differences in the physiological correlates of relaxation and coherence, but the associated psychological states are also quite different. Relaxation is generally a dissociative state, conducive to rest or sleep, in which attention is primarily drawn away from cognitive and emotional processes. In contrast, coherence generally involves the active experience of positive emotions. This mode promotes a calm, balanced, yet alert and responsive state that is conducive to everyday functioning, including problem-solving, decision-making, and the performance of tasks requiring mental acuity, focus, coordination, and discrimination [1, 16].

21.6
Revisiting the HeartMath Techniques: A Repatterning Process

When the Freeze-Frame and Heart Lock-In techniques were first introduced in the earlier part of this chapter, we focused on a simple description of the steps the individual uses to implement the tools. Now, with an understanding of the psychophysiological processes involved in the generation of emotion, the key role of the heart in the emotional system, and the distinctive physiological changes accompanying positive emotions, we are in a position to better understand how these tools work, as well as their larger implications for health and well-being.

In essence, the significance of the HeartMath tools is that they offer the individual a systematic and reliable means by which one can intentionally feed forward out of a state of emotional unease or stress into a new positive state of emotional calm and stability. This occurs as result of a process in which the individual intentionally creates a new positive emotional state as the system's future target and activates changes in patterns of psychophysiological activity that enable the system to achieve and maintain that new state.

Intervening at the level of the emotional system, HeartMath techniques utilize the heart as a point of entry into the psychophysiological networks that underlie emotional experience. The model of emotion discussed in this chapter highlights the brain's role as a pattern-identification and -matching system and underscores the importance of afferent bodily input in establishing the familiar patterns that are critical in determining emotional experience. As a principal and consistent source of rhythmic information patterns that impact the physiological, cognitive, and emotional systems, the heart thus provides an access point from which system-wide dynamics can be quickly and profoundly affected [12, 16].

We have found that the process of coupling an intentional shift in attention to the physical area of the heart with the self-induction of a sincere heartfelt positive emotional feeling appears to excite the system at its resonant frequency, thus facilitating the natural emergence of the psychophysiological coherence mode (Fig. 21.2). This shift to coherence, in turn, results in a change in the pattern of afferent cardiac signals sent to the brain, which is of significance for several reasons. First, at the physiological level, this shift serves to interrupt or prevent the triggering of the body's normal stress response. Second, at the emotional level, the movement to a more organized pattern of cardiac afferent input that accompanies a coherent heart rhythm pattern is one that the brain associates with feelings of security and well-being, resulting in a pattern match with positive emotional experience. This shift in the pattern of the heart's input to the brain, thus, serves to reinforce the self-generated positive emotional shift, making it easier to sustain. Through consistent use of the HeartMath tools, the coupling between the psychophysiological coherence mode and positive emotion is further reinforced. This subsequently strengthens the ability of a positive feeling shift to initiate a beneficial physiological shift towards increased coherence, or a physiological shift to facilitate the experience of a positive emotion.

A further outcome of the shift to a state of psychophysiological coherence manifests at the cognitive level, as a result of the change in the pattern of cardiac afferent information reaching the brain's higher cognitive centers. Our own and others' research has shown that changes in input to the brain from the cardiovascular system can modify the brain's electrophysiological activity and can also lead to significant changes in perceptual and cognitive processing (for a revew see [16]). Indeed, this relationship may provide a physiological basis for research findings demonstrating a link between positive emotions and improved creativity, cognitive flexibility, and innovative problem-solving, faculties that are also frequently enhanced during or following the generation of the psychophysiological coherence mode. We postulate, therefore, that the activation of positive emotions and the coherence mode leads to a state in which higher cognitive faculties are facilitated [16].

Thus, in the Freeze-Frame technique, although attention is initially drawn away from stressful perceptions and feelings, once individuals have activated a positive emotion and a consequent shift to coherence, they then return to address the original stressor from the vantage point afforded by this new psychophysiological state. Our experience indicates that this nearly always leads to a change in perception, feeling, or attitude about the stressor, and the ability to address it from a more objective, discerning, and resourceful perspective. In this way, individuals are actually able to *transform* the source of their stress in real time, replacing an automatic, emotionally draining, self-limiting, response with a proactive, creative one.

While the process of activating the psychophysiological coherence mode clearly leads to immediate benefits by helping to transform stress in the moment it is experienced, it can also contribute to long-term improvements in emotion regulation abilities and emotional well-being that ultimately affect many aspects of one's life. This is because each time individuals intentionally arrest and override the psychophysiological and behavioral patterns associated with stress by self-generating a state of psychophysiological coherence, the "new" coherent patterns – and "new" repertoires for responding to challenge – are reinforced in the neural architecture.

With consistency of practice, these patterns become increasingly familiar to the brain. Thus, through a feedforward process, these new, healthy patterns become established as a new baseline or reference, which the system then strives to maintain. It is in this way that HeartMath tools facilitate a *repatterning process*, whereby the maladaptive patterns that underlie the experience of stress are progressively replaced by healthier physiological, emotional, cognitive, and behavioral patterns as the "automatic" or familiar way of being.

This repatterning process is greatly facilitated by use of the Heart Lock In technique, which is specifically designed to reinforce or lock-in the coherent psychophysiological patterns associated with positive emotional states. By building the capacity to sustain heartfelt positive emotions and psychophysiological coherence for longer periods, consistent practice of this tool plays a critical role in the feedforward process that helps establish coherence as a new reference pattern. Our research supports the proposition that this process promotes increased emotional stability, mental acuity, and physiological efficiency as a new familiar baseline, thus diminishing the future likelihood of experiencing prolonged stress. Moreover, even when stress or emotional instability is subsequently experienced, the familiar, coherent state is more readily accessible, enabling a quicker and more enduring emotional shift.

The occurrence of such a repatterning process is supported by both physiological and psychological data. At the electrophysiological level, ambulatory recordings demonstrate a greater frequency of spontaneous (without conscious practice of the tools) periods of coherence in the heart rhythm patterns of individuals practiced in the HeartMath techniques in comparison to the general population. There are also data linking the practice of HeartMath tools with favorable changes in hormonal patterns. Specifically, a significant increase in the DHEA/cortisol ratio was demonstrated in individuals who consistently used the HeartMath tools for 30 days. This finding, which has recently been independently replicated, is interpreted as evidence of a repatterning process occurring at a fundamental level, given that there is normally little physiological variability in levels of these hormones from month to month [19].

The physiological changes observed with use of these interventions typically occur in conjunction with significant changes in psychological patterns. Reductions in measures of emotional distress, including anxiety, depression, anger, hostility, guilt, and burnout, have been consistently observed in many different populations with practice of the HeartMath tools (see [1, 11] for a summary). These observations suggest that the interventions are effective in helping to modify the habitual emotional patterns that are a major source of stress.

21.7
Heart Rhythm Coherence Feedback Training: Facilitating Coherence

We have found that the learning and effective use of HeartMath positive emotion-focused tools can be significantly facilitated by heart rhythm coherence feedback training. This technology provides real-time physiological feedback that serves as a powerful aid and objective validation in the process of learning to self-generate increased psychophysiological coherence [20].

Technologies have recently been developed that enable heart rhythm coherence, the key physiological marker of the psychophysiological coherence mode, to be objectively monitored and quantified. One such device is the Freeze-Framer heart-rhythm-monitoring and coherence-building system (Quantum Intech, Boulder Creek, California). This interactive hardware/software system monitors and displays individuals' heart rate variability patterns in real time as they practice the positive emotion refocusing and emotional restructuring techniques taught in an included tutorial. Using a fingertip sensor to record the pulse wave, the Freeze-Framer plots changes in heart rate on a beat-to-beat basis. As people practice the techniques, they can readily see and experience the changes in their heart rhythm patterns, which generally become more ordered, smoother, and more sine-wave-like as they feel positive emotions. This process reinforces the natural association between the coherence mode and positive feelings. The real-time physiological feedback helps to take the guesswork and randomness out of the process of self-inducing a positive emotional state, resulting in greater consistency, focus, and effectiveness in practicing emotional shifts. The software also analyzes the heart rhythm patterns for coherence level, which is fed back to the user as an accumulated score or success in playing one of three games designed to reinforce the emotion refocusing skills. This heart rhythm coherence feedback technology is available on two platforms: a personal computer based version and a newly developed handheld version.[1]

Because this technology uses a fingertip pulse sensor and involves no electrode hook-up, it is extremely versatile, time-efficient, and easy to use in a wide variety of settings (e.g., workplaces, homes, schools, etc.). Heart rhythm coherence feedback training and the positive emotion-focused tools discussed in this chapter have been successfully used in diverse contexts by mental health professionals, physicians, law enforcement personnel, educators, athletes, and corporate executives to decrease stress, anxiety, depression, and fatigue; promote improved academic, work, and sports performance; reduce physical and psychological health risk factors; and facilitate improvements in health and quality of life in patients with numerous clinical disorders [1, 11, 20].

21.8
Conclusions and Implications

With continually rising stress levels now a problem of global proportions, it is imperative, for both individual and societal health, that practical and effective strat-

---

[1] Newly updated versions of this technology, in both personal computer-based and handheld formats, will be released in 2006 under the name emWave™. For additional information on this technology, see www.emwave.com.

egies for reducing and transforming stress be made available to all people. Here we have argued that understanding and directly addressing the internal *emotional* source of stress provides an important key.

Heart-based techniques that enable the self-activation of positive emotions show promise as a simple and powerful means to modify engrained emotional patterns that contribute to the experience of stress and its debilitating effects on health and well-being. We have shown that use of such techniques gives rise to psychophysiological coherence, a highly efficient and regenerative functional mode that appears to have wide-ranging benefits. By virtue of the brain's pattern-matching function, the intentional generation of positive emotions and psychophysiological coherence enables individuals to activate a feedforward process whereby stress-producing psychophysiological and behavioral patterns engrained through past experience are progressively replaced by new, healthier patterns of activity. Thus, through the establishment of a new reference pattern, individuals effectively create an *internal* environment that is conducive to the maintenance of physiological efficiency-mental clarity, and emotional stability-one that is resilient and adaptive as we respond to life's inevitable challenges.

The use of positive emotion-based interventions to address stress and its deleterious repercussions has been shown to be effective in a wide range of contexts, including health care, business, and education. Moreover, there is evidence that such an approach can provide benefits that extend beyond stress reduction. Interventions that cultivate positive emotions also appear to be effective in enhancing creativity and performance in both individuals and work teams; in improving organizational climate; in decreasing risky behaviors and improving academic performance among students; and in facilitating enduring improvements in health. Furthermore, psychotherapists have found that a positive emotion-based emotional restructuring approach is not only an effective therapeutic tool in dealing with stress and trauma, but also significantly enhances the quality of the client's life. This has also been the experience of individual practitioners of positive emotion-focused techniques, in that many report that the use of these tools has enabled them to intentionally infuse their daily experiences with greater emotional quality, leading to lasting positive changes in their attitudes, social relationships, world view, and sense of personal empowerment and fulfillment.

In short, these findings collectively suggest that positive emotions are not merely *markers* of good health and optimal functioning, but are in fact active *agents* in the processes by which these states can be achieved. The correlates of the coherence mode we have identified may provide an important key to elucidating the psychophysiological basis of the effects of positive emotions on health, cognition, and psychosocial functioning that have been increasingly documented by research. Further studies on the use of positive emotion-focused interventions conducted with larger samples and longer follow-up are needed to replicate and extend the findings obtained thus far. Such research will deepen scientific knowledge of the repatterning that can be facilitated by these interventions, including its long-term effects on the health and well-being of the individual and society.

From a broader perspective still, a new approach to addressing stress, grounded in a scientific understanding of the psychophysiological basis of emotion, may well lead us through the doorway to a new era. From our emergence more than half a million years ago, emotions have played an enormous role not only in the everyday lives of individuals but also in affecting the course of historical events of monumental importance for human civilization. But because the genesis of emotions was poorly understood, humankind has relied primarily on social regulation and constraint, and more recently pharmacological and psychotherapeutic interventions, to modulate and direct the enormous power of emotional energy. Now, with the beginnings of an understanding of how emotions are generated by specific psychophysiological processes, we are not only significantly closer to a more complete understanding of human function and behavior, but we also have effective and accessible tools, based on scientific knowledge, that individuals can use to regulate and intentionally change their inner states. Rather than remaining at the mercy of emotions and their individual and societal consequences, we can now be proactive in willfully generating positive emotional states to effect a healthier, happier, and more functional life.

Acknowledgements

We would like to express our appreciation to Dr. Raymond Bradley, whose insightful comments and helpful suggestions greatly benefited this chapter.

Note

HeartMath, Freeze-Frame, and Heart Lock-In are registered trademarks of the Institute of HeartMath. Freeze-Framer is a registered trademark and emWave is a trademark of Quantum Intech, Inc.

References

1 R. McCraty, D. Childre. 2004. The grateful heart: The psychophysiology of appreciation. In: The Psychology of Gratitude. R.A. Emmons, M.E. McCullough (eds.) Oxford University Press, New York, pp 230–255.

2 D. Childre, D. Rozman. 2005. Transforming Stress. New Harbinger, Oakland, CA.

3 J. LeDoux. 1996. The Emotional Brain: The Mysterious Underpinnings of Emotional Life. Simon and Schuster, New York.

4 P. Niedenthal and S. Kitayama (eds.) 1994. The Heart's Eye: Emotional Influences in Perception and Attention. Academic, San Diego.

5 C.R. Snyder, S.J. Lopez (eds.) 2002. Handbook of Positive Psychology. Oxford University Press, New York.

6 L.G. Russek and G.E. Schwartz. 1997. Feelings of parental caring predict health status in midlife: A 35-Year Follow-up of the Harvard Mastery of Stress Study. J Behav Med 20:1–13.

7 D.D. Danner, D.A. Snowdon, W.V. Friesen. 2001. Positive emotions in early life and longevity: Findings from

the nun study. J Pers Soc Psychol 80:804–813.

8 A.M. ISEN. 1999. Positive affect. In: Handbook of Cognition and Emotion. T. DALGLEISH, M. POWER (eds.) Wiley, New York, pp 522–539.

9 B.L. FREDRICKSON. 2002. Positive emotions. In: Handbook of Positive Psychology. C.R. SNYDER, S.J. LOPEZ (eds.) Oxford University Press, New York, pp 120–134.

10 D. CHILDRE, H. MARTIN. 1999. The HeartMath Solution. HarperSanFrancisco, San Francisco.

11 R. MCCRATY, M. ATKINSON, D. TOMASINO. 2001. Science of the Heart: Exploring the Role of the Heart in Human Performance. HeartMath Research Center, Institute of HeartMath, Publication No. 01-001, Boulder Creek, CA.

12 R. MCCRATY. 2003. Heart–Brain Neurodynamics: The Making of Emotions. HeartMath Research Center, Institute of HeartMath, Publication No. 03-015, Boulder Creek, CA.

13 K.H. PRIBRAM, F.T. MELGES. 1969. Psychophysiological basis of emotion. In: Handbook of Clinical Neurology. P.J. VINKEN, G.W. BRUYN (eds.) North-Holland, Amsterdam, pp 316–341.

14 K.H. PRIBRAM. 1991. Brain and Perception: Holonomy and Structure in Figural Processing. Lawrence Erlbaum, Hillsdale, NJ.

15 J.A. ARMOUR, G.C. KEMBER. 2004. Cardiac sensory neurons. In: Basic and Clinical Neurocardiology. J.A.

ARMOUR, J.L. ARDELL (eds.) Oxford University Press, New York, pp 79–117.

16 R. MCCRATY, M. ATKINSON, D. TOMASINO, R.T. BRADLEY. 2006. The Coherent Heart: Heart–Brain Interactions, Psychophysiological Coherence, and The Emergence Of System-Wide Order. HeartMath Research Center, Institute of HeartMath, Boulder Creek, CA.

17 R. MCCRATY, M. ATKINSON, W.A. TILLER, G. REIN, A.D. WATKINS. 1995. The effects of emotions on short-term power spectrum analysis of heart rate variability. Am J Cardiol 76:1089–1093.

18 R. MCCRATY, M. ATKINSON, G. REIN, A.D. WATKINS. 1996. Music enhances the effect of positive emotional states on salivary IgA. Stress Med 12:167–175.

19 R. MCCRATY, B. BARRIOS-CHOPLIN, D. ROZMAN, M. ATKINSON, A.D. WATKINS. 1998. The impact of a new emotional self-management program on stress, emotions, heart rate variability, DHEA and cortisol. Integr Physiol Behav Sci 33:151–170.

20 R. MCCRATY, D. TOMASINO. 2004. Heart rhythm coherence feedback: A new tool for stress reduction, rehabilitation, and performance enhancement. In: Proceedings of the First Baltic Forum on Neuronal Regulation and Biofeedback, Riga, Latvia, Nov. 2–4, 2004. (Also available at http://www.heartmath.org/research/research-papers/HRV_Biofeedback2.pdf).

22

Stress Systems in Aging – Cognitions and Dementia

Nicole C. Schommer and Isabella Heuser

22.1
Introduction and Overview

The United Nations note that in 2000, 10% of the world's inhabitants were 60 years or older and in 2050 one out of five persons will be at least 60 years old. In this population the diagnosis of multiple chronic disorders is common, with women having a higher risk for Alzheimer's disease (AD) than men despite a lesser average life expectancy in men. One simple definition of aging is the gradual loss of functional capacity and resiliency in physiological as well as psychological systems. These changes occur, however, with a great variation in degree and progression of deterioration across individuals, ranging for instance from "normal" age-related cognitive changes via mild cognitive impairment to severely demented states. Many factors might be responsible for age-related brain alterations with immune, metabolic and neuroendocrine changes as potential pathogenetic variables. It is well-known that aging is accompanied with a decrease in the ability to maintain homeostasis and with a reduced resiliency when the system is stressed. The neuroendocrine stress-system with its cortical and peripheral components plays a pivotal role in these processes. The concept of "allostatic load" hypothesizes that differences in the aging process result from an accumulation of wear and tear by daily experiences and major life events that interact with genetic constitution, and predisposing early life events. In this context the neuroendocrine, autonomic nervous and immune systems are considered mediators of adaptation to challenges of daily life. Many disorders in older age are associated with a dysregulation of one or all of the above mentioned systems. This chapter will first focus on activity and reactivity of the major neuroendocrine stress-regulating system, the hypothalamus–pituitary–adrenal (HPA) system in the elderly. Additional remarks will be made about sex steroids and dehydroepiandrostendione (DHEA) and their relationship to cognitive functioning. Aging processes will be described in healthy elderly individuals, and then the involvement of the HPA system in patients suffering from disorders ranging from mild cognitive impairment to dementia like Alzheimer's disease will be discussed.

Stress in Health and Disease. Edited by Bengt B. Arnetz and Rolf Ekman
Copyright © 2006 WILEY-VCH Verlag GmbH & Co. KGaA, Weinheim
ISBN: 3-527-31221-8

22.2
Endocrine Systems in the Healthy Elderly

22.2.1
Basal Activity of the HPA System

For this chapter basal activity of the HPA system will be considered as the un-stimulated HPA activity along the diurnal cycle. Most papers have reported no or only small age effects concerning basal HPA parameters. While there are only little changes in daytime basal ACTH and cortisol levels (for overview see [1]), the circadian rhythm seems to advance with age with flattened diurnal amplitudes [2, 3] possibly due to a reduced mineralocorticoid receptor (MR) capacity [4]. In a study with 16 young men and 20 elderly men and women, adrenocorticotropic hormone (ACTH) and cortisol profiles were investigated during undisturbed nocturnal sleep; significant higher cortisol levels during the first part of the night in the elderly and heightened ACTH levels during the entire night were observed. A reanalysis of six studies with a total of 177 subjects aged 20–80 years with different parameters of basal HPA activity resulted in an increase of mean plasma cortisol levels by 20–50% over the years and nocturnal nadir was shortened and mean levels of nadir were higher in aged than in young adults. Additionally, in elderly women, early morning cortisol rise was enhanced compared to the young subjects.

In summary, in healthy aged subjects, circulating glucocorticoid levels show a relative constancy over time with no or only subtle changes with age during the daytime while during nighttime glucocorticoid concentration is clearly enhanced.

22.2.2
Stimulated Reactivity of the HPA System

Age-related alterations of HPA dysregulations are more prominent after various challenge tests, including pharmacological and psychosocial stress tests. Different pathways of the HPA system are activated, depending on the nature of a stimulus: While psychological stressors activate the HPA system by stimulation of the para-ventricular nucleus (PVN) of the hypothalamus through the limbic system [pre-frontal cortex (PFC), hippocampus, amygdala], a more direct pathway to the PVN is reached by pharmacological/physiological stressors. Whereas most pharma-cological HPA system stimulation tests primarily act at the pituitary or adrenal level, psychological stressors certainly require processing at higher brain levels (Fig. 22.1). With respect to pharmacological tests one has to consider the possibility that different doses of a drug change the main target of the chosen test. For exam-ple, by administration of a small dose of synthetic ACTH the sensitivity of the ad-renal cortex can be addressed, while administration of a larger dose of synthetic ACTH would assess its maximum capacity. Thus, seemingly contradictory results concerning age (and sex)-related effects could possibly be attributed to differences in the applied HPA system stimulation procedures.

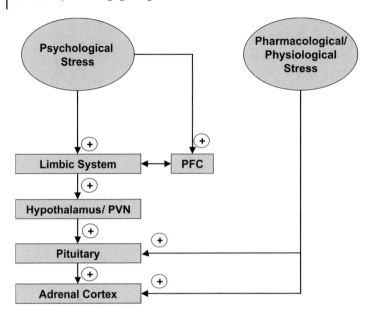

Fig. 22.1. Different pathways in stimulation of the
hypothalamus–pituitary–adrenal (HPA) system by
psychological versus pharmacological or physiological
challenge. *PFC* Prefrontal cortex, *PVN* paraventricular nucleus.

A large numbers of human studies applying neuroendocrine challenge tests in
elderly compared to young subjects have repeatedly showed age-related alterations
of HPA reactivity after different well-known pharmacological stimulation tests like
the corticotropin-releasing hormone (CRH), the combined vasopressin and CRH
or the dexamethasone (DEX)–CRH tests (the latter being CRH after premedication
with DEX). Outcomes in these tests show mostly higher HPA responses in aged
subjects than in young adults. Results concerning HPA feedback sensitivity after
the DEX suppression test (DST) in aged subjects are contradictory: some studies
report higher cortisol levels in the elderly after DEX which would reflect an impaired feedback mechanism, while others fail to demonstrate these outcomes.
However, the combined DEX–CRH test, reported to be distinctly more sensitive
in detection of HPA dysregulations, shows mostly higher cortisol responses in the
elderly.

With respect to non-pharmacological stimulation conditions, like psychosocial
stress tests, few studies so far have investigated age effects. Although in one study
age-related differences in HPA responses using a psychosocial stress task were reported, the computer-based stress protocol employed may have been inappropriate
for induction of comparable psychosocial stress in both age groups. Other

studies employing standardized psychosocial stress protocols in elderly subjects either failed to evoke a significant endocrine stress response or did not include a young comparison group (for overview see [5]). In two well-designed double-blind and placebo-controlled studies to investigate age and sex steroid effects on psychosocial stress as well as a pharmacological challenge (DEX–CRH test), Kudielka and colleagues [6] studied a group of healthy elderly receiving hormonal replacement with estrogens (women) and testosterone (men), one age-matched group of healthy elderly treated with a placebo and one group of healthy young adults. The authors observed no influence of age or hormonal replacement on HPA reactivity following a psychosocial stress test consisting of a free speech and mental arithmetic. However, after the DEX–CRH test, the untreated older women showed significantly higher free and total cortisol responses and a tendency towards higher ACTH reactivity in comparison to the young group. Substitution with estrogens for 2 weeks resulted in attenuated cortisol responses compared to the placebo-treated elderly, but still with higher responses than the young controls (Fig. 22.2).

A similar outcome is observed in men after a bolus injection of 250 mg testosterone 5 days before testing. Placebo-treated elderly males showed markedly higher total plasma cortisol responses and a trend towards increased free cortisol and ACTH responses and again testosterone-substituted men showed attenuated HPA reactivity compared to the placebo group.

Recently Otte et al. [7] performed a meta-analysis of 45 studies investigating stimulated cortisol responses in healthy elderly compared to young controls with a total of 1295 subjects (670 young subjects, mean age 27.8 years; 625 elderly subjects, mean age 69.1 years). Studies conducting pharmacological ($n = 39$) and psychological/psychosocial challenge tests ($n = 6$) were included and there was a large variety of different pharmacological stimulation paradigms, like administration of ACTH, CRH, DEX, epinephrine, insulin, naloxone, somatostatin, ghrelin, growth-hormone-releasing hormone, metyrapone, physiostagmine, etc. All studies used between-group designs and included only healthy, nonhospitalized subjects. The analyses revealed significantly larger cortisol responses to challenge tests in the elderly compared to younger controls with an effect size of $d = 0.42$; $p < 0.001$. Furthermore the authors investigated possible gender effects based on a total of 26 studies. They found a highly significant impact of gender in relation to age and HPA responses, with a threefold higher age effect in women than in men (Fig. 22.3).

Beside age effects, gender effects are also well-documented. In elderly men, higher total plasma cortisol responses than in women were observed after a test battery composed of the Stoop color word task, a mental arithmetic test, an anagram test, the cold pressure test, and a psychological stressor. In contrast, Seeman et al. [8] reported higher plasma cortisol reactivity in elderly women than in elderly men employing a driving simulation challenge. Recently, these observations were corroborated by the same group using a 30-min cognitive challenge paradigm. However, a closer look at the results of these two studies reveals that in the first study no significant gender effects were observed in mean plasma cortisol re-

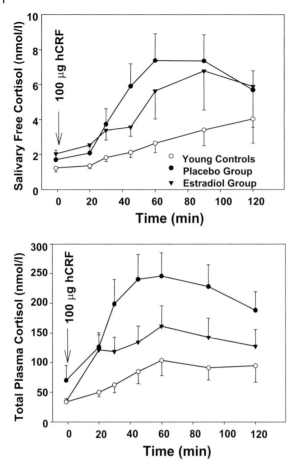

Fig. 22.2. Salivary free and total plasma cortisol levels in young untreated, elderly placebo-treated and elderly estradiol-treated individuals before and after corticotropin- releasing hormone (*CRH*) injection (100 μg human CRH (hCRH) after premedication with 1.5 mg dexamethasone (DEX). Figure reprinted from Kudielka with permission of Cuvillier.

sponses in terms of (a) maximal increase, (b) area under the curve, and (c) repeated measures ANOVA, but solely in simultaneously elevated ACTH and cortisol responses above the respective sample median. In the second study, the reported effect of elevated saliva cortisol responses in older women compared to older men were based on only two subjects in the group of elderly female responders (non-responders were excluded by the authors). In a study investigating HPA stress responses following the Trier psychosocial stress test (TSST), which mainly consists of a free speech and a mental arithmetic task of 15 min duration performed in front of an audience, 102 healthy subjects between the ages of 9 and 76 years were investigated [5]. Results showed that the stress task induced significant HPA

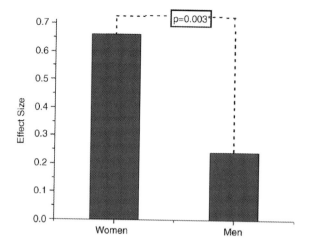

Fig. 22.3. Effect of age on cortisol response in women and men. Effect size is shown as Cohen's *d*. Differences of effect sizes were analyzed by one-way ANOVA. Figure reprinted from Otte et al. [7] with permission from Elsevier.

system responses in all subjects. While in children and younger adults data revealed no gender differences in free cortisol responses, elderly men showed larger salivary free cortisol responses than aged women. This effect was not attributable to the subjectively perceived stress load to the TSST. Likewise, for total plasma cortisol, the response patterns did not differ between age and gender groups. However, total plasma cortisol concentrations were generally heightened in elderly women. For ACTH, the response was higher in younger men. The observed ACTH and total plasma cortisol response patterns in younger and older adults suggest that a heightened hypothalamic drive in younger men decreases with age, resulting in similar ACTH responses in elderly men and women and that younger adult females have a higher adrenocortical sensitivity to ACTH signals. This is in accordance with earlier reports on greater ACTH pulses in middle-aged men and a higher sensitivity to ACTH of the female adrenal cortex.

Concerning heightened stress reactivity in aged women compared to young controls, in a recent study the degree of aerobic fitness in the elderly was shown to be a relevant impact variable on HPA reactivity. The degree of aerobic fitness was determined with a continuous, inclined treadmill test and based on individual maximal oxygen consumption (VO_{2max}) older women were classified as "old–unfit" in case of a VO_{2max} below the average for the respective age group, whereas women with a VO_{2max} above the average were classified as "old–fit" women. A combination of mental, physical and psychological stress resulted in all three groups in significant cortisol and ACTH stress responses. However, unfit older women showed significantly higher cortisol responses and ACTH baseline and peak levels compared to the old–fit women and the young controls; the latter two groups did not differ from each other. So the authors concluded that higher aerobic fitness among older women is able to attenuate or prevent age-related changes in HPA stress reactivity.

Finally, besides stress-related or pharmacological induced cortisol increases time-to-baseline seems to be an important index and therefore, more fine-grained analyses of recovery should be provided in future stress studies. In their informative and still relevant review on aging and HPA system response to challenge in humans, Seeman and Robbins [1] underscore this idea by defining stress resilience as "the overall pattern of HPA responses to challenge, encompassing the rate of initial response to challenge, the magnitude of the response, and the rate of recovery of the HPA system to the basal state."

Even more than 10 years later there is still a lack of comprehensive studies investigating these topics in healthy and nonhealthy elderly.

Concerning mechanisms accounting for the above reported age effects there are several hypotheses to be considered.

According to the glucocorticoid cascade hypothesis [9], increasing cortisol responses in aged subjects are caused by loss of both mineralo- and glucocorticoid receptors in the hippocampus resulting in a reduced normal inhibitory impact of the hippocampus on the HPA system. While the heightened cortisol levels in turn further desensitize hippocampal glucocorticoid receptors, a maladaptive feedforward circle is started. In this context, Lupien and coworkers [10] demonstrated an association between decreased hippocampal volume and increased cortisol levels.

Another theory addressing the change of glucocorticoid receptor activity from protective to harmful is the Receptor Balance Theory [11]. This theory assumes a balance between hippocampal mineralocorticoid receptor (MR) and glucocorticoid receptor (GR) activities. Current data suggest that the MR controls the stress system reactivity, while the GR, however, facilitates the systems recovery by restraining further stress responses. In case of a disproportionate capacity, the corticosteroid receptors may lose their ability to terminate stress responses, and target tissues are thus exposed for a prolonged time to elevated glucocorticoid levels. This hypercortisolism is thought to promote feedforward feedback loops, and consequently, a further aggravation of stress system imbalance occurs. The theory postulates, that a balance in these stress-regulating corticosteroid receptors is necessary for maintenance of homeostasis and thus for health.

Finally, a recent hypothesis suggests that, with age, the proinflammatory cytokines, such as interleukin-6 that strongly stimulates hypothalamic CRH release, are increased and this might result in age-associated increased basal HPA system activity.

HPA reactivity is heightened in aged compared to young adults, with a more pronounced age effect in elderly women than in men. However, summarizing results on pharmacological and psychosocial stimulation tests the age effect is more clearly demonstrated after pharmacological challenge. It would be very interesting to perform meta-analyses separately for these different kinds of challenge tests.

Nevertheless there is a substantial heterogeneity in age-related HPA activity and re-activity: while some individuals show considerable changes, others maintain HPA function similar to that of young individuals.

22.2.3
DHEA, Estrogen, and Testosterone

22.2.3.1 Dehydroepiandrostendione

The adrenal steroid dehydroepiandrostendione (DHEA) and its sulfate (DHEA-S) show, in contrast to the more discrete changes of basal glucocorticoid secretion, a marked reduction in secretion rate in the elderly compared to young adults. Peak levels occur in the mid-twenties and approach a nadir with about 80% of reduction in the late sixties. On the other hand, in about 15% of males, DHEA-S levels increase with age. DHEA has a variety of "functional antagonistic" effects upon the actions of glucocorticoids. Functional antagonistic effects refers to its ability to counteract some actions of glucocorticoids and does not imply a direct interaction via binding to GRs. DHEA counteracts, for instance, the memory and long-term potentiation inhibiting effects of glucocorticoids (for overview see [12]).

Human studies and DHEA impact on cognition are contradictory. Most comparison studies between young and elderly reported significant inverse relationships between DHEA-S-to-cortisol ratios and DHEA-S levels alone and cognitive performance (e.g., tests involving automatic processing; semantic memory). In elderly subjects with a greater decrease in DHEA-S-to-cortisol ratio over a 2-year period, a more pronounced cognitive decline was observed while DHEA-S levels alone were not significantly correlated to cognitive decline. In contrast, in another study, cognitive impairment in chronically stressed females was associated with higher DHEA-S levels. On the other hand, short-term substitution studies investigating healthy elderly subjects revealed no significant improvement on cognitive function, either in spatial or in verbal explicit or implicit memory tasks.

With respect to dementia several studies reported lowered DHEA-S levels in Alzheimer's disease (AD) patients compared to age-matched healthy controls, while others failed to observe these effects. In one study, significantly lower DHEA levels were observed but not correlated with severity of AD. On the other hand, even higher levels of DHEA in AD patients were found to be associated with poorer cognitive performance. In most cases, treatment studies also failed to show cognitive-performance-enhancing effects of DHEA in demented patients. Small, transient improvements were only observed in one study after 3 months of DHEA substitution in cognitive performance tests, but not in global ratings.

In summary, it is reasonable to hypothesize that the greater the decline in DHEA-S respective to the DHEA-S-to-cortisol ratio, over time the less successful aging will be in terms of cognitive performance. On the other hand the theoretically assumed beneficial effects of DHEA-S supplementation for healthy, or even for "anti" aging processes are far from being proven to date. This is also true for DHEA-S treatment in AD patients.

22.2.3.2 **Estrogen**

A steep decline in estrogen levels after menopause, a decrease in bone mineral density and a higher prevalence for cardiovascular diseases is well-established for postmenopausal women. However "cognitive consequences" of low estrogen concentrations are less clear. Possible mechanisms by which estrogens may impact on cognition are not well-known; however, suggestions refer to estrogen-induced alterations in neurotransmitter activity that may have relevant implications for prevention and maybe treatment of AD. However, a large-scale study has been unable to show beneficial effects of two different doses of additional estradiol treatment in patients with AD who were also treated with acetycholesterase inhibitors.

In healthy nondemented humans, the effects of estrogens on cognition, mostly hormonal replacement therapy (HRT), are ambiguous: Beneficial as well as no effects on cognitive performance in retrospective and in prospective studies are reported. Two large prospective studies with age- and education-matched comparison groups revealed no advantageous effects of HRT on cognitive tests, whereas other, smaller, randomized HRT trials, reported an improvement in cognitive function in the estrogen groups. In a recent meta-analysis small beneficial effects of HRT on several aspects of cognitive function such as memory, attention, reaction time, and abstract reasoning were observed. However, these effects were somewhat inconsistent. In a recent study with short-term transdermal HRT in cognitively unimpaired healthy postmenopausal women only in measures of reaction time an improvement could be observed. Performance in all other cognitive tests, like immediate and delayed word recall, digit vigilance, visual tracking, picture and face recognition, were unaffected by HRT.

In many cases, study results are difficult to evaluate due to methodical problems like multiple cognitive tests with only one ore two significant differences, noncontrolled study groups (e.g., for depression, education and general health status) or very small sample seizes. Studies investigating the risk for developing dementia (AD as well as vascular dementia) in women receiving HRT also showed very contradictory results. Some report a reduced risk, others no effect, and in some cases even a nonsignificant trend towards a higher risk for developing dementia in elderly women treated with estrogen was seen. A meta-analysis published by Yaffe and coworkers [13] revealed a 29% reduced risk for developing dementia in HRT users. Concerning preventing effects of HRT for cognitive impairment or development of dementia, Gibbs and Gabor [14] concluded, based on animal and human data, that HRT will in fact provide substantial benefit to age-related cognitive decline, provided estrogens are administered in an appropriate regimen with only estrogen and not combined estrogen/progesterone replacement and initiated as early as possible following loss of ovarian function. Some smaller studies treating women suffering from AD with estrogen reported improvement in some dementia scales compared to untreated women. However, the above mentioned large HRT study does not support a beneficial effect of HRT on progression of AD.

Summarizing these results, decreases in estrogen levels seem to have a negative impact on cognitive function in menopausal women and HRT may have a protective effect on the development of dementia. However, once a dementia disorder like AD has developed, estrogens do not seem to have antidementive efficacy. In this context Mulnard et al. [15] concluded in a recent review that based on current evidence there is no role for HRT in treatment or prevention of AD or cognitive decline. Similar conclusions can been drawn from *The Canadian Study of Health and Aging* investigating in a prospective analysis risk factors for AD [16] and *The Rotterdam Study*, likewise a population-based, prospective cohort study in elderly investigating occurrence and determinations of chronic disease in later life [17]. Both studies are based on a very large sample size with nearly 8000 and 4600 participants respectively. Thus, there is no support for the hypothesis of an association between high endogen- or exogen-induced estradiol levels and a lowered risk for AD, in women or in men.

22.2.3.3 Testosterone

A decrease in androgen, especially testosterone levels, in aging males is well-established. However, compared to reduction of estrogens in women after menopause, the decline of testosterone in men is more subtle and shows a more pronounced interindividual variability. Testosterone is converted into estrogens and due to this conversion, estrogen levels in aged men are maintained at fairly constant levels. With respect to modulation of cognitive processes, influences of testosterone has been less well-studied than estrogens and existing results are even more conflicting and confusing. Since (young) men perform better in visual–spatial tests than women, it is speculated, that testosterone is involved in this ability. Results in young as well as in aged males revealed that there is a curvilinear relationship between testosterone and visual–spatial performance, due to a negative correlation between very high testosterone levels and visual–spatial performance in males. Testosterone substitution in elderly men was shown to improve visual–spatial cognitive performance. However, from animal studies it has been derived that high peripheral testosterone levels in males correspond to high brain levels of estrogens. Thus it is reasonable to assume that it is the central estrogen that impacts on cognitive performance.

The association between testosterone and AD is vividly discussed in the literature. *In vitro* studies have demonstrated that testosterone reduces the formation of ß-amyloid from the amyloid precursor molecule and the hyperphosphorylation of tau protein, the two hallmarks of AD. Also in older healthy men carrying the ε4 allele of the apolipoprotein E (APOE), known to increase the risk for AD, testosterone levels are lowered. In the Baltimore Longitudinal Study of Aging, a prospective study, 574 men aged at baseline 32–87 years and without dementia were followed up over a mean of 19 years. While AD development was significantly inversely associated with the free testosterone index (FTI), the ratio of total testosterone to sex hormone binding globulin (SHGB), neither total testosterone nor SHBG levels were significant predictors of AD. For each 10 nmol ml^{-1} increase in FTI, risk for AD was decreased about 26%. Similar observations were reported with normal total testosterone levels but elevated SHBG levels in male and female AD patients.

Heightened SHBG reduces both estrogens and testosterone and thus has implications for both genders. On the other hand, in the Rotterdam Study mentioned, in men no clear association between estradiol levels and risk of dementia could be observed [17].

Concerning hypogonadal but otherwise healthy elderly men it seems reasonable to assume beneficial effects of testosterone substitution on AD risk. However, randomized clinical studies to clarify this issue are lacking.

22.3
Cognitive Function in the Healthy Elderly and Impact of Endocrine Stress Reactivity

There is common agreement about a general, although highly variable, decline in memory performance from youth to senescence. However, while decrements in implicit memory tasks, e.g., priming or short-term memory tasks, are typically slight, age-related losses in tasks including cued or free recall or those asking for an original context of an event as well as a "prospective memory" task such as remembering future actions, are more affected. The hippocampus as part of the limbic system is not only critically involved in the feedback regulation of the HPA system but also in declarative memory processes, more specifically in memory formation and retrieval processes. Declarative or explicit memory includes conscious semantic memory (facts and words) and episodic memory (events). Glucocorticoids modulate declarative memory function biphasically. While basal, i.e., lower levels enhance formation of memories concerning emotionally charged events, (higher) stress levels suppress memory processing. This is mainly due to the ratio or balance of hippocampal MR and GR occupation. Under normal, unstressed conditions glucocorticoids bind mainly to MRs, facilitating hippocampal long-term potentiation (LTP), a cellular mechanism that is thought to induce formation of new memories. Under stressful conditions, that is, excessive cortisol levels, the GR becomes fully occupied, which is associated with inhibition of hippocampal LTP [11]. Over time, periods of repeated stressful events with markedly increased glucocorticoids may result in atrophy of neuronal structures subserving memory function. Clinical and research evidence overwhelmingly suggests that hypercortisolism can be detrimental to hippocampal functions.

In the Douglas Hospital Longitudinal Study a set of very interesting studies with respect to age, changing cortisol levels and alterations in cognitive performance were conducted. In a sample of aged healthy elderly women ($n = 17$) and men ($n = 34$) basal cortisol levels were measured once a year for 24 h over a period of 3–6 years [10]. An individual cortisol slope was calculated for each subject based on at least three cortisol profiles via regression analyses. Subjects were divided in two groups of cortisol history: (1) subjects showing an increase of cortisol levels over the years (~85%) and (2) those showing a decline (decreasing group; ~15%). A second classification was made within the first group dividing individuals in those who had reached cortisol levels comparable to levels seen in patients with AD (increasing/high group), and those participants who had only had moderate increases over the years (increasing/moderate group). In the last year of the study the authors conducted a battery of cognitive tests including short-term memory test (digit span test), long-term memory tests with immediate and delayed recall (paragraph recall, visual reproduction and associate learning), implicit (word completion) versus explicit (cued recall) long-term memory tests, selective and divided attention as well as language testing (verbal fluency and picture naming). Correlational analysis revealed two main results: only explicit memory functions and selective attention tasks were significantly associated with increasing glucocorticoid levels and second, according to cortisol measurements, cognitive function was only related to the cortisol slope over time, i.e., the higher the increase of cortisol levels over time had been, the worse subjects performed on explicit memory tasks ($r = -0.60$) and the longer the reaction time in selective attention tasks had been ($r = 0.57$). Taken together, these results support the notion of a neuropsychological dissociation between explicit and implicit performance in the elderly at least partially dependent upon increases in cortisol concentrations over time. In two subsets of the above described groups magnetic resonance imaging (MRI) was performed focussing on hippocampal volume. The increasing/high group showed, aside from impaired hippocampal-dependent memory performance, a 14% smaller hippocampal volume compared to the decreasing group. Moreover, the hippocampal volume was strongly correlated with both the degree of cortisol elevation over time, and the current basal cortisol level. In a third study the authors investigated whether the impairment of memory performance in the increasing/high cortisol group was related to the current high cortisol levels or to the long-term high cortisol exposure. Therefore current cortisol levels were modulated by a hormonal removal–replacement protocol. First, glucocorticoid levels were lowered by metyrapone, a potent inhibitor of glucocorticoid synthesis, and afterwards cortisol was restored by infusion of hydrocortisone and memory performance was tested after each condition and compared to a placebo day. If the memory deficit in the increasing/high cortisol group is caused by current high cortisol levels, memory performance should improve after metyrapone and again become impaired after hydrocortisone administration. However, in the subjects of the increasing/high cortisol group, no effect of cortisol modulation on memory performance could be observed. In contrast, in the increasing/moderate group, memory performance could be modulated by the acute pharmacological manipulation of glucocorticoids. In conclusion, the chronic exposure to high cortisol levels is responsible for the observed cognitive impairment in the increasing/high group. All results are summarized in Fig. 22.4.

In a recent study by McLullich and coworkers [18] these results were partly replicated. In 97 aged men (65–70 years) cortisol levels were measured in the morning and afternoon and a low dose of DEX (0.25 mg) was administered. Additionally, cognitive function was tested and MRI scans of hippocampus, temporal and frontal lope volumes were performed. Higher plasma cortisol levels in the morning

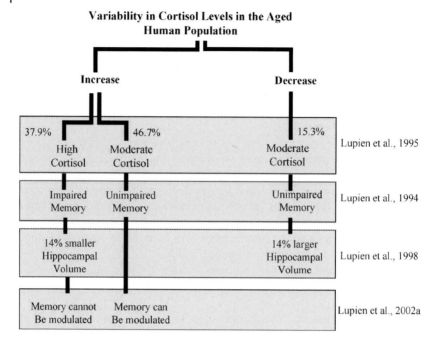

Fig. 22.4. Schematic representation of the data obtained in aged subjects followed over a period of 3–6 years (The Douglas Hospital Longitudinal Study of Normal and Pathological Aging). Figure reprinted from Lupien et al. [10] with permission from Elsevier.

were associated with a worse cognitive function represented by a "general cognitive factor," which accounted for 51% of variance in cognitive function. In contrast to the results reported by Lupien et al. [10], this association was not mediated by differences in brain volumes. The pituitary glucocorticoid feedback sensitivity measured by the DST was associated neither with neuroimaging variables nor with cognitive functioning.

Some interesting results from a more psychological point of view were observed by investigating individual distress proneness and cognitive decline in a large group of older men and women as part of the Chicago Health and Aging Project [18]. Cognitive testing (immediate and delayed recall, perceptual speed and Mini Mental State Examination (MMSE)) was conducted twice at 3-year intervals. Distress proneness was measured by a neuroticism scale. Decline in global cognitive score, based on the above-mentioned tests, was 30% faster over the years in subjects highly prone to distress (subjects above the 90th percentile in neurotics scale) compared to subjects with low distress proneness (below the 10th percentile) and this effect was unchanged after controlling for level of cognitive activity or baseline cognitive impairment. On the other hand, controlling for depressive symptoms reduced the significant relationship to a trend. The authors assume that chronic psychological distress eventually compromises neuronal systems involved in the regulation of the HPA system.

22.4
Stress Systems and Dementia

Mild cognitive impairment (MCI) is considered to be a transitional state between the normal cognitive changes in human aging and very early dementia and is recognized as a risk factor for the development of AD. MCI patients have memory impairment exceeding that expected for their age, although a diagnosis of dementia can not be made (yet). In neuroimaging studies, reduced hippocampal volumes as well as qualitative hippocampal atrophy have been observed in aged MCI subjects.

The two most common forms of dementia are AD and the vascular forms of dementia (VD) with a large overlap between the two. Most data about dysregulated stress reactive systems, especially the HPA system, refer to these two major forms of dementia and most data are available about AD.

Diagnostic criteria for dementia according to the Diagnostic and Statistical Manual of Mental Disorders (DSM-IV) are development of multiple cognitive deficits manifested by both, first, memory impairment (impairment in learning new information or in recall of previously learned information) and second, at least one of the following cognitive disturbances: aphasia, apraxia (impaired ability to carry out motor tasks despite intact motor function), agnosia (failure to recognize or identify objects despite intact sensory function) or disturbance in executive functioning (e.g., planning, organizing abstracting). The cognitive deficits described above cause significant impairment in social or occupational functioning and represent a relevant decline to previous levels of functioning. In case of AD the course of disease is characterized by gradual onset and continuing cognitive decline. The type of dementia, AD or VD (or others), is mainly defined by the existence or absence of other medical factors, such as hypertension, history of stroke and imaging studies (i.e., white matter lesions). The diagnosis of VD is made by the presence of focal neurological signs or laboratory evidence of cerebrovascular disease that are judged to be etiologically relevant for the impairment. In a recent review, several evidences for AD as a primarily vascular disorder were discussed, since AD and VD share many risk factors, overlapping clinical symptoms and evidence for parallel cerebrovascular and neurodegenerative pathology. Among others, here is convincing evidence for some biological markers to be involved in the etiology of sporadic AD and pathogenesis, such as increased tau protein in cerebrospinal fluid (CSF) or presence of the apolipoprotein $\varepsilon 4$ (APOE) allele. Also, patients with AD have early loss of hippocampal volume. Taken together, however at this time, there is no universally accepted biological marker for AD.

Since this chapter focuses on involvement of HPA system in dementia, the above-listed possible pathogenetic factors are only mentioned in case they have a significance for HPA system dysregulation.

To the best of our knowledge, to date only one study has been conducted on the activity of the HPA system in subjects with MCI. Wolf et al. [19] measured in 16 MCI patients, 28 healthy elderly and 14 young controls circadian profiles of salivary cortisol at six time points between 9 a.m. and 11 p.m. Within the group of elderly participants, MCI patients showed no differences in overall cortisol levels compared to the healthy elderly and no differences in circadian rhythms. However, in comparison to the young control group, MCI patients had lower morning cortisol levels at 9 a.m. In the discussion of these somewhat unexpected results the authors mention several methodological points: First, due to the small sample size, particularly in the MCI group, negative findings could reflect a lack of power. As ambulatory saliva sampling does not allow control for potential impact variables like activity, diet, etc., more standardized laboratory sampling may reveal different results. The low morning cortisol levels in MCI patients compared to the young controls may reflect the earlier wake-up time in these subjects, which may put them ahead in their circadian cycle. Taken together, futures studies investigating HPA activity in MCI patients are necessary, especially those applying pharmacological and/or psychological challenge tests to investigate changes in HPA activity in these patients.

Insulin-induced hypoglycaemia, as a pharmacological stimulation test of the HPA system, resulted in a blunted ACTH response in patients with mild AD compared to healthy elderly controls. However, cortisol peaks were not different between the groups. Moreover, since AD patients reached peak levels faster, they seemed to have an adrenal hyperresponsiveness. Results supporting this notion were also observed after CRH stimulation in AD patients. These patients had blunted ACTH but higher cortisol responses relative to the amount of ACTH release compared to age-matched controls. Also, after a cold pressure test, another standardized stress system provocation test, AD patients had increased cortisol responses compared to controls, while ACTH reactivity did not differ between the groups. By applying only a low dose of ACTH, a more reliable assessment of adrenal sensitivity can be achieved. When this test is used in AD patients, they show significantly higher cortisol peak levels as well as a larger area under the response curve (AUC) compared to healthy elderly subjects. Furthermore cortisol AUCs were significantly positively correlated with age and inversely associated with cognitive performance.

In VD and in AD, higher cortisol levels along with impaired feedback sensitivity in the DST were often described. In a longitudinal study using the DST in AD patients and healthy controls, in the patients' group cortisol levels at baseline (= initial DST) were significantly higher before and after dexamethasone. While all healthy controls showed a sufficient suppression, after DEX only in the patients group nonsuppressors were observed. Cortisol levels were negatively correlated to MMSE scores. A second and third DST was applied after 9 and 18 months. Despite a higher rate of nonsuppression, overall there was no change in pre- or post-DEX cortisol levels over time. Moreover, no correlation between cognitive decline and change in post-DEX cortisol could be observed. In contrast, several other studies found a positive correlation between cortisol reactivity and hippocampal atrophy in AD patients. Finally, cortisol increases in patients with AD seem to be a sensitive marker of the progressive rate of their cognitive decline.

It is suggested that conventional cortisol measures underestimate the degree of hypercortisolism in AD patients due to the observation of a reduction of levels of corticoid binding globulin (CBG) of about 30% in these patients. Ferrari and colleagues [2] studied circadian cortisol rhythms during daytime (every 4 h) and nighttime (every 2 h) under unstimulated conditions and after administration of 1 mg dexamethasone at 11 p.m. in healthy elderly, demented elderly (AD and VD patients) and a group of young healthy adults. Amongst others, the cortisol profiles of demented patients were significantly more flattened than those of the healthy elderly group. These changes were associated with the degree of dementia as measured with the MMSE.

In 64 AD patients and 34 nondemented age-matched controls cortisol levels were measured in CSF. Additionally subjects were genotyped with respect to APOE allele subtype. First, CSF cortisol levels were significantly higher in AD patients and second cortisol levels in the CSF were significantly related to apolipoprotein $\varepsilon 4$ (APOE-$\varepsilon 4$) allele in AD patients with highest cortisol levels in the homozygote $\varepsilon 4$ genotype ($\varepsilon 4/\varepsilon 4 > \varepsilon 3/\varepsilon 4 > \varepsilon 3/\varepsilon 3$). In normal older controls cortisol levels were highest in the $\varepsilon 3/\varepsilon 4$ and lowest in the $\varepsilon 2/\varepsilon 3$ genotype. The authors conclude that increased cortisol concentrations are associated with APOE-$\varepsilon 4$ frequency, which is a well-known genetic susceptibility factor.

Summarizing the results from the literature, in most, but not in all studies, patients with AD have higher basal and/or stimulated cortisol levels than healthy age-matched controls and a flattened circadian cortisol profile. Especially after DST, AD patients show higher post-DEX cortisol concentrations and higher rates of non-suppressors, indicating impaired negative feedback sensitivity on the level of the pituitary. An increased adrenocortical sensitivity is also well-documented. Taken together, an increased activity and reactivity of the HPA system in patients suffering from dementia can be considered as a well-established phenomenon, and many studies suggest that the amount of HPA activity is negatively associated with cognitive performance (for overview see [20]). With regard to the cumulative evidence for HPA overactivity in dementia and the observation that hippocampal atrophy – a hallmark of dementia – is promoted by elevated cortisol and associated to the degree of cognitive dysfunction, therapeutic trials with antiglucocorticoids may be an option in hypercortisolemic dementia. For example, mifepristone (RU486), a potent GR antagonist, improved rodents' spatial learning and memory function significantly. One pilot study with administration of 200 mg mifepristone in five AD patients compared to four placebo-treated patients resulted in an improvement in word recall performance, orientation and word recognition [20]. Owing to the very small sample size, results are inconclusive. However, these preliminary results need to be explored further.

Within this context, it is also interesting that in patients with hypercortisolemic depression the adjunctive administration of a GR antagonist was shown to improve depression-related cognitive deficits. Currently GC-receptor antagonists are tested for efficacy in hypercortisolamic depression.

22.5
Summary and Conclusion

In this chapter, changes in the activity and reactivity of the HPA system in the elderly, possible consequences with respect to cognitive functioning, and potential mediating mechanism were described. In particular, AD and its association to altered HPA activity was the second main focus. Taken together, the activity of the HPA system is altered with age, while changes in basal activity are less pronounced. An age-associated hyperactivity can be documented after pharmacological or psychological challenge. Moreover, in older females these changes are more pronounced. The most prominent hypothesis connecting HPA hyperactivity and cognitive decline are the Glucocorticoid Cascade Hypothesis and the Receptor Balance Theory, both referring to loss of hippocampal volume due to centrally heightened glucocorticoid concentrations. HPA hyperactivity in demented patients is well-documented and many results suggest a negative association between HPA activity and cognitive performance. However, it is still unknown to what extent increased glucocorticoids can be regarded as a risk factor for accelerated aging or development of AD or VD. A major task for future studies is the integration of this knowledge into prevention and/or therapy of aging stigmata or dementia.

References

1 T.E. SEEMAN, R.J. ROBBINS. 1994. Aging and hypothalamic–pituitary–adrenal response to challenge in humans. Endocr Rev 15:233–260.

2 E. FERRARI, L. CRAVELLO, B. MUZZONI, D. CASAROTTI, M. PALTRO, S.B. SOLERTE, M. FIORAVANTI, G. CUZZONI, B. PONTIGGIA, F. MAGRI. 2001. Age-related changes of the hypothalamic–pituitary–adrenal axis: pathophysiological correlates. Eur J Endocrinol 144(4):319–329.

3 M. DEUSCHLE, U. GOTTHARDT, U. SCHWEIGER, B. WEBER, A. KÖRNER, J. SCHMIDER, H. STANDHARD, C.-H. LAMMERS, I. HEUSER. 1997. With aging in humans the activity of the hypothalamus–pituitary–adrenal system increases and its circadian rhythm flattens. Life Sci 61:2239–2246.

4 I. HEUSER, M. DEUSCHLE, A. WEBER, A. KNIEST, C. ZIEGLER, B. WEBERAND, M. COLLA. 2000. The role of mineralocorticoid receptors upon the circadian activity of the human hypothalamus–pituitary–adrenal system: effect of age. Neurobiol. Aging 21:585–589.

5 B.M. KUDIELKA, A. BUSKE-KIRSCHBAUM, D.H. HELLHAMMER, C. KIRSCHBAUM. 2004. HPA system responses to laboratory psychosocial stress in healthy elderly adults, younger adults, and children: impact of age and gender. Psychoneuro-endocrinology 29:83–98.

6 B.M. KUDIELKA, A.K. SCHMIDT-REINWALD, D.H. HELLHAMMER, C. KIRSCHBAUM. 1999. Psychological and endocrine responses to psychosocial

stress and Dex-CRF in healthy postmenopausal women and young controls: the impact of age and a two-week estradiol treatment. Neuroendocrinology 70:422–430.

7 C. Otte, S. Hart, T.C. Neylan, C.R. Marmar, K. Yaffe, D.C. Mohr. 2005. A meta-analysis of cortisol response to challenge in human aging: importance of gender. Psychoneuroendocrinology 30(1): 80–91.

8 T.E. Seeman, B. Singer, P. Charpentier. 1995. Gender differences in patterns of HPA system response to challenge: Macarthur studies of successful aging. Psychoneuroendocrinology 20:711–725.

9 R.M. Sapolsky. 2003. Stress and plasticity in the limbic system. Neurochem Res 28(11):1735–42.

10 S.J. Lupien, A. Fiocco, N. Wan, F. Maheu, C. Lord, T. Schramek, M.T. Tu. 2005. Stress hormones and human memory function across the lifespan. Psychoneuroendocrinology 30(3):225–242.

11 E.R. De Kloet. 2004. Hormones and the stressed brain. Ann N Y Acad Sci 1018:1–15.

12 B.S. McEwen. 2003. Interacting mediators of allostasis and allostatic load: towards an understanding of resilience in aging. Metabolism 52(10):10–16.

13 K. Yaffe, G. Sawaya, I. Lieberburg, D. Grady. 1998. Estrogen therapy in postmenopausal women: effects on cognitive function and dementia. J Am Med Assoc 279(9):688–95.

14 R.B. Gibbs, R. Gabor. 2003. Estrogen and cognition: applying preclinical findings to clinical perspectives. J Neurosci Res 74:637–643.

15 R.A. Mulnard, M.M. Corrada, C.H. Kawas. 2004. Estrogen replacement therapy, Alzheimer's disease, and mild cognitive impairment. Curr Neurol Neurosci Rep 4(5):368–373.

16 J. Lindsay, D. Laurin, R. Verreault, R. Hebert, B. Helliwell, G.B. Hill, I. McDowell. 2002. Risk factors for Alzheimer's disease: a prospective analysis from the Canadian Study of Health and Aging. Am J Epidemiol 156(5):445–453.

17 M.I. Geerlings, L.J. Launer, F.H. de Jong, A. Ruitenberg, T. Stijnen, J.C. van Swieten, A. Hofman, J.C. Witteman, H.A. Pols, M.M. Breteler. 2003. Endogenous estradiol and risk of dementia in women and men: the Rotterdam Study. Ann Neurol 53(5):607–615.

18 A.M. MacLullich, I.J. Deary, J.M. Starr, K.J. Ferguson, J.M. Wardlaw, J.R. Seckl. 2005. Plasma cortisol levels, brain volumes and cognition in healthy elderly men. Psychoneuroendocrinology 30(5):505–515.

19 O.T. Wolf, A. Convit, E. Thorn, M.J. de Leon. 2002. Salivary cortisol day profiles in elderly with mild cognitive impairment. Psychoneuroendocrinology 27(7):777–789.

20 N. Pomara, W.M. Greenberg, M.D. Branford, P.M. Doraiswamy. 2003. Therapeutic implications of HPA system abnormalities in Alzheimer's disease: review and update. Psychopharmacol Bull 37(2):120–134.

23
Stress and Addiction

Bo Söderpalm and Anna Söderpalm

23.1
Introduction

Since ancient times human beings have used different substances to experience euphoria, stimulation and satisfaction. Early on, these substances were discovered in nature and were in that sense natural products, but in more recent years substances synthesized by man have also been introduced. Well-known examples of natural drugs are ethanol, tobacco (nicotine), opium (morphine) and cocaine. These drugs have often been used in connection with various rites and not uncommonly for the purpose of putting the mind into an ecstatic state. Many substances have, on the other hand, just as often been used for the opposite reasons, that is to calm down or reduce anxiety. Alcohol is for many reasons one of the most interesting drugs, partly because it has both stimulatory and anxiolytic, sedative properties, usually depending on dose, and partly because alcohol abuse, besides nicotine abuse, is the most common type of substance abuse and that which has the greatest impact on human health and the community. The text below will therefore to some extent focus on alcohol. It should already be noted that the abovementioned psychoactive substances are dependence-producing, i.e., the use of them easily escalates and becomes uncontrollable.

23.2
Stress, Alcohol and Nicotine

It is commonly known that alcohol and nicotine often are consumed in connection with stress. Most smokers can probably testify about how when stressed, as in the face of difficult tastes, a heavy workload, family problems, etc., they often increase their nicotine consumption. Some alcohol users, perhaps especially heavy consumers, can probably report the same phenomenon with respect to their alcohol consumption. Under these circumstances most drug users find that they use the drug in order to calm down, to focus or to relax, and it has been proposed that ethanol intake during stress represents a type of self-medication ("tension reduction hypothesis"). In large groups this is probably also the purpose of using alcohol

Stress in Health and Disease. Edited by Bengt B. Arnetz and Rolf Ekman
Copyright © 2006 WILEY-VCH Verlag GmbH & Co. KGaA, Weinheim
ISBN: 3-527-31221-8

and nicotine on the completion of significant work or performances, and on Friday nights after a week filled with heavy work. It is likely that drug consumption for individuals with this more controlled, limited drug intake also represents a form of reward for various achievements.

It has long been suggested that not only use but also misuse and abuse of different dependence-producing drugs are related to stress and that the individual's risk for lapsing into e.g., nicotine and alcohol abuse is increased when stressed. Probably both smokers and ethanol-dependent individuals could readily accept this idea. There are several testimonies on how stressful situations, e.g., difficulties at work or in the family, or significant losses, have produced relapses into nicotine or ethanol abuse even after several years of abstinence. There is also scientific evidence available supporting the view that stressful events such as the above trigger relapse [1], even though they are not, of course, a prerequisite for this. Many alcoholics can bear witness that they have relapsed at times when they have been feeling unusually well, and other, often periodic drinkers, may even plan their relapses, i.e., that may decide on what day they will start drinking again. It is, however, for several reasons very difficult, or maybe even impossible, to perform prospective, controlled studies on the role of stress for alcohol and drug consumption in man, not least because of the difficulties met when trying to standardize the stressors. There are large individual differences with respect to how stressors are perceived. Most human studies available are instead retrospective and correlative, and may show some possible associations, but they do not tell us anything about the underlying mechanisms. For example, it has been reported that post traumatic stress disorder (PTSD), which often is a consequence of long-term or intermittent periods of stress, may be followed by development of alcohol dependence. Moreover, there appears to be a positive correlation between alcohol consumption and the degree of PTSD. It is possible that this relationship is due to self-medication, since PTSD patients report amelioration of their symptoms after consumption of alcohol, heroin, cannabis or benzodiazepines. Lately, several well-controlled, experimental studies on the influence of stress on the subjective experience of drug intoxication have been published. These will be discussed in more detail at the end of this chapter.

23.3
What Are the Biological Underpinnings?

Even if it is accepted that there is some kind of connection between stress and drug abuse, the relationship remains to be understood from a biological point of view. Environmental stress thus has the ability to direct behavior towards e.g., alcohol intake in a way that sometimes escapes control. Since all sensations, thoughts, decisions, and behaviors, according to our present understanding, are products of the activity of millions of neurons and other cells in the brain, stress has to use these components to change behavior from that characterizing an abstinent alcoholic to that of a relapsing one. Ethanol by itself, when consumed, will of course contribute to the behavioral change and most likely also to the escalating loss of control (see below). How stress and alcohol act in concert to influence neurobiological pro-

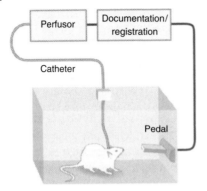

Fig. 23.1. Picture of self-administering rat.

cesses that produce behaviors associated with substance dependence (see Table 23.1) is an extremely complicated issue to study. Recent developments in experimental neuroscience have, however, made it possible to sense the vague contours of these phenomena. Below some of the hypotheses that have been generated in studies applying mainly experimental animals are described.

Tab. 23.1. Diagnostic criteria for substance dependence according to the DSM IV.

Maladaptive drug consumption causing clinically significant functional loss or distress with at least three of the following symptoms appearing within a 12 month period:

1. Tolerance, defined by one of these conditions:
   a) evidently larger quantities of the substance are needed to experience intoxication or any other desired effect
   b) the same quantity of the substance consumed produces an evidently diminished effect.

2. Abstinence, manifested by one of these signs:
   a) abstinence symptom typical for the substance consumed
   b) same (or similar) substance is taken for the purpose to alleviate or avoid abstinence symptom.

3. The substance is frequently consumed in larger quantity, or over a longer period than intented.

4. There is a sincere desire, or an attempt has failed to cut down or control drug consumption

5. Much time is spent getting hold of the substance (e.g., seeing several doctors to get a prescription), consuming the substance (e.g., chain-smoking), or, recovering from drug consumption effects.

6. Important social activities, professional or spare time activities, are given up or reduced in favor of drug consumption.

7. Drug misuse is continued in spite of the knowledge that intake of the substance is likely to cause or aggravate physical or emotional disorders (e.g., repeated cocaine intake though knowing about cocaine-induced depression; continuous drinking though knowing that alcohol might make stomach pains worse).

23.3.1
Animal Experimental Models

The possibility of using experimental animals to study neuronal mechanisms of importance for substance dependence may be better than that of using animals to study any other behavioral alteration of relevance for psychiatric disorders. This statement is based on the fact that experimental animals of various kinds, such as rats, mice and monkeys, regularly can be trained to self-administer drugs of abuse but not other, nonabused drugs [2]. This is for example true with respect to ethanol, nicotine, heroin, morphine, cocaine and amphetamine (Fig. 23.1). Moreover, drug self-administration is very stable and is thus not easily distracted by the presentation of e.g., natural rewards. A cocaine-dependent rat will for instance continue to self-administer the drug in favor of eating, drinking or engaging in sexual acts, if given the opportunity; a phenomenon called ursurpation [2]. This is reminiscent of the neglectful attitude of a drug abuser, when former interests, work, family and friends are given up in favor of the drug. Another similarity between the animal models and the human situation is the fact that renewed exposure to the drug or drug-related stimuli often produces a rapid relapse in dependent animals that have been withdrawn from the drug for some time [3]. Moreover, as in man, there is great interindividual variation in the self-administering behavior in heterogeneous, outbred rat or mouse lines, while on the other hand, inbred rat lines with higher or lower propensity to self-administer ethanol or other drugs of abuse are available. The latter indicates that, just as in man, the susceptibility for substance dependence, including ethanol dependence, is inheritable. Another similarity with the human situation is the fact that stress also appears to be of importance for self-administration of dependence-producing drugs in experimental animals.

23.3.2
**Stress and Self-Administration of Dependence-Producing Drugs
in Experimental Animals**

Several studies have shown that the doses required are lower and that drug self-administration is more rapidly established if the experimental animal is stressed before or during the establishment of the behavior. Moreover, several different kinds of stressors, both physical, e.g., exposure to foot-shocks, and "psychic", e.g., witnessing physical stress being inflicted on another rat, produce similar results. Also exposure to an aggressive conspecific facilitates drug self-administration, regardless of whether the subject is protected from direct physical contact or not. Social stress, in the form of living in mixed colonies (males and females) with high social competition, also facilitates self-administration of psychostimulants in males, as does social isolation. Furthermore, exposure of pregnant dames to stress will increase the offsprings' self-administration of amphetamine when adult, and recently a number of studies have been pusblished indicating that stress early in life, for example neonatally or during adolescence facilitates drug self-administration later in life. Food restriction, which is one of the most powerful stressors in terms of increasing plasma corticosterone levels in the rat, also consistently increases self-administration of various dependence-producing drugs.

As already described in this book the neurohumoral stress reaction is complex. However, several studies indicate that corticosterone release (the rat hormone that corresponds to cortisol in man) is important for mediating the above-described effects of stress on self-administration behavior. For example, all the stressors mentioned above increase corticosterone release, whereas suppression of adrenal function, either by surgery (adrenalectomy) or by administration of a corticosterone synthesis inhibitor, may inhibit the effects of stress on the behavior [4]. Furthermore, repeated, passive injections of corticosterone by itself also increases the propensity to self-administrate dependence-producing drugs. However, it is not known whether the corticosterone effects are primarily produced via interactions in the periphery or via direct interactions with mechanisms in the central nervous system. Neither is it known whether the effects are produced via the classical intracellular type I and type II receptors or via different cell-membrane effects of corticosterone or its metabolites [5]. Results from a study on the establishment of cocaine self-administration indicate, however, that simultaneous activation of type I and II receptors may be required. Both these receptors are also activated when stress increases endogenous corticosterone levels. The further enhancement of the self-administrating behavior that was observed after even higher corticosterone levels could, however, be produced via other mechanisms. Such detailed knowledge may seem unnecessary, but if the exact mechanisms involved in mediating the effects of stress can be revealed the possibility of finding effective pharmacological treatments to prevent them will increase.

Several studies using different types of stressors show that the motivation to take the drug, which can be measured by different sophisticated techniques, is also enhanced when a self-administrating behavior has already been established. As regards the effects of stress on alcohol intake in experimental animals, these have been studied mainly in animals that have already established a high alcohol intake and preference. In such animals ethanol intake increases if the animals are exposed to chronic crowding stress, and in some studies stress also enhances the alcohol deprivation effect (an enhancement of ethanol intake after a period of abstinence), whereas in others this effect is instead weakened by stress. These effects appear, however, to vary depending on what rat strain is studied, i.e., whether alcohol-preferring rat strains or outbred rats are used. In regular laboratory rats of the Wistar strain both surgical and pharmacological adrenalectomy decrease alcohol intake and preference, but the effect is temporary, since the animals gradually increase their ethanol consumption after surgery [6]. It is not known if this "relapse" is associated with reemergence of endogenous corticosterone production from e.g., ectopic adrenal tissue, or if it is due to compensatory mechanisms. Nor has the possibility been excluded that these effects are due to alterations of alcohol metabolism, meaning that in adrenalectomized rats lower ethanol doses may produce similar ethanol concentrations and biological effects as in controls. In these studies it was, however, noted that corticosterone substitution, but not substitution with type I or II receptor agonists, not only prevented the effect of adrenalectomy but also further increased ethanol consumption above the normal level, both in adrenalectomized rats and in sham-operated controls [6]. These interesting results indicate that the corticosterone effect in this context is mediated via other mechanisms than the classical intarcellular receptors.

Several studies have been published in which the effects of stress and stress hormones on relapsing to drug intake has been examined in experimental animals that have been withdrawn from drugs. Such withdrawal can, for example, be produced by exchanging the cocaine solution to a saline solution, so that the rat receives saline instead of cocaine when pressing the cocaine-associated lever. After a number of sessions the rat will stop pressing the lever, i.e., an extinction of the drug self-administering behavior is obtained. This extinction appears, however, labile and the behavior is quickly reestablished after stress exposure. Furthermore, and surprisingly, stress appears to be more efficient than passive drug administration with respect to producing a relapse. Interestingly, pharmacological adrenalectomy may prevent stress-induced relapse, indicating that corticosterone secretion may be involved in mediating this effect. Since the substance used in these experiments is also available in the clinic these results open up an interesting possibility to test the same strategy in patients with substance dependence. Whether the relapse-producing effects of corticosterone are mediated via intracellular corticosterone receptors (type I and/or type II) or via other mechanisms remains to be established. Stress or stress-related stimuli have also been demonstrated to precipitate relapse in ethanol-withdrawn rats, and, interestingly, the stress effect appears additive to the relapse-precipitating effects of other conditional stimuli.

In these studies performed in experimental animals it has become clear that the manner of applying the stress also is of importance. If the stress is predictable or if the stress intensity is too low, drug self-administration will not be altered. The duration of the stress and the relationship between the stressor and the self-administration situation is also of importance [5]. If the stress episodes are short it is mandatory that they are in close proximity with the self-administrating situation, while if the stress is more chronic, even if it has consisted of repeated short stress episodes, it may be interrupted several weeks before commencement of the self-administration studies and still produce a facilitation of the behavior.

Taken together, it is clear that stress, and especially the stress hormone corticosterone, is involved in modulating drug self-administration in experimental animals, both during establishment of the behavior and in relapse mechanisms. As judged from the findings presented above regarding the conditions required for the effects produced by acute and chronic stress, it seems likely that several different stress-related mechanisms are involved. Considering corticosterone, both acute and chronic effects of the hormone appear to play a role (see further below). Whether the animals, as suggested for man, self-administer drugs in these situations in order to reduce tension is difficult to judge. It appears, however, unlikely that this would be the primary reason for animals self-administering amphetamine or cocaine in these situations, since these drugs normally do not produce anxiolysis but rather the opposite. Considering alcohol, it is, however, possible that the intake produces anxiolysis and other beneficial effects to the animal, at least in the short-term perspective. As early as 1946, Masserman and Yum performed experiments in the cat suggesting such beneficial effects of ethanol in stressful situations. A cat with a relatively high social rank in a cat colony was subjected to an aversive stimulus every time it approached its food tray. This stressful situation caused the cat to quickly lose its position in the group. When the cat was administered low doses of alcohol it resolved the stressful situation and regained its position in the group.

23.3.2.1 Drugs of Abuse and the Hypothalamic–Pituitary–Adrenocortical Axis

A complicating fact is that most dependence-producing drugs increase corticosterone release by themselves, when acutely administered. This is true for psychostimulants, nicotine and ethanol. For some of these drugs, e.g., nicotine, tolerance often develops to this effect, but not for others. It is well-known that many alcoholics present clinical signs ("pseudocushing") similar to those observed in patients that have received long-term treatment with high doses of cortisol or that have a hormone-producing tumor along the hypothalamic–pituitary–adrenocortical (HPA) axis. It has also been suggested that the concomitant drug-induced corticosterone secretion is of great importance for the establishment of self-administration of, e.g., cocaine. Indeed, it has been suggested that corticosterone by itself is dependence-producing, and rats do self-administer corticosterone both orally and intravenously. These findings represent another similarity to the human situation, since abuse of cortisol-containing pharmaceuticals is a well-known clinical phenomenon. It is not farfetched to suggest that addictive effects of corticosterone could be involved in mediating some of the nonpharmacological "addictions", such as pathological gambling and sensation seeking.

23.3.3
Neurobiological Correlates to Stress-Induced Drug Intake

23.3.3.1 The Mesocorticolimbic Dopamine System

The fact that experimental animals so strenuously self-administer drugs of abuse indicates that these substances, via their neurochemical effects, influence one or several neuronal systems in the brain of importance for motivation and reward. Neurochemical research has demonstrated that drugs of abuse influence a number of neuronal systems in the brain, and especially those using biogenic amines as neurotransmittors. Among these multiple effects there is, however, one common denominator for the most important drugs of abuse (ethanol, nicotine, opiates, cocaine, amphetamine, cannabis) – they all activate the mesolimbic dopamine system [2] and increase extracellular dopamine levels in the ventral striatum (nucleus accumbens in the rat). This happens both after passive injections of the drug and when the rat self-administers the drug. Moreover, and even more important, this dopamine activation appears to be important for initiating and maintaining drug self-administration in experimental animals [2].

23.3.3.2 Sensitization

Increased mesolimbic dopamine activity is often associated with locomotor stimulation in experimental animals [7]. This effect is most obvious after psychostimulants such as cocaine and amphetamine, but can also be observed after nicotine if the animals have first been adapted to the test environment or after low doses of ethanol, at least in the mouse. Interestingly, repeated administration of all drugs of abuse produces a progressive increase, or sensitization, of the locomotor stimulatory effects of the drugs [8]. It has been suggested that this increase may be due to the development of a tolerance to the inherent sedative effects of e.g., ethanol or morphine, which would disclose the stimulatory effects, and a contribution by such phenomena cannot be excluded. Studies on different mice strains have, however, demonstrated that the enhanced stimulation after alcohol is most likely a phenomenon of its own, since there is no correlation between the degree of tolerance development to the sedative effects on the one hand and the development of behavioral sensitization on the other. That is, both phenomena may develop simultaneously but independently from each other (Fig. 23.2). Furthermore, continuous cocaine administration produces tolerance to the stimulatory effect of the drug, whereas the same total amount of drug given intermittently produces sensitization. This raises an important question: does a "binge-drinking" tradition (as in, e.g., Sweden), with repeated high ethanol consumption, pose a higher risk for behavioral sensitization and for development of dependence and crossdependence (see below)?

In order to maintain homeostasis organisms usually try to overcome stressors by means of adaptation. While tolerance development, the opposite of sensitization, can be understood from this perspective, sensitization may superficially appear an inappropriate phenomenon. However, considering that mesolimbic dopamine neurons are involved in motivational learning, the conclusion reached may be different. Memory processes make use of neurobiological phenomena that enhance information flow, e.g., long-term potentiation phenomena in synapses, which in that sense represent a type of sensitization. Since the mesolimbic dopamine system appears to have a role in associating stimuli in the environment to consummatory behaviors that facilitate the survival of the individual and the species [9], it is thus

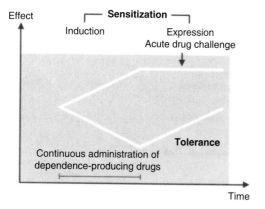

Fig. 23.2. Tolerance vs. sensitization – independent phenomena.

likely that dependence-producing drugs make use of natural, preformed potentiating mechanisms. The sensitization phenomenon as such may thus not be inappropriate but rather the fact that the dependence-producing drugs have such powerful effects on the system, perhaps because they generally release dopamine more powerfully than natural rewards or because they destroy other homeostatic mechanisms. It is also possible that dopamine release after drugs of abuse is qualitatively different from that produced by natural rewards and that this contributes to the strong association between environmental cues and dopamine activation that is typical for dependence-producing drugs (see below).

The sensitization phenomenon has two phases, the induction of the phenomenon and its expression, that is when the phenomenon develops and when the drug interacts with the sensitized system. Both the induction and the expression consist of a conditioned component, that is dependent on the integrity of the environment, and an unconditioned component, where the enhanced drug effect can be observed also in the test tube. For some drugs, e.g., cocaine, the conditioned component is very strong. Thus, one single injection of cocaine may potentiate the drug effect already on the next day, provided that both injections are given in the same environment.

Behavioral sensitization to dependence-producing drugs has its neurochemical basis in an enhancement of the sensitivity both of pre- and postsynaptic mechanisms in the mesolimbic dopamine system, as a consequence of a protein-synthesis-dependent reconstruction of the system (Fig. 23.3 [10]).

The reconstructed dopamine system is hyperreactive in two ways. Drugs that activate the system will stimulate it even more, and internal and external stimuli

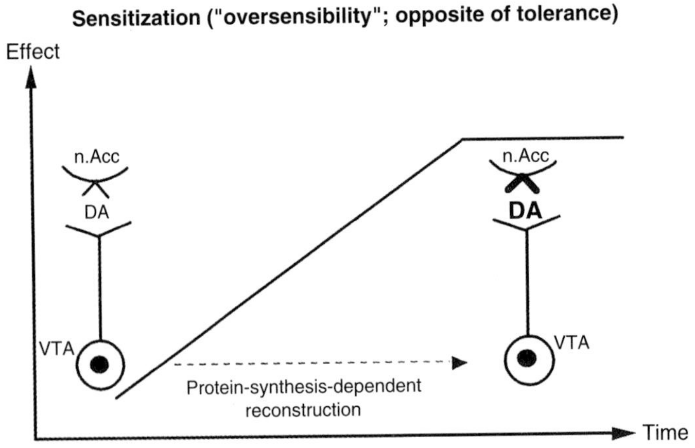

Fig. 23.3. Sensitization – neurochemical effects in the mesolimbic dopamine (*DA*) system and their behavioral correlates are enhanced upon repeated exposure to dependence-producing drugs.

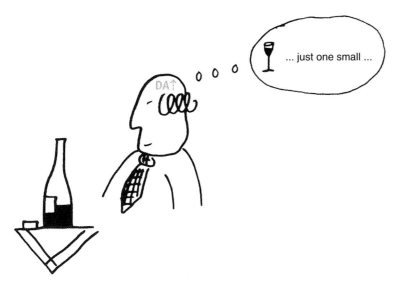

Fig. 23.4. It has been suggested that the sensitized mesolimbic dopamine system is activated by various conditioned stimuli, which attract the individual's attention and trigger new drug consumption. As pharmacological effect, the drug increases dopamine levels, which explains why, e.g., an acoholic will find it difficult to stop drinking before he/she has emptied the bottle.

that previously have been associated with intake of these dopamine-activating drugs will now activate the system by themselves [11]: a conditioned dopamine release is obtained upon exposure to such stimuli (Fig. 23.4). Interestingly, advanced brain-imaging techniques have recently shown that, e.g., cocaine abusers who are exposed to pictures of cocaine paraphernalia report an enhanced craving in parallel with an enhancement of brain activity in limbic brain regions.

It has been suggested that the sensitized, hyperreactive mesolimbic dopamine system via internal and external conditioned stimuli provides the incentive to take the drug ("wanting"; "craving") while the pleasure of using the drug ("liking") would be mediated via other systems [11]. The sensitization would thus mean an isolated increased craving for the drug, despite the fact that the dependent individual no longer experiences a positive effect of the drug. This hypothesis would explain why the drug career often is characterized by a loss of the positive drug effects ("subjective pleasure") over time, while the propensity to take the drug is paradoxically increased. Other reasons to suspect that the sensitization phenomenon could be related to the behavioral problems observed in the clinic are that the phenomenon is very long-lasting, maybe even permanent, and that cross-sensitization readily deveolps between different dependence-producing drugs, a phenomenon that at least partly could underlie polydrug abuse (for discussion see [11]).

23.3.4
Stress, Sensitization and the Mesocorticolimbic Dopamine System

It was early found that administration of electric shocks to experimental animals produces behavioral sensitization to amphetamine, i.e., that cross-sensitization between stress and psychostimulants readily develops [12]. Also repeated, passive injections of corticosterone produce sensitization to the locomotor stimulatory effects of amphetamine. Conversely, bilateral adrenalectomy inhibits the development of amphetamine and nicotine sensitization in the rat, and in both cases a lack of steroid type II, but not type I, activation is of importance. On the other hand, adrenalectomy of already-nicotine-sensitized animals does not influence the expression of the phenomenon after passive injection of the drug. The adrenal glands thus appear to be of importance for induction of nicotine sensitization but not for its expression upon passive drug delivery. As is evident from the above, the findings with respect to stress, corticosteroids and sensitization are very similar to those that have been reported with respect to drug self-administration.

Against the above background the question arises as to whether these stress effects can be observed also neurochemically in the mesolimbic dopamine system. It is well-known that stress activates the mesocorticolimbic dopamine system (for references see [4]) and enhances dopamine release, not only in the nucleus accumbens but also in the amygdala and the prefrontal cortex, but it is not clear if these stress-induced effects require the presence of corticosteroids. However, corticosterone may by itself increase dopamine release in the mesolimbic dopamine system in the rat brain, possibly via a membrane-bound effect not invoking the classical type I and II receptors. Corticosterone also increases the number of dopamine D2 receptors, while adrenalectomy instead decreases it. Accordingly, it was recently reported that adrenalectomy prevents the development of postsynaptic dopamine receptor hypersensitivity in response to repeated nicotine administration, whereas dopamine release is not affected. However, corticosterone could very well be involved in activation of the sensitized mesolimbic dopamine system in response to conditional stimuli (Fig. 23.5). Such a dopamine activation could explain why stress increases self-administration of e.g., cocaine in drug-withdrawn but still probably sensitized animals.

23.4
Stress and Inhibitory Control

A wealth of evidence suggests that the mesolimbic dopamine system is a motivating and behavioral activating neuronal system in the brain. This system in itself, as well as the neuronal consequences of its activation, are under inhibitory control from other neuronal systems. In this way enough time is normally provided for higher cortical centers to process information in order to allow selection of the most appropriate behavior in a given situation. By the 1970s, brain serotonin neu-

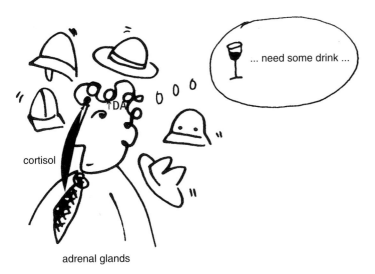

Fig. 23.5. In response to stress, the adrenal glands secrete the hormone cortisol, which is transported via the blood stream to the brain. There – as indicated by animal experiments – the hormone increases dopamine (DA) release. This dopamine signal is considered to cause the addict's craving for the drug.

rons were already implicated in such a control function. One of the most consistent findings in biological psychiatry is that signs of deficient serotonin function are associated with a decreased inhibitory control, which probably explains at least part of the deviant behaviors observed in low-serotonergic individuals. Both human and animal studies indicate that decreased serotonin function increases self-administration of alcohol and other drugs of abuse, and several studies indicate that there is a positive correlation between the degree of impulsivity in rats and their alcohol consumption. Interestingly, recent results indicate that repeated nicotine or amphetamine exposure besides producing locomotor sensitization also produces behavioral disinhibition, and the latter phenomenon is more strongly correlated to the ensuing increase in alcohol intake than the former [13]. Another neurotransmitter that has been suggested to influence inhibitory control is the amino acid gamma-aminobutyric acid (GABA). Both benzodiazepines, barbiturates, certain neurosteroids and ethanol, which all are positive modulators of GABA$_A$ receptors, decrease inhibitory control in low doses, whereas they produce sedation in higher doses.

That stress increases the risk for acting spontaneously and without consideration is trivial, but the biological mechanisms that are involved remain to be elucidated. Animal studies have, however, indicated that corticosterone may decrease the ability of serotonin to reduce alcohol intake in rats. Also, the GABA system is heavily influenced by stress: stressors increase the activity of the system, probably mostly via different forms of directly acting steroid metabolites, so-called neurosteroids. Animal experiments also indicate that there is a close interplay between the serotonin system, the GABA system and corticosteroids in the regulation of inhibitory control.

23.5
Stress-Sensitivity and Risk for Excessive Drug Self-Administration

Given that stress, or rather corticosterone secretion, is so intimately associated with drug self-administration and activation of the mesolimbic dopamine system, the question arises whether stress-sensitive individuals, or rather, individuals that respond with a high secretion of corticosterone when stressed, are more prone to drug self-administration than others. Studies in rats have shown that animals responding with high locomotor activity when exposed to a new environment are more inclined to drug self-administration than those responding with lower activity. These high-responding animals also release more corticosterone in a novel environment, and if the adrenal glands are removed the difference between groups disappears [14]. These animals also show a larger reactivity in their mesolimbic dopamine system in response to stress, another difference that disappears after adrenalectomy. Furthermore, young monkeys responding with high corticosterone secretion when separated from their mothers are those that in adulthood will consume the most ethanol in a free choice between ethanol and water. These animal studies thus strongly argue for the notion that individuals with a high stress responsivity are at a greater risk for developing drug dependence.

23.6
Human Studies

As indicated above, epidemiological studies show an association between stress and drug intake. For instance, people going through a divorce or having financial problems report increased alcohol consumption, and patients with anxiety or affective disorders, which are associated with stress, are at greater risk for developing drug dependence. But there are also experimental studies in humans available that may support the association. For example, acute stress or stress imagery activate both the HPA axis and the sympatho–adreno–medullary system and increases craving for cocaine [15].

Another avenue of investigations is whether the subjective qualitative experience of drugs are altered by stress. Underlying these studies is the hypothesis that the way the drug is perceived and/or how it interacts with the present mood or state is of importance for the risk of recurrent use. An individual experiencing euphoria or other positive drug effects is more likely to use a drug than one not experiencing positive drug effects. Sensitive and reliable methods to estimate mood alteration and the subjective effects of drugs have been developed. These methods are sensitive for different pharmacological (different drugs and doses) and environmental variables, as well as social circumstances, expectations, family history of alcoholism and hormonal status. Therefore studies of subjective experiences of drug effects may become an important method to investigate why some drugs are abused by some individuals but not by others.

These methods have been applied in studies of stress and show that stress may dampen the subjective experiences of drugs. Thus, acute stress has a sobering effect on alcohol-intoxicated individuals and dampens the euphoric effects of laughing gas, fentanyl (an opioid analgesic), and several of the subjective effects of morphine. It has further been demonstrated that acute stress may enhance the sedative effects of alcohol and reduce the stimulatory effects of methamphetamine. While these studies indicate that stress and stress hormones can influence the subjective experience of alcohol and other drugs of abuse, they do not, however, address whether stress in fact increases drug intake, as has been the case in animal studies.

The biological mechanisms underlying the association between stress and drug craving or intake have not been studied much in humans and the results obtained are contradictory. In one study, cortisol administration was shown to enhance cocaine craving in cocaine-dependent individuals, while in another investigation the cortisol response to cocaine cues was not related to subjective craving. In the latter study a pharmacological agent attenuated the adrenocortical response to cocaine cues, but, if anything, enhanced the subjects' ratings of the likelihood of cocaine use.

With respect to ethanol one study has investigated the responsiveness of the HPA axis to stress and the effect of ethanol on the stress response in subjects at high and low risk of alcoholism [16]. Those at high risk showed lower basal adrenocorticotropic hormone (ACTH) but not cortisol levels and a lower stress-induced elevation of ACTH levels than low-risk subjects. The high-risk subjects also displayed a delayed recovery of ACTH and cortisol levels. Ethanol intake attenuated (ACTH) or abolished (cortisol) the stress-induced increases of these hormones in both groups. Thus, even though the response of the HPA axis to stress differed between high- and low-risk individuals, ethanol had a similar effect on this response in both groups. In another study high-risk subjects had higher baseline values of pulse and systolic blood pressure and lower plasma beta-endorphin levels than low-risk subjects [17]. Stress induced a small increase in cardiovascular activity, an effect that was not prevented by alcohol. Stress, but not alcohol, also increased plasma beta-endorphin levels. Low-risk subjects presented a higher stress-induced increase in plasma beta-endorphin and a faster recovery than high-risk subjects. Alcohol attenuated the stress-induced increase in plasma beta-endorphin in both groups, but the effect was stronger in low risk subjects. Thus, there are differences in the stress response, in the response of beta-endorphin to stress and in the effect of ethanol on stress responses, as a function of family history of alcoholism.

It is interesting to note that healthy sons of male alcoholics also show an increased autonomic reactivity to both aversive and nonaversive stimuli and an enhanced alcohol-induced dampening of these reactions [alcohol-induced stress response dampening (SRD)]. Since this phenomenon appears to be robust among high-risk individuals it has been suggested that SRD could be a marker of genetic vulnerability for alcoholism. On the other hand, studies of alcoholics and healthy sons of alcoholics indicate that they have a rigid and exhausted, rather than hyperreactive, HPA axis [18].

23.6.1
Stress and Gender

Women may be more sensitive to social stress than men and they are more afflicted with the psychiatric disorders associated with stress, e.g., major depression and PTSD. The risk of developing depression in response to stressful life events is approximately three times higher in women than in men. Both the physiologic/endocrine response to and the subjective experience of acute stress differ between men and women, and the response in women varies with the menstrual cycle. A number of studies also indicates that the association between stress and drug use is stronger in women than in men. For example women appear to experience a stronger sense of "heaviness" and "coasting" after morphine, and are more sensitive to the conditional aspects of nicotine and cocaine than men. Thus there appears to be complex gender differences with respect to stress and drugs, which may depend on the type of stress exposed for, the drug and dose of drug and the variables studied. However, despite these findings, which would put women at greater risk for drug abuse than men, it should be noted that drug abuse is more common among men than women, indicating that besides stress, a number of other factors contributes to the risk of developing drug abuse.

23.6.2
Sensitization in Humans?

With the exception of a few studies mentioned above there is not much evidence available from human experiments that lend support to the hypothesis that stress via stress hormones produces its drug intake enhancing effect via acute or chronic (sensitization) interference with brain mesolimbic dopamine neurons. However, there is accumulating evidence that psychostimulants and alcohol indeed release dopamine in the ventral striatum of humans and that this effect is related to euphoria/stimulation as well as to a wish to consume the drug. In addition a recent study indicates that these effects correlate positively to a concomitant increase in plasma cortisol levels [19].

Whereas behavioral sensitization is well-documented in experimental animals, this phenomenon has not yet been demonstrated beyond doubt in humans. This is partly because it is ethically difficult to administer repeated doses of e.g., psychostimulants to healthy volunteers, and drug addicts would probably already be sensitized. This is illustrated by a study failing to demonstrate sensitization after two intravenous injections of cocaine in cocaine experienced individuals. In healthy volunteers the findings are contradictory. Thus in several different studies Strakowski and coworkers (e.g., [20]) have found that repeated injections with low doses of d-amphetamine progressively increase the effects of amphetamine on activity level/energy, mood, talkativeness and eye-blink frequency. However, in a study performed by another research group repeated administration of d-amphetamine did not increase the response in healthy volunteers. No studies have been published comparing e.g., the amphetamine response in healthy volunteers to that in drug abusers.

If sensitization develops in humans it is not clear how this would be manifested. Indeed, if the counterpart to behavioral sensitization in rodents would be a sensitization of the incentive properties of drugs of abuse, as suggested by Robinson and Berridge [11], the mere development of additive phenomena with loss of control over drug intake would in a sense prove its existence. Another possibility is that the increased risk for development of psychosis and/or hallucinosis that is associated with repeated intake of most drugs of abuse reflects sensitization of the mesolimbic dopamine system. A third possibility is that the increased choreatic movements often observed in, e.g., amphetamine abusers reflect sensitization of brain dopamine systems.

23.7
Summary

Corticosteroids, which are typical transcription factors that instruct the genome about what genes should or should not be transcribed, thus seem to be involved in a protein-synthesis-dependent reconstruction of the mesolimbic dopamine system, which follows upon repeated exposure to drugs of abuse or stress. This reconstructed system could be the neurochemical underpinning to craving. One consequence of this hypothesis is that intake of dependence-producing drugs in a stressed state, which probably is very common, could be especially disadvantageous from the perspective of dependence development. Corticosteroids could also be involved in stress-induced activation of the reconstructed, hyperreactive dopamine system and thereby precipitate relapse.

Environmental factors such as stressors thus may make the reward systems more sensitive both for the reinforcing effects of drugs of abuse and for environmental signals associated with earlier drug intake. Thus both the vulnerability for developing dependence and the risk for relapse may be increased. These new findings of how stress hormones influence the brain reward system exemplifies how the environment, via a hormonal mediator, can affect complex neurobiological events and thereby the behavior.

References

1 BRADY KT, SONNE SC. 1999. The role of stress in alcohol use, alcoholism treatment, and relapse. Alcohol Res Health 23:263–271.

2 KOOB GF. 1992. Drugs of abuse: anatomy, pharmacology and function of reward pathways. Trends Pharmacol Sci 13:177–184.

3 STEWART J. 2000. Pathways to relapse: the neurobiology of drug- and stress-induced relapse to drug-taking. J Psychiatry Neurosci 25:125–136.

4 PIAZZA PV, LE MOAL M. 1998. The role of stress in drug self-administration. Trends Pharmacol Sci 19:67–74.

5 McEWEN BS, DE KLOET ER, ROSTENE W. 1986. Adrenal steroid receptors and actions in the nervous system. Physiol Rev 66(4):1121–1188.

6 FAHLKE C. 1994. Alcohol consumption in the rat: modulation by adrenal steroids and mesotelencepahlic dopamine. Thesis, Göteborg University, ISSN 1101–718X.

7 ENGEL J. 1977. Neurochemical aspects of the euphoria induced by dependence-producing drugs. Excerpta Med Int Congr Ser 407:16–22.

8 KALIVAS PW, SORG BA, HOOKS MS. 1993. The pharmacology and neural circuitry of sensitization to psychostimulants. Behav Pharmacol 4:315–334.

9 SCHULTZ W, DAYAN P, MONTAGUE PR. 1997. A neural substrate of prediction and reward. Science 275:1593–1599.

10 NESTLER EJ. 1994. Molecular neurobiology of drug addiction, Neuropsychopharmacology 11:77–87.

11 ROBINSON TE, BERRIDGE KC. 1993. The neural basis of drug craving: an incentive-sensitization theory of addiction. Brain Res Rev 18:247–291.

12 ANTELMAN SM, EICHLER AJ, BLACK CA, KOCAN D. 1980. Interchangeability of stress and amphetamine in sensitization. Science 207:329–331.

13 OLAUSSON P, ENGEL JA, SÖDERPALM B. 2002. Involvement of serotonin in nicotine dependence: processes relevant to positive and negative regulation of drug intake. Pharmacol Biochem Behav 71:757–771.

14 PIAZZA PV, MACCARI S, DEMINIERE JM, LE MOAL M, MORMEDE P, SIMON H. 1991. Corticosterone levels determine individual vulnerability to amphetamine self-administration. Proc Natl Acad Sci U S A 88:2088–2092.

15 SINHA R, TALIH M, MALISON R, COONEY N, ANDERSON GM, KREEK MJ. 2003. Hypothalamic–pituitary–adrenal axis and sympatho–adreno-medullary responses during stress-induced and drug cue-induced cocaine craving states. Psychopharmacology 170:62–72.

16 DAI X, THAVUNDAYIL J, GIANOULAKIS C. 2002. Response of the hypothalamic–pituitary–adrenal axis to stress in the absence and presence of ethanol in subjects at high and low risk of alcoholism. Neuropsychopharmacology 27:442–452.

17 DAI X, THAVUNDAYIL J, GIANOULAKIS C. 2002. Differences in the responses of the pituitary beta-endorphin and cardiovascular system to ethanol and stress as a function of family history. Alcohol Clin Exp Res 26:1171–1180.

18 RASMUSSEN DD, BOLDT BM, BRYANT CA, MITTON DR, LARSEN SA, WILKINSON CW. 2000. Chronic daily ethanol and withdrawal: 1. Long-term changes in the hypothalamo–pituitary–adrenal axis. Alcohol Clin Exp Res 24:1836–1849.

19 OSWALD LM, WONG DF, McCAUL M, ZHOU Y, KUWABARA H, CHOI L,

Brasic J, Wand GS. 2005. Relationships among ventral striatal dopamine release, cortisol secretion, and subjective responses to amphetamine. Neuropsychopharmacology 30:821–832.

20 Strakowski SM, Sax KW, Setters MJ, Keck PE Jr. 1996. Enhanced response to repeated d-amphetamine challenge: evidence for behavioral sensitization in humans. Biol Psychiatry 40:872–880.

Index

Stress in Health and Disease. Edited by Bengt B. Arnetz and Rolf Ekman
Copyright © 2005 WILEY-VCH Verlag GmbH & Co. KGaA, Weinheim
ISBN: 3-527-30785-0